S0-BCP-499

THE BODY IN BRIEF
Essentials for Healthcare

Rebecca Rayman, R.N.C., B.S.N.

Illustrated

Skidmore-Roth Publishing, Inc.
Aurora, Colorado

SR
Skidmore-Roth

Cover Design: Robert Pawlak
Developmental Editor: Wendy Thompson

Copyright© 1989, 1993, 1997 by Skidmore-Roth Publishing, Inc. All rights reserved. No part of this book may be copied or transmitted in any form or by any means without written permission of the publisher.

Notice: The author and publisher of this volume have taken care to make certain all information is correct and compatible with the standards generally accepted at the time of publication.

Library of Congress Cataloging-in-Publishing Data

Rayman, Rebecca.
The body in brief. 3rd ed.

Includes bibliographies and index.
1. Nursing — Outlines, syllabi, etc. I. Title.
[DNLM: 1. Anatomy — nurses' instruction. 2. Nursing Assessment.
3. Physiology — nurses' instruction.

ISBN 0-944132-76-6

THE BODY IN BRIEF

Table of Contents

This book is dedicated:

In loving memory to my father, John G. Wessel

and to

my father-in-law, Richard A. West

I love you both,
Becky

I would also like to mention

George K. Rayman

Charles K. Rayman

Christopher M. Rayman and

Jeremy J. Rayman

The other "men" in my life.

HOW TO USE THIS BOOK

The Body in Brief, Essentials for Health Care, was designed as a quick reference to provide information on topics which are needed in the every day clinical practice. The book is designed with portability in mind, so that it would fit into the pocket of a lab coat, backpack or purse. Topics for inclusion were chosen carefully, concentrating on information that would be useful to the student as well as the practitioner.

This is the third edition which has been greatly expended and revised. Procedures and conditions have been separated out into their own sections to provide for more convenience. New laboratory and diagnostic tests have been added. All sections have been reviewed and revised to provide current information.

The book is divided into nine chapters based on major organ systems of the body. Each chapter is further divided into subsections to reduce the time spent in locating information. The subsections are:

I.   Overview
II.   Assessment
III. Laboratory and diagnostic tests
IV.   Procedures
V.   Conditions
VI.   Diets
VII. Drugs
VIII. Glossary

How to Use Each Section

Section I — OVERVIEW

The overview of each chapter contains information on the primary functions of the organic system being reviewed. The components that make up the organ system are then discussed along with their functions. Drawings of the components are included. This section also includes some basic concepts of the organ system. The purpose of this section is to provide a review of the system. Where appropriate, flow sheets are included to provide a visual progression of the material discussed.

Section II — ASSESSMENT

This section includes two subsections, the health history and the physical assessment. This section is designed to aid the clinician, whether a beginner or with experience, in performing a thorough assessment of the system. The health history and physical assessment forms are provided as an assessment tool. The health history assessment forms include open-ended questions to assess the patient's health beliefs. A space to write notes is included.

Section III — LABORATORY AND DIAGNOSTIC TESTS

The section on laboratory and diagnostic tests provides information on the tests used in the system. The tables include information on expected results, why the test may have been ordered (indications), collection information, and what abnormal results may signify. The diagnostic test information tables provide the expected results, indications, and what should be done before and after the procedure.

Section IV — PROCEDURES

The procedure section contains information about common nursing procedure that pertain to this system. Information here was chosen based on what would be helpful to students or nurses in the clinical setting. Procedures range from the routine to complex. In the previous two editions, this section was combined with conditions.

Section V — CONDITIONS

This section contains information about common conditions or disorders that affect the organ system. For each condition, the definition, prevalence, etiology, and signs and symptoms are given. This section also includes the components of an initial examination to help the student or practiced nurse perform a complete assessment. This portion of the section includes information on the medical history, physical examination, and laboratory and diagnostic tests that are an important part of the assessment. The last component of this section involves the treatment of the condition.

Section V — DIETS

This section provides information on diets that may be ordered for the patient with problems involving this system. Each diet includes a general description, why it would be ordered (indications), what foods are allowed or restricted, nutritional value, and comments or interventions for that diet. This section should be helpful when the patient wants a snack or when the patient asks about allowed foods.

Section VI — DRUGS

This section has been revised to include more classes of drugs, more information about each class of drugs, and more examples of drugs within the class. The section still includes information on the action and indications for each class of drugs. New to the section is an expanded look at an example drug to include route, pharmacokinetics, contraindications, adverse effects, and interventions that the nurse should be aware of.

Section VII — GLOSSARY OF TERMS

Included to help decipher unfamiliar words within the text or to look up words that are unfamiliar when reading medical reports or charts.

A special thanks to Wendy Thompson, my editor at Skidmore-Roth Publishing, for her help in the preparation of this third edition.

Rebecca J. Rayman, R.N., B.S.N.

Cardiovascular System

CARDIOVASCULAR SYSTEM

Table of contents

Section I — THE OVERVIEW

Primary functions
- Transport oxygen, nutrients and other substances to the cells
- Transport and remove carbon dioxide, produced by cellular metabolism via the lungs and cellular wastes via the kidneys
- Aid in the regulation of body temperature

Components
The primary components of the cardiovascular system are the heart and blood vessels of the body. Figure 1A shows the heart and Figure 1D shows the primary blood vessels.

Heart
- Primary organ of the circulatory system
- A two-sided pump that forces blood throughout the body, the right side and the left side are separated by the interventricular septum

Components of the Heart

Vena cavae
- Two major veins that lead into the heart from the body, all blood returning to the heart enters through one of these veins
- There are no valves where these veins empty into the right atrium

Superior vena cava
Returns unoxygenated blood from the head and upper portion of the body to the heart

Inferior vena cava
Returns unoxygenated blood from the lower portion of the body to the heart

Chambers
- Four chambers; two on each side
- Chambers which receive the blood are the atria
- Chambers that expel the blood are the ventricles

STRUCTURE OF THE HEART

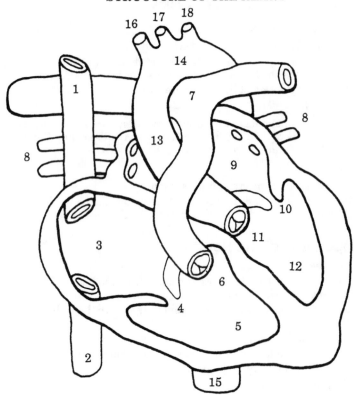

1. Superior vena cava
2. Inferior vena cava
3. Right atrium
4. Tricuspid valve
5. Right ventricle
6. Pulmonary valve
7. Pulmonary artery
8. Pulmonary veins
9. Left atrium
10. Bicuspid (mitral) valve
11. Aortic valve
12. Left ventricle
13. Ascending aorta
14. Aortic arch
15. Decending thoracic aorta
16. Brachiocephalic artery
17. Left common carotid artery
18. Left subclavian artery

Figure 1A

Atria
- No valves at the entry points to the atrial chambers so blood flows in continuously (passive blood movement)
- Have the capacity to hold about 57ml or almost 2 oz of blood

Right atrium
Unoxygenated blood flows into the right atrium from both vena cavae
Larger and its wall is thinner than the left atrium

Left atrium
Oxygenated blood flows into the left atrium from the pulmonary veins on its way back from the lungs

Ventricles
- Receive blood from the atria via the atrioventricular or AV valves (tricuspid and bicuspid)
- Force the blood out through the semilunar valves (pulmonary and aortic) into arteries
- Ventricles walls are thicker and they are able to generate and withstand more pressure than atrial walls (active blood movement)
- Have the capacity to hold 85ml or about three ounces

Right ventricle
Tricuspid valve at its entrance
Pulmonary valve (semilunar) at its exit
Unoxygenated blood flows through it on the way to the lungs

Left ventricle
Bicuspid valve at it's entrance
Aortic valve at it's exit
Oxygenated blood from the lungs is pumped out to the body

Heart valves
- Blood travels through the heart in only one direction because of one-way valves at the exit point of each chamber
- The valves open and close passively in response to pressure changes in the chambers

AV valves
- Valves between the chambers on either side of the heart are the atrioventricular valves or AV, valves

Tricuspid valve

The AV valve on the right side has three cusps or flaps
When these triangular cusps are open blood flows into the
right ventricle

Bicuspid or mitral valve

The AV valve on the left side of the heart has two cusps

Semilunar valves

- Located in the arteries at the exit point of the ventricles
- Prevent the blood from flowing back to the heart

Pulmonary valve

Located between the pulmonary artery and the right
ventricle

Aortic valve

Located between the aorta and the left ventricle

Concepts

Blood flow and the heart

General information review

- The heart is a 4-chambered, 2-sided pump; each side pumps
simultaneously, the atria contract just prior to the contraction of
the ventricles
- Right side forces oxygen-deficient blood through the lungs where
the blood picks up oxygen molecules
- Left side forces oxygen-rich blood (returning from lungs) to the
body where the oxygen will be used by cells
- Blood flows in one direction because the heart valves open and
close with the contraction and relaxation of the chambers

Cardiac output

- *Systole* is the period of time when the ventricles contract
- *Diastole* is the relaxation phase of the ventricles
- *Stroke volume (SV)* is the amount of blood ejected by a ventricle
during systole (averages 70cc)
- *Cardiac output (CO)* equals the amount of blood ejected from the
left ventricle into the aorta per minute

CO = SV x HR, therefore, average CO equals:
CO = 70cc x 72 bpm (average heart rate)
CO = 5,040 cc/min or approximately 5 liters of blood

CIRCULATION OF BLOOD THROUGH THE HEART

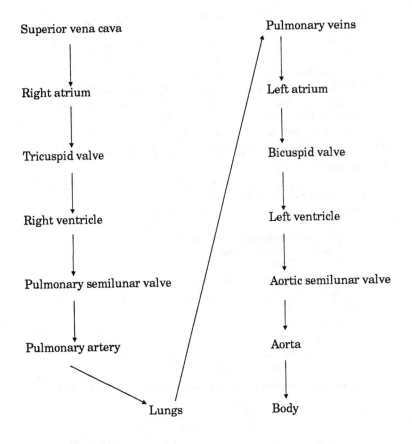

Figure 1B

Heart sounds

- AV valves are open during diastole and closed during systole
- The AV valve closure makes the 1st heart sound (S1) heard as lubb
- Semilunar valves are open during systole and closed during diastole
- The semilunar valve closure makes the second heart sound heard as dubb

Coronary Arteries

- The heart requires a constant supply of oxygenated blood
- Blood to heart is supplied from the coronary arteries which branch from the aorta to the myocardium (heart muscle)
- These small branches encircle the heart

The heart's electrical conduction system

- Initiates the cardiac cycle
- Cardiac cycle is the period from the beginning of one heart beat to the beginning of the next heart beat
- The components of the electrical conduction system are:
    Sinoatrial node (SA node)
    Atrioventricular node (AV node)
    Bundle of His (AV bundle)
    Purkinje fibers

Initiation of the cardiac cycle

- SA node is the pacemaker of the heart, the cardiac cycle begins when this node fires (depolarizes)
- The electrical impulse (depolarization wave) generated by the SA node travels through the atrial tissue to the AV node
- This same impulse stimulates the atria to contract
- When the atria contract, blood is forced into the ventricles
- Once the impulse reaches the AV node there is a short delay before it is rapidly transmitted to the Bundle of His
- The Bundle of His divides into the left and right bundle branches which pass down the interventricular septum
- From the bundle branches the impulse is transmitted to the Purkinje fibers which penetrate into deeper myocardium
- When the impulse reaches the ventricular muscle, contraction occurs and the blood is forced out of the heart to the lungs or body

The Heart's Electrical Conduction System

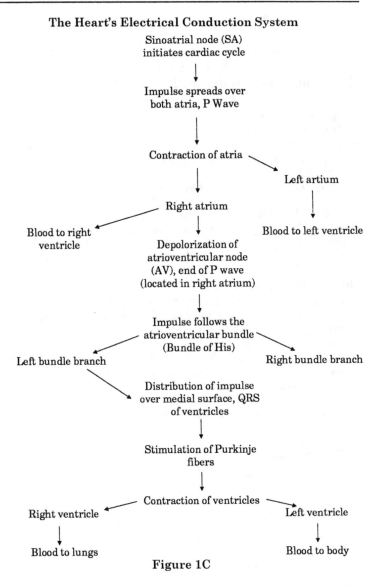

Sinoatrial node (SA)
initiates cardiac cycle

Impulse spreads over
both atria, P Wave

Contraction of atria

Left artium

Right atrium

Blood to right
ventricle

Blood to left ventricle

Depolorization of
atrioventricular node
(AV), end of P wave
(located in right atrium)

Impulse follows the
atrioventricular bundle
(Bundle of His)

Left bundle branch

Right bundle branch

Distribution of impulse
over medial surface, QRS
of ventricles

Stimulation of Purkinje
fibers

Contraction of ventricles

Right ventricle

Left ventricle

Blood to lungs

Blood to body

Figure 1C

- The cardiac cycle is complete, and the SA node is again ready to fire
- If the SA node does not function, the AV node takes over the initiation of the cardiac cycle but at a slower rate

Blood flow within the body

Regulation of blood flow

- The amount of blood needed by the tissues and organs is variable depending on the body's demand for oxygen
- The amount of blood flowing through the body can be regulated to meet the body's needs (e.g., an increased need for oxygen during exercise)
- Blood flow can be increased by increasing the heartrate (HR) and/or stroke volume (SV), this would increase the volume and rate at which blood is circulated through the system
- Blood flow can also be increased by regulating the amount of blood any one organ receives, such as increasing the blood flow to vital organs (heart, brain) and simultaneously decreasing flow to non-essential organs (skin, stomach)

Blood vessels (Figure 1D)

- Two types of blood vessels: arteries and veins
- Arteries carry blood from the heart to the tissues; all arteries except pulmonary arteries carry oxygenated blood
- Larger arteries lead into smaller arterioles and then finally to capillaries where the exchange of most nutrients and wastes occur
- Veins return blood to the heart; all veins except pulmonary veins carry unoxygenated blood
- Blood flow back to the heart begins in the capillaries, then passes into the venules and finally into the larger veins

The Major Arteries of the Body

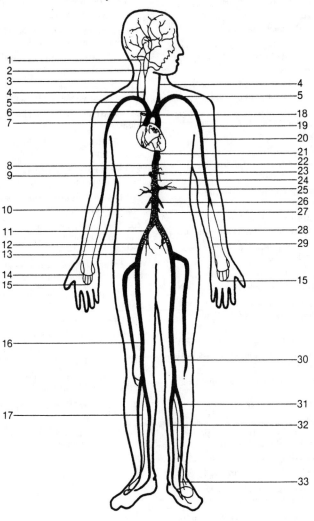

Figure 1D

1.   **Internal carotid** —supplies blood to the brain, eyes, and nose.

2.   **External carotid** —supplies blood to the neck, face and skull.

3.   **Vertebral** —supplies blood to the muscles of the neck, vertebrae, spinal cord and brain.

4.   **Common carotid** — supplies blood to the neck and thyroid.

5.   **Subclavian arteries** — supply blood to the brain, meninges, spinal cord, neck and arms.

6.   **Brahiocephalic** — supplies blood to right common carotid and the subclavian arteries.

7.   **Ascending aorta** — supplies blood to the heart.

8.   **Celiac** — supplies blood to the liver, stomach, pancreas and spleen.

9.   **Common hepatic** — supplies blood to the liver.

10. **Abdominal aorta** — supplies blood to the celiac artery and the legs.

11. **Common iliacs** — supply blood to the pelvis, abdominal wall and the legs.

12. **Internal iliacs** — supply blood to the uterus, bladder, and muscles to the buttocks and thighs.

13. **External iliacs** — supply blood to the abdominal walls, external genitalia (sex organs) and lower extremities.

14. **Deep palmar arch** — supplies blood to the palm and fingers.

15. **Superficial palmar arch** — supplies blood to the palm and fingers.

16. **Femoral** — supplies blood to the external genitalia, abdomen and legs.

17. **Peroneal** — supplies blood to the muscles of the calf and ankle.

18. **Arch of the aorta** — supplies blood to the brachiocephalic, carotids and subclavian arteries.

19. **Axillary** — supplies blood to the underarm and the brachial artery.

20. **Brachial** — supplies blood to the upper arms.

21. **Thoracic aorta** — supplies blood to the chest muscles and esophagus.

22. **Gastric** — supplies blood to the stomach.

23. **Splenic** — supplies blood to the spleen, pancreas and stomach.

24. **Superior mesenteric** — supplies blood to the intestines and colon.

25. **Renal** — supplies blood to the kidneys and ureters.

26. **Testicular/Ovarian** — supplies blood to the ureters, epididymis and testes, or the ovaries and uterine tubes.

27. **Interior mesenteric** — supplies blood to the colon and rectum.

28. **Radial** — supplies blood to the forearm and palm arteries.

29. **Ulnar** — supplies blood to the forearm, wrist and hand.

30. **Popliteal** — supplies blood to the knees and calf.

31. **Anterior tibial** — supplies blood to the leg, ankle and foot.

32. **Posterior tibial** — supplies blood to the leg, foot and heel.

33. **Dorsalis pedis** — supplies blood to the ankle and food.

Section II — ASSESSMENT

HEALTH HISTORY

Chief complaint

- Common chief complaints for this system include:
  - Chest pain
  - Shortness of breath
  - Rapid or slow pulse, heart palpitations
  - Dizziness, fainting, intolerance to exercise
  - High blood pressure

Family and personal history

- Family history is a significant factor in heart disease
- Obtain specific diagnoses and age at diagnosis when known
- Obtain ages and causes of death in immediate family members
- Assess for presence and past treatment of the following:
  - High blood pressure
  - Rheumatic fever (including presence of valve damage)
  - Heart attack
  - Congestive heart failure
  - Surgery on heart or major blood vessels (type)
  - Varicose veins
- If above condition exists assess for required life style changes and current treatment of condition to include medications

Chest pain

- A common chief complaint
- Does not always indicate a Myocardial Infarction (MI or heart attack), although chest pain is the most significant symptom
- Pain that is severe, crushing or persistent may indicate MI
- If present assess location, severity, duration, and if pain radiates to other areas such as shoulder and jaw
- Pain that is deep, dull, and not localized may be angina, MI, tumor, aortic aneurysm, pulmonary embolism, or gallbadder disease
- Intermittent pain is more likely to be angina
- Pain that is sharp and well localized may be pleurisy, pneumothorax, pericarditis, hiatal hernia, breast lesions, rib fracture, or gallbadder disease
- Pain that intensifies with deep breathing or coughing and can be localized may be: pleurisy, broken ribs, or a torn muscle

Shortness of breath

* Indicates heart's failure to pump adequately, usually present in MI or other acute cardiac conditons

Heart palpitations

* Rapid throbbing or fluttering of the heart

Cardiovascular system testing

* Assess for tests completed or ordered and patient's knowledge and understanding of any test procedures or results

CARDIOVASCULAR ASSESSMENT

Chief complaint

Patient's statement_____ Onset_____

Frequency_____ Duration_____ Other areas affected_____

Have you had this before?_____ Date of last episode_____

What treatment was given?_____

What do you think caused this?_____

What changes have been made in lifestyle because of this problem?_____

_____

Personal and family history

	Patient	Family member		Patient Only Current	Past
High B/P			Palpitations		
MI			Shortness of		
Rheumatic fever			breath		
Heart surgery			Swelling in		
type_____			feet/ankles		
_____			Arm/leg pain		
Blood clots			Numbness		
Varicose veins			in extremity		
Leg ulcers			Syncope		
Blood clots			Chest pain		
			Where		
			Severity		
			Frequency		
			Duration		

Describe_____

Cardiovascular system testing

Electrocardiogram_____ Echocardiogram_____ Coronary arteriogram_____

Angiogram_____ Cardiac cath_____ Stress test_____ Holter monitor_____

Venogram_____ Ultrasound_____ Chest X-ray_____ Blood tests_____

Current treatments/medications

Medication: _____ Dose_____ Frequency_____ Route_____

Use of oxygen_____ How much_____ Frequency_____

Cigarettes/day_____/_____yrs. Alcohol/kind_____ Amountyrs._____/_____

Usual weight_____ Type of exercise_____ Frequency_____

What is your usual pulse?_____ Blood pressure_____/_____

How far can you walk comfortably?_____

PHYSICAL ASSESSMENT

- Cardiovascular assessment is done in the following order:
  1. Inspection
  2. Palpation
  3. Auscultation
- Assessment includes examination of the heart, abdominal aorta, peripheral pulses and blood pressure
- Patient is undressed to the waist for this exam and should be assessed in supine, left lateral and sitting positions

INSPECTION

General appearance

- Assess patient's chosen positioning — Patient who is short of breath may best tolerate a sitting position
- Assess current comfort level — Patient having chest pain may have hand on their chest or even be splinting the chest with a pillow
- Appearance — Patient experiencing acute chest pain or heart failure will appear anxious, restless and/or complain of weakness or feeling faint

Skin

- Color — Pallor or cyanosis may be present
- Pale, cool, moist skin with frank sweating (diaphoresis) is a cardinal sign of a heart attack when chest pain is present
- Cyanosis can occur in heart failure or other disorders where there is a lack of oxygen; assess mucous membranes and nailbeds for cyanosis
- Flushed skin can occur with any condition that leads to vasodilation including some forms of shock
- Clubbing of fingers is related to chronic heart or lung disease
- Varicose veins may be observed on the lower extremities Indicates stretching of the vascular wall due to increased venous pressure from poorly functioning venous valves that would normally prevent back flow and pooling of blood

Apical impulse inspection

- Apical impulse is a visible pulsation in the area of the midclavicular line in the fifth left intercostal space produced by the contraction of the left ventricle during a heart beat (evident in about one-half of adults)

- During examination stand to the right side and observe the chest for pulsations, heaves or lifts; note location
- Heaves or lifts indicate the heart is working harder than normal

PALPATION

- Assist patient to supine position
- Warm hands to avoid startling patient

Chest palpation

- Use the fingertips or the ball of your hand to palpate the chest beginning at the midclavicular line in the fifth intercostal space on the left side
- Apical impulse may be felt over the apex at the midclavicular line (feels like a faint tap), palpable in one-half of adults
- A *cardiac thrill* is palpable vibrations (described like the purring of a cat) often related to a loud cardiac murmur, always indicative of pathology
- Record the precise location of any palpable findings

Pulse checks

- Assess pulse points to include; radial, carotid, femoral, popliteal, and dorsalis pedis
- Are pulse points equal bilaterally? What is the rate?
- Often recorded as follows: Radial R>L 80bpm

Auscultation

- Diaphragm picks up high pitched sounds best like S1,S2, the bell is for low pitched sounds like S3 and S4
- Apply the bell lightly, the diaphragm firmly
- It may be necessary to auscultate with the patient in more than one position to determine the presence of murmurs

Apical pulse

- Auscultate at the 5th intercostal space near the midclavicular line for one full minute
- The first heart sound, S1 (lubb) is made at the closure of the bicuspid and tricuspid valves
- The second heart sound, S2 (dubb) is made at the closure of the aortic and pulmonic valves
- Assess rate, regularity and intensity of heartbeat
- If irregular, assess for a pattern (Does it vary with respirations?)

Apical/radial pulse

- Indicated when the radial pulse is irregular
- Taken by two people simultaneously. One assesses the apical pulse, the other the radial pulse for one full minute
- Any variance between rate is called the pulse deficit

Heart valves

- Auscultate using stethoscope diaphragm then bell at each of the four valve locations, record which heart sound is louder S1 or S2, also note any extra heart sounds

S3/S4

- The third heart sound or S3 is best heard at the apex of the heart with the bell of the stethoscope
- S3 follows S2 and is normal in some children and young adults
- The fourth heart sound is heard best at the apex of the heart and occurs shortly before S1; it is best heard with the bell and when present may indicate coronary artery disease and/or hypertension

Murmurs

- Occurs when blood flow through the heart is abnormal
- Common cause is a malfunctioning valve which allows blood to flow backwards into a heart chamber
- A murmur will last longer than the heart sounds normally heard
- If found grade the intensity

1	=	Very faint, difficult to hear
2	=	Quiet
3	=	Moderate
4	=	Loud
5	=	Very Loud
6	=	Heard with stethoscope just off chest wall

- Determine the timing, is it at diastole or systole
- Determine the pitch, is it high, medium or low
- Determine the quality, is it blowing, rumbling, harsh or musical

Blood pressure (BP) measurement

- Use the stethoscope bell as the sounds are low in pitch
- Take on each arm in lying, sitting and standing position

CARDIOVASCULAR PHYSICAL ASSESSMENT FORM

Inspection

General appearance/posture_____

General skin color _____ Cyanosis: Mouth_____ Nail beds_____

Clubbing of fingers_____ Skin ulcerations_____

Chest symmetrical_____ Visual pulsations/location_____

Varicose veins_____

Palpation

Apical impulse_____ Cardiac thrills/location_____

Radial pulse_____ Femoral pulse_____ Popliteal pulse_____

Dorsalis pedis pulse_____ Carotid pulse_____ Homan's sign_____

Auscultation

Apical pulse_____ Rhythm_____ Intensity_____

S3_____ S4_____ Apical/radial_____

Aortic valve (2nd intercostal space RT) S2 S1_____ S1=Lubb

Pulmonic valve (2nd intercostal space LT) S2 S1_____ S2=Dubb

Tricuspid valve (lower LT sternal border at 5th) S1 S2_____

Mitral valve (5th intercostal space) S1 S2_____

Murmurs_____ Location_____ Systolic_____ _ Diastolic_____

Murmur intensity_____ Pitch_____ Quality_____

Rate change with inspiration_____ expiration_____

Rt. Blood pressure: _____/_____Lying _____/_____Sitting _____/_____Standing

Lt. Blood pressure: ____/_____Lying _____/_____Sitting _____/_____ Standing

Jugular venous distention_____ Bruits carotid artery_____

Assessment notes:

_____

_____

_____

_____

_____

Section III — LABORATORY & DIAGNOSTIC TESTS

In the following section traditional laboratory values and SI units values are given, it is important to recognize that "normal" values vary from laboratory to laboratory. Check the normal values at the agency or institution where a test is performed. Most labs print their normal values on the laboratory reporting slip or page.

Table of Common Laboratory Tests

Test Name	Indications	Comments
Aspartate aminotransferase (AST) Blood test **Normal:** 4-36 µ/ml (SI)	Acute myocardial infarction Angina pectoris Liver disease or damage Suspected damage to heart muscle	**Regarding collection:** Use red-top tube; collect 5-10 ml List any IM injections and all drugs patient is taking on lab slip **Results:** Level above 40 within 6-12 hrs of cardiac damage, peaks 24-48 hrs Increase peak at 3-5 times normal Levels return to normal 4-6 days Usually ordered daily for 3 days and then repeated in 1 week
Cholesterol Blood test **Normal:** <200 mg/dl <5.20 mmol/L (SI)	High blood pressure Heart disease Family history of high cholesterol or heart disease	**Regarding collection:** Low-fat diet prior to testing then NPO for 12 hrs; check agency policy Water allowed; no alcohol day prior Use red-top tube, collect 5-10 ml Usually done as part of lipid tests **Results:** >200 mg/dl usually indicates need for dietary and lifestyle changes
Creatin Phosphokinase — CPK or Creatin kinase (CK) Blood test **Normal:** Male 12-70 µ/ml 55-170 µ/L (SI) Female 10-55 µ/ml 30-135 µ/L (SI)	Acute myocardial infarction (MI) Angina pectoris Suspected heart muscle damage Skeletal muscle disease or damage Cerebral vascular disease or damage	**Regarding collection:** Use red-top tube, collect 5 ml List any IM injections in last 1-2 days on lab slip List drugs taken on lab slip **Results:** Level increase 3-6 hrs after damage Peak levels within 18-24 hrs Normal levels after 2-3 days CPK-MB elevated in cardiac disease MI, cardiac surgery or Reyes

Test Name	Indications	Comments
CPK — cont'd **CK Isoenzymes** CPK-MM 100% CPK-MB 0% CPK-BB 0%		CPK-BB elevated in cerebral or lung disease, shock or seizures CPK-MM elevated in muscular disease or trauma, muscular dystrophy, IM injections, surgery, seizures
Cryoglubulin Blood test **Normal**: No cryoglobulins	Vascular disease with Raynaud's Endocarditis Rheumatoid arthritis Malignancies	**Regarding collection**: NPO for 8 hrs; check agency policy Use red-top tube that has been pre-warmed to body temp; collect 10 ml **Results**: <1mg/ml endocarditis, mononucleosis, viral hepatitis, arthritis 5-10mg/ml malignancies
Lactic dehyrogenase (LDH) Blood test **Normal**: 45-90 µ/L 115-225 IU/L 0.4-1.7 µmol/L (SI) **Isoenzymes** LDH-1 17-27% LDH-2 27-37% LDH-3 18-25% LDH-4 3-8% LDH-5 0-5% LDH-2 > the other four LDH enzymes	Acute mycardial infarction (MI) Congestive heart failure Anemia Heart muscle damage Skeletal muscle damage	**Regarding collection**: Use red-top tube; collect 7-10 ml List pt diagnosis on lab slip List drug taken on lab slip Do not shake tube, avoid hemolysis **Results**: Level increases 24-72 hrs after damage occurs (MI), peaks 3-4 days and normal levels return in 14 days LDH > LDH-2 strongly suggests MI (known as flipped LDH), when the LDH-2 > LDH-1 it rules out MI LDH-1 mainly in heart & vessels LDH-2 reticuloendothelial system LDH-3 lungs, LDH-4 kidney, pancrease LDH-5 liver and striated muscle
Lipoproteins Blood test **Normal**: HDL Male >45mg/dl >0.75 mmol/L (SI) Female >55 mg/dl >0.91 mmol/L (SI) LDL 60-180mg/dL 3.37 mmol/L (SI) VLDL 25-50% HDL ratio to total cholesterol 1:3-5	High blood pressure Cardiac disease High cholesterol Arterial disease	**Regarding collection**: NPO for 12 hours except water No alcohol day prior to testing Use red-top tube, collect 5-10ml **Results**: Low-density lipoproteins (LDH) deposit cholsterol in artery walls High-density lipoproteins (HDL) take cholesterol from cells and transport it to the liver for disposal. Low HDL and high LDL are risk factors for arteriosclerosis Very low-density lipoproteins carry blood triglyceride

Test Name	Indications	Comments
Myoglobin Blood test **Normal**: 90-85ng/ml 0-85 nmol/L (SI)	Acute mycardial infarction (MI) Heart muscle damage	**Regarding collection**: Use red-top tube, collect 5ml List on lab slip any IM injections **Results**: Increased MI or cardiac damage
Renin assay Blood test **Normal**: Pt upright and Na+ restricted 2.9-24.0 ng/ml/hr in ages 20-39 yrs; 2.9-10.8 ng/ml/hr in ages 40 plus Pt upright without dietary changes 0.1-4.3 ng/ml/hr in ages 20-39 yrs; 0.1-3.0 ng/ml/hr in ages 40 plus	Hypertension Hyperaldosteronism	**Regarding collection**: Medications are usually restricted for several weeks prior to testing; check with primary care provider Low-salt diet for 3 days prior NPO for 12 hours prior to testing Patient must sit or stand for 2 hrs before blood is drawn; check policy Use lavender-top tube, collect 12ml Tube should be chilled List diet, medications, pt's position & time of day on slip Place ample on ice, to lab ASAP **Results**: Increase in hypertension, Adisons disease, Bartter's syndrome
Triglycerides Blood test **Normal**: Male 40-160 mg/dl 0.45-1.81 mmol (SI) Female 35-135 mg/dl 0.40-1.52 mmol (SI)	Hypertension Arterial diseases Hyprlipoproteinemia Uncontrolled diabetes	**Regarding collection**: NPO for 12 hrs except water No alcohol day prior to testing Use red-top tube, collect 5-10ml List sex & age on lab slip **Results**: High levels indicate need for dietary and lifestyle changes

Table of Diagnositic Tests

Test Name	Indications	Comments
Angiography X-ray with contrast dye **Normal** femoral vascular anatomy Also known as Arteriography of lower extremities	Arteriosclerosis Suspected emboli Suspected neoplasm Aneurysm	Pre-procedure: Signed consent form is required Assess for allergy to iodine dye Radiopaque dye will be injected Coagulation studies may be ordered NPO for 8 hrs prior to testing Assess and mark peripheral pulses Pre-procedure sedative may be given Procedure takes from 1-3 hrs

Test Name	Indications	Comments
Angiography — cont'd		**Post-procedure:** Monitor VS and peripheral pulses Assess neuro status (R/O stroke) Observe puncture site for bleeding Maintain pressure at site (sandbag) Assess for numbness, tingling, pain, pallor or loss of motor function Administer analgesic as ordered Encourage fluids
Cardiac catheteriza-tion X-ray with contrast dye **Normal** anatomy and heart-muscle function, normal intracardiac volumes & pressure	Coronary artery disease Assess heart size and structure Determine cardiac & pulmonary pressures Assess cardiac output	**Pre-procedure:** Signec consent form is required NPO 4-8 hrs prior to testing Assess for iodine alergy Radiopaque dye will be injected Prepare insertion site as ordered Establish IV site as ordered Pre-procedure drugs will be ordered Procedure takes about 1 hour **Post-procedure:** Monitor VS and peripheral pulses Maintain pressure on puncture site Assess site for bleeding Bed rest for 6-8 hours Encourage fluids
Cardiac Scan Nuclezr scan **Normal** coronary perfusion and ejection fration	Determine cardiac funtion Cordonary bypass surgery Past infarction Heart disease	Pre-procedure: Non-infasive procedure Procedure takes about 30 mins May be NPO, check orders or policy **Post-procedure:** Encourage fluids
Carotid duplex scanning Ultrasound **Normal** Patent carotid artery with no occlusive disease	Suspected narrowing or occlusion of the carotid artery	Non-invasive procedure No special preparations or care required
Digital subtraction angiography (DSA) X-ray with contrast dye **Normal** vasculature	Arterial aneurysm Vascular anomalies Arterial occlusion Stroke	Pre-procedure: Signed consent form is required NPO for 2 hrs prior to testing Assess for allergies to iodine Radiopaque dye will be injected Check for pt use of anticoagulants **Post-procedure:** Assess vital signs Monitor puncture site for bleeding Encourage fluids

Test Name	Indications	Comments
Echocardiogram Ultrasound **Normal** cardiac size, position & movement of heart muscle, normal blood flow	Hypertension Heart disease Heart failure Heart anomaly Narrowed vessels	Pre-procedure: Non-invasive, no special preparation is required Color Doppler echocardiography may be done to map and determine velocity and blood turbulence Transducer will be guided over all of chest with slight pressure
Electrocardiogram (ECG or EKG) **Normal** heart rate and rhythm	Abnormal cardiac patterns Assess electrical activity of heart	Pre-procedure: Non-invasive, no special preparation is required See also Cardiac monitoring
Exercise stress testing **Normal** No ECG rhythm changes noted with exercise	To assess heaert's response to physical stressors	Pre-procedure: NPO for 4 hrs prior to testing No smoking 4 hrs prior to test Record baseline VS Pre-test ECG is usually done Informed consent is required
Holter monitoring Normal heart rate and rhythm	Suspected cardiac rhythm disturbance	**Pre-procedure**: Non-invasive procedure Holter monitor is worn 24-48 hrs See alco Cardiac monitoring
Positron-emission tomography (PET) **Normal** tissue metabolism	Mycardial infarction Determine the metabolism of the heart or brain	**Pre-procedure**: Signed consent form may be required No alcohol, caffeine or tobacco for 24 hrs prior to testing 2 IV lines are required, 1 for radioisotope and 1 for blood sample No special care after procedure
Venography of lower extremities X-ray with contrast dye No evidence of pathology	Venous thrombosis Venous obstruction	**Pre-procedure**: Signed cosnent form is required Assess for allergies to iodine dye Pre-procedure analgesic or fluids may be ordered **Post-procedure**: Monitor site for bleeding Monitor VS for tachycardia, chills, elevation in temp (R/O infection) Encourage fluids as ordered

Section IV — PROCEDURES

BLOOD PRESSURE MEASUREMENT

- Blood pressure (BP) is the amount of pressure the blood exerts on the inside wall of a vessel

Equipment needed:

- Stethoscope with bell (for low-pitched sounds)
- Sphygmomanometer with proper size cuff. Cuff width should be about 40% of the arm circumference or about 12-14cm in the average adult. A too narrow cuff will give a false-high reading. The cuff bladder length should almost encircle the arm

Proper placement of arm and cuff:

- Arm should be free of clothing and slightly flexed to promote relaxation
- Lower cuff border should be about 2.5cm above the antecubital space, at the level of the heart
- A cuff placed too low will give a false-high reading
- A cuff placed too high will give a false-low reading
- Fit cuff on snugly, too loose will result in false-high reading
- Support the cuffed arm or allow it to rest on a surface to prevent a false-high reading from muscular contraction used to sustain arm

Measurement of blood pressure:

- Place manometer dial so it is level and facing you
- Locate the brachial artery above the antecubital space and near the biceps tendon
- Palpate brachial pulse and inflate the cuff to 30mm Hg above where you feel the pulsations stop (palpatory systolic pressure)
- Slowly deflate cuff feeling for the last pulsation
- Wait 30 seconds
- Place stethoscope bell over brachial artery and inflate cuff to 30mm Hg above palpatory systolic pressure
- Deflate slowly (about 3mm Hg per second), note reading when you hear two consecutive beats (systolic pressure)
- Continue deflation until no beats are heard (diastolic pressure)
- Let remaining air out rapidly until reading is zero
- Record and repeat on the other extremity as required

- Pressure should be taken in three positions (lying, sitting and standing) if cardiac problems or syncope are present

What do the readings mean?

- BP greater than 140/90 is considered to be high
- BP greater than 140/90 on at least three separate occasions may indicate hypertension (See also hypertension under conditions)

CARDIAC MONITORING

- Used to detect abnormalities in the rhythm of the heart
- Examination may be routine as in physical examination or pre-surgical work-up
- May be done to rule out cardiovascular disease or as part of work-up for chest pain or MI
- May be performed in physician's office, out patient clinic or hospital setting

Electrocardiogram (ECG)

- Most commonly used clinical cardiac evaluation
- Standard 12-lead monitoring system has 10 electrodes
  - 6 leads are attached to the chest
    V1 in the 4th ICS at right sternal border
    V2 in the 4th ICS at left sternal border
    V3 midway between V2 and V4
    V4 in 5th ICS at the midclavicular line
    V5 at the left anterior axillary line at level of V4 horizontally
    V6 at the left midaxillary line on the level of V4 horizontally
    (ICS = intercostal space)
  - 4 leads are attached to the extremities
    limb leads are placed one on each limb
- Have patient lie supine and still, no talking during procedure
- The heart's electrical activity is recorded on a galvanometer
- The ECG takes about 5-15 minutes
- Any medications taken should be listed on ECG request form
- The ECG tracing is assessed for abnormal rhythms, computer interpretation of the ECG is available, however, all ECG's should be reviewed by the care provider.

The ECG Strip of a Normal Heart Beat

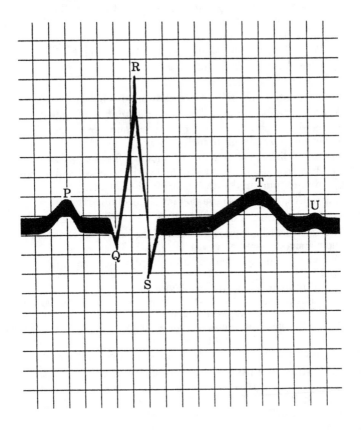

Figure 1E

Holter monitoring
- Noninvasive 24-48 hour continuous ECG recording
- Three-lead system with three electrodes applied to the chest that monitor the heart's deflections and record them in a small portable unit worn by the patient
- Apply electrodes as follows:
  - White lead to right side of chest (white on right)
  - Black lead to left side of chest
  - Green below chest and to one side
- Instruct patient not to bathe or shower with holter unit
- A record is kept of physical/emotional activity during test
- A record is kept of any symptoms or unusual occurrence experienced by patient to include time of day
- Record or diary is turned in with monitor for evaluation
- The ECG tracing record is matched with the diary and accounts of pain are compared with concurrent ECG tracing
- Entire ECG tracing is assessed for abnormal rhythms

Basic interpretation of the rhythm strip (Figure 1E)
- The electrocardiogram is a record of the heart's electrical activity and consists of several waves: P, Q, R, S, T
- The wave forms are recorded on a graph which contains large and smallboxes
        Each small box equals 0.04 seconds
        Each large box equals 0.2 seconds and has 5 smaller boxes
        5 large boxes equal 1 second
        15 large boxes equal 3 seconds (every 3 seconds is a divider)
        30 large boxes equal 6 seconds
- A 6-second strip is used to determine heart rate (HR) and rhythm

Identification of a normal heart beat tracing
- The tracing consists of a series of waves and complexes labeled as P, PR, QRS, and QT
- P wave represents depolarization of the atrial muscle tissue
- QRS complex represents depolarization of the ventricles
- T wave represents repolarization of the ventricles

Reading the ECG
1   **Determine the PR interval**
    - Should be greater than 0.11 seconds (3 small boxes)
    - Should be less than 0.20 seconds (1 large box)

- No P wave or flattened P wave in hyperkalemia

2   Determine the QRS interval
- Should be less than 0.12 seconds (3 small boxes)
- Prolonged wave may occur with quinidine and procainamide therapy or in hyperkalemia

3   Determine the QT interval
- Should be less than 0.43 seconds
- Usually increases with decreasing HR

4   Determine the rate
- Count the number of QRS cycles in a 6-second strip tracing
- Multiply the count by 10 to equal the approximate HR
- If rate is less than 60, bradycardia is present (adult)
- If rate is greater than 100, tachycardia is present (adult)

5   Check the T wave
- Inverted in myocardial infarction or ischemia
- Narrow, peaked T wave in hyperkalemia

TABLE OF RHYTHMS AND SIGNIFICANCE

Rhythm	Possible cause
SINUS RHYTHMS	
Sinus tachycardia Rate 100-180 bpm Normal rhythm pattern Each T wave is followed by a P wave Rhythm begins in sinus node	Anxiety Fever Hypotension Hyperthyroidism COPD Drugs: Atropine Epinephrine
Sinus bradycardia Rate less than 60 bpm Normal rhythm pattern Each T wave is followed by a P wave Rhythm begins in sinus node	Athlete Hypothyroidism Drugs: Digitalis Proranolol
Sinus Arrhythmia Rate is somewhat irregular Rate increases with inspiration Rate decreases with expiration Rhythm begins in sinus node	Normal variation

ATRIAL ARRHYTHMIAS

Rhythm	Possible cause
Premature Atrial Complexes (PACs) Rhythm begins in atrium Rhythm is premature, occurs before next expected sinus beat Rhythm is irregular PR interval may be prolonged QRS interval may be normal or widened	Stress Caffeine Tobacco Alcohol Hypoxia Drugs: Digitalis intoxication
Paroxysmal atrial tachycardia (PATs) Rate 160-240 bpm Atrial rhythm is regular Ventricular rhythm is usually regular P wave may not be identifiable PR interval normal or prolonged ARS interval normal or prolonged Run of PACs (greater than 3)	Heart disease Drugs: Digitalis intoxication
Atrial fibrillation Atrial rate 400-700 bpm (uncountable) Ventricular rate 160-180 bpm Irregular rhythm No P waves ARS interval is usually normal	Heart disease Pericarditis Mitral valve disease Pulmonary embolism Congestive heart failure May occur without any heart disease
Atrial flutter Atrial rate 220-350 Atrial rhythm is regular Ventricular rhythm is regular or irregular P waves resemble a "sawtooth" PR interval is regulr but may vary QRS is variable	Valvular disease Pulmonary emboli Coronary heart disease Cor pulmonale

VENTRICULAR ARRTHYTHMIAS

Premature ventricular complex (PVCs) Rhythm irregular Rhythm is premature, occurs before next expected sinus beat Originates in the ventricle P wave is obscure Wide QRS interval greater than 0.12 seconds (may be notched) ST segment in opposite direction of QRS Isolated PVC or repetitive PVCs	Caffeine Anxiety Heart Disease Hypoxia Hypokalemia Acidosis Anemia Digitalis toxicity
Ventricular tachycardia Rate 100-220 bpm Rhythm usually regular, may be irregular P waves may not be recognizable Wide QRS interval greater than 0.12 seconds (may be notched) May lead to ventricular fibrillation	Same as for PVCs

Rhythm	Possible cause
Ventricular fibrillation Rate is very rapid and disorganized Rhythm is irregular Wave forms vary in size and shape No P wave, QRS, ST segment or T wave Life-threatening	Cardiac arrest No cardiac output noted
Ventricular asystole No ventricular electrical activity No cardiac output noted	Cardiac arrest Complete heart block

STARTING AN INTRAVENOUS INFUSION
Steps in starting an intravenous infusion
Equipment:
- Tourniquet
- Antiseptic (Alcohol or betadine solution)
- Catheter — Angiocath or butterfly in appropriate size
- Gloves
- Tape, dressing (Op site or gauze)
- Ordered IV solution or heparin lock device
- Tubing
- IV pump or stand

Steps:
- Check physician's orders against solution
- Flush tubing or heparin lock device
- Select insertion site
    - When possible, use nondominant hand or lower arm
    - Assess veins before attempting insertion
- Put on gloves (universal precautions)
- Cleanse site well and allow to dry
- Apply tourniquet 4-6 inches above site
- Insert needle 1 cm below vein at 20-45 degree angle
- Advance catheter into vein, insert up to 1/4 inch
- Watch for blood return
- Advance only the catheter while maintaining positon of needle
- Advance needle if using butterfly
- Release tourniquet
- Remove needle and connect tubing to catheter

- Open up tubing and start pump
- Observe site for swelling, burning or redness
- Remove catheter if swelling or pain occurs
- Tape securely and apply dressing according to agency policy

Common problems and solutions:

- *Tape sticks to gloves*

    Tape the fingertips of the gloved hand before starting

- *Poor venous distention*

    Lower the extremity to increase venous distention while having the patient contract and relax hand

    Strike the vein lightly with 2 fingers

    Apply a warm pack to promote venous distention

- *Veins roll*

    Enter from the top of the vein not the side

    Hold vein in place with free hand once skin is punctured to stablize the vein

- *Small fragile veins*

    Try a butterfly needle or a smaller gauge angiocath (#24)

- *Complaints of pain*

    Check agency policy for use of 1% lidocaine or buffered lidocaine to provide local anesthesia prior to attempting IV

    Use a smaller gauge needle if possible

- *Need blood sample*

    During IV insertion, once blood return is noted, connect syringe to catheter hub and withdraw sample slowly to prevent venous collapse; once sample is obtained, connect IV tubing

- *Difficulty taping the IV*

    Place a small narrow piece of tape (sticky side up) beneath the catheter hub prior to insertion; after tubing is connected, fold tape over catheter mounts

- *Blood drips out when trying to connect tubing*

    Quickly place your thumb over the vein just below the insertion site

- *Slow flow of solution*

    Is clamp open? Pump on? Tubing properly placed in pump? IV site positional (turn extremity)? IV site patent?

CENTRAL VENOUS LINES
Purpose
- Introduction of intravenous fluids and/or medications
- Introduction of nutrition (hyperalimentation)
- Measurement of central venous pressure (CVP)
- Measurement of heart's pumping ability and parameters

Equipment
- Requires signed informed consent
- Assemble equipment or prepackaged CVP tray
  The following should be included:
    - Minor procedure tray (check agency policy)
    - Antiseptic solution prep
    - Gloves
    - Sterile drape for sterile field
    - Syringe (25 gauge needle) with anesthetic (lidocaine)
    - Suture needle of specified gauge and appropriate silk
    - Occlusive dressing (Op site) or ordered dressing
    - Instrument tray
    - Masks for everyone (check agency policy)
    - Gowns (check agency policy)
    - Central venous catheter, check orders for type:
      Intracath, Hickman, Broviac, Sawn-Gantz
    - Solution ordered with flushed IV line tubing or flushed
      heparin lock

Immediately prior to procedure
- Position patient in trendelenburg to prevent air embolism
- A rolled towel can be placed between shoulder blades to assist
  physician in correct catheter placement
- Place mask on patient and instruct them to turn their head
  opposite of placement site
- Use strict sterile technique in assisting physician
- Be ready to draw up lidocaine as directed
- Assess patient for distress during procedure, monitor VS
- Be ready with tubing and solution or heparin lock cap

After the procedure:
- Apply dressing and antiseptic ointment

- Call for chest x-ray to verify placement and R/O pneumothorax
- Adjust rate of intravenous solution flow to ordered amount
- Assess periodically for complications of CVP line placement

Discontinuing a CVP line:

- Remove dressing using antiseptic technique
- Clamp off IV tubing
- Remove sutures
- Withdraw catheter applying steady, gentle pressure
- Apply pressure with sterile 2x2 for 2-5 minutes
- Apply sterile dressing and antiseptic
- Assess periodically for bleeding or signs of infection

MAJOR COMPLICATIONS OF CENTRAL PRESSURE LINES

Complications	Signs & Symptoms	Prevention
Infection	Fever, chills, redness, swelling, pain, tenderness, or drainage at site Tachypnea Increased WBCs	Aseptic technique Change tubing q48 hrs Change TPN tubing q24 hrs Provide discharge teaching
Thrombosis	Edema of arm Pain in neck or arm Jugular venous distention	Monitor site carefully for redness or heat Monitor PT and PTT Check for resistance to flushing, report if present
Air embolism	Confusion, anxiety, tachypnea, pallor, unresponsiveness, tachycardia or hypotension	Check for leaks in catheter Tape catheter connections Restrain confused patients For catheter placement, position in Trendelenburg Keep clamp at bedside in case of accidental damage to catheter lumen Flush tubing of all air
Infiltration return	No blood return Pain or swelling at site	Always check for blood leaking and swelling at site prior to infusion
Pneumothorax	Dyspnea, shock, sudden sharp chest pain, respiratory failure	Occurs at insertion in about 2% of pts Instruct pt of the importance to lie still during insertion Obtain chest x-ray to assess for pneumothorax

Central venous pressure (CVP) monitoring
- Measures right ventricular filling pressure
- Used to assess the ability of the right side of the heart to fill and pump blood
- Requires CVP intravenous catheter with two or more lumens inserted into the subclavian vein or internal jugular
- A manometer and IV solution bag must be attached to one of the lumens

Reading the CVP
- Place zero mark on manometer at the phelebostatic axis
- Phelebostatic axis is the cross point of a line from the fourth intercostal space at a point where it joins the sternum, and a line midpoint between the anterior and posterior surface of the chest
- Mark phelebostatic axis for subsequent readings
- Head of bed should be flat unless contraindicated
- Manometer should fluctuate with respirations
- Normal CVP readings are between 4-10 cm H20
- A high CVP reading may indicate CHF, Corpulmonale, or COPD or ventricular failure
- A low CVP reading may indicate hypovolemia
- Ventilators will alter readings; alteration is due to changes in intrathoracic pressure; when possible remove patient from ventilator when taking readings

Management of a code arrest
- Cardiopulmonary resuscitation (CPR) is required when the heart stops to prevent permanent organ damage and death

Cardiopulmonary resuscitation
- Artificial respiration (breaths) and circulation (compressions)
- Compressions without breaths are useless as no oxygen is given

Cardiac arrest in the acute care setting
- Review agency policy on codes and know how to call in code
- Know location of resuscitation masks, ambu bag, code cart
- Practice assembly and use of ambu bag
- Familiarize yourself with code (resuscitation) cart

One person adult CPR:
- Assess the situation, determine cause of arrest if possible
- Assess level of consciousness (if conscious, CPR is not needed)

- If unresponsive, call for help (use emergency call bell)
- Position on back with firm surface underneath (bed headboard)
- Open the airway by head-tilt/chin lift method
- Assess for respirations (look, listen, and feel for 3-5 seconds)
- No respirations, position mask (if available) over patieht's face
- Give 2 full breaths lasting 1-1.5 seconds
- Assess carotid pulse for 5-10 seconds
- No pulse, begin compressions
- Compress 1.5-2 inches (adult) deep, at a rate of 80-100per minute (count — one and two and three and ... fifteen)
- If cracking of ribs occurs, reposition hands and continue
- Give 15 compressions followed by 2 full breaths (1 full cycle) then relocate hand position and repeat compressions
- Recheck pulse after 4 full cycles:
  If pulse is present, stop compressions, monitor VS, give rescue breathing as needed
  If no pulse. continue CPR, recheck pulse every 3-4 minutes
- If after 1 minute, no help has arrived, interrupt CPR and call in the code from patient's telephone, then continue CPR
- DO NOT LEAVE THE PATIENT UNATTENDED TO GET HELP

When help arrives:
- Have second rescuer call in code if this has not been done
- Send second recuer for resuscitation cart
- If more help arrives, continue CPR using two person method

Two-person adult CPR
- First rescuer completes assessment steps and performs rescue breathing, second rescuer does the compressions
- During compressions, first rescuer monitors carotid pulse
- Compression:ventilation ratio is 5:1, 1 breath after every 5 compressions; check carotid pulse after 10 cycles
- When switching roles, second rescuer completes 5 compressions, calls for change; first rescuer gives breath then switches roles while second rescuer checks pulse

Additional rescuers in hospital code:
Staff nursing personnel (2-4 present at code arrest)
- Obtain bag/mask setup (ambu bag) and connect oxygen
  Ventilation is then provided via ambu bag until patient is intubated

- Establish and/or maintain IV lines for fluid and medications
- Place pt on cardiac monitor and record ECG activity continuously
- Continue CPR until primary care provider orders or pt has pulse
- Administer medications as ordered by primary care provider
  Calls out name and dose of all medications as administered
- May defibrillate (if ACLS certified)
- Records all events
    - Type of arrest — respiratory or cardiac
    - How arrest was recognized; if witnessed, name of witness
    - Time resuscitation effort was begun, by whom and how
    - Time code was called
    - Time of primary care provider's notification and response
    - Type of artificial ventilation used (ambu bag, ET)
    - Time of intubation, size of tube and by whom
    - VS readings and times
    - Time of defibrillation and watts/second
    - Medications given: name, dosage, route, time
    - Time spontaneous heartbeat and breathing began
    - Time consciousness was restored
    - Time that resuscitation efforts were stopped
- Collects all ECG strips and lab slips

Equipment needed for cardiac arrest
- Resuscitation cart should contain the following:
    - Airways in various sizes
    - Bag/mask setup, also known as ambu bag
    - Oxygen flow meter and tubing
    - Intravenous catheters, tubing and solutions
    - Intravenous cutdown set
    - Laryngoscope and endotracheal tubes
    - Tracheostomy set
    - ECG machine (usually part of defibrillator)
    - Suction wall unit and tubing
    - Defibrillator
    - Emergency drugs
    - Syringes, needles, gloves and tapes

Remember ...

* During defibrillation, stand clear of pt and bed to prevent
  electrical shock
* When defibrillating, be sure the synchronizer switch is off
* After defibrillating, check the monitor for rhythm pattern
* Use defibrillating pads, saline soaked guaze or electrode gel to
  prevent burns to pt
* Discard needles in proper container to avoid needle sticks to pt
  and hospital personnel

ASSESSMENT OF ARRTHYMIAS DURING RESUSCITATION

Rhythm	Intervention	Comments
Ventricular fibrilation or pulseless ventricular tachycardia	Precordial thump	If arrest is witnessed
	CPR begun	If no pulse after thump
	Intubation-oxygen	100% concentration
	Defibrillation	200 Joules, if no response
	Defibrillation	200-300 Joules, if no response
	Defibrillation	Up to 360 Joules, if no response
	E pinephrine	1:100,000, 0.5-1.0 mg IV push, repeat every 5 min if no response
	Defibrillation	Up to 360 Joules, if no response
	Lidocaine bolus	1mg/kg IV push, may be repeated at 0.5 mg/kg every 8 min to a total dose of 3 mg/kg
	Defibrillation	Up to 360 Joules, if no response
	Bretylium	5mg/kg IV push, if remains unresponsive
	HCO₃ (consider use)	If unresponsive after 10 min, 1mg/kg IV push slow (questionable value); may be repeated at 0.5 mg/kg every 10 min
	Defibrillation	Up to 360 Joules, if no response
	Bretylium	10 mg/kg IV push
	Defibrillati on	Up to 360 Joules, if no response
	Repeat lidocaine or betrylium	
	Defibrillation	Up to 360 Joules
Asystole	CPR	
	Intubation-oxygen	100% concentration
	Epinephrine	1:10,000, 0.5-1.0 mg IV push, repeat every 5 min if no response
	Atropine	1.0 mg IV push slowly, repeat dose in 5 min
	HCO₃ (consider use)	If unresponsive after 10 min, 1mg/kg IV push slow (questionable value); may be repeated at 0.5 mg/kg every 10 min

Rhythm	Intervention	Comments
Ventricular tachycardia with pulse	Oxygen Lidocaine bolus	1mg/kg IV push, may be repeated at 0.5mg/kg every 8 min if not resolved, to a total dose of 3mg/kg
	Procainamide	20 mg/min until resolved up to 1,000 mg
	Cardioversion* Cardioversion C ardio version Cardioversion	50 Joules, if unresolved 100 Jules, if unresolved 200 Joules, if unresolved Up to 360 Joules
	Lidocaine Drip	2gm in 500cc D5W 30-50cc/hr

*if unstable, sedate then begin cardioversion

Rhythm	Intervention	Comments
Premature ventricular complexes	Lidocaine bolus Lidocaine drip	1mg/Kg IV push 2gm in 500cc D5W, 30-60cc/hr
Bradycardia and hypotension	Atropine	0.5mg IV push slowly, may be repeated at 5 min intervals until HR is 60 bpm or greater
	Isuprel drip	2mg in 500cc D5W, 30cc/hr For severe bradycardia only Unresponsive to atropine Titrate to blood pressure
Hypotension (systolic less than 90 mmHg)	Dopamine drip	2-5µg/kg/min initially, rate increased until BP is improved

Section V — CONDITIONS

Hypertension

Definition

- Sustained elevation of systemic blood pressure (BP)
- Arbitrary BP levels have been established to define those at risk of developing serious cardiovascular disease or events
- BP should be measured at least twice during two separate examinations after an initial elevation is found to confirm hypertension

Diastolic blood pressure (mmHg)	Systolic Blood Pressure (mmHg)		
	Less than 140	140-159	160 or greater
Less than 85	Normal blood pressure	Borderline isolated systolic hypertension	Isolated systolic hypertension
85-89	High normal blood pressure		
90-104	Mild hypertension		
105-114	Moderate hypertension		
115 or greater	Severe hypertension		

From the National Committee on Detection, Evaluation and Treatment of High Blood Pressure, 1984 Report

Prevalence

- Most prevalent cardiovascular disorder in the United States
- Affects over 60 million Americans
- More than half of population over 60 years has hypertension
- 40% of all black adults have hypertension

Etiology

- Two types of hypertension: Essential and secondary hypertension
- Essential hypertension makes up 95% of all cases
- Essential hypertension is also known as primary
- Essential hypertension is unrelated to any identifiable cause
- Secondary hypertension may be caused by:
  - Renal disorders

- Endocrine disorders (adrenal gland problems, hyperpara-thyroidism, and acromegaly
- Pregnancy-induced hypertension
- Coarctation of the aorta
- Neurologic disorders (quadriplegia, increased ICP)
- Some medications

Risk factors associated with development of essential hypertension

- Risk factors that cannot be changed
    - Heredity or family history of hypertension
    - Gender, hypertension more common in males than females
    - Race, hypertension affects 10-29% of whites and 20-38% of blacks
      Blacks also have 3X more cases of severe hypertension
    - Advancing age, blood pressure usually increases with age
    - Salt sensitivity, 60% of hypertensives are particularly responsive to sodium intake
- Risk factors that can be changed
    - Smoking, increases heartrate and causes vasoconstriction of the vessels leading to high blood pressure
    - Alcohol (Ethanol) consumption
    - High blood levels of LDL cholesterol, forms deposits on artery walls which narrow or block them
    - Obesity
    - Inactivity
    - Stressful occupation and/or lifestyle
    - High fat diet

Symptoms of hypertension

- Usually asymptomatic — often called the "silent killer"
  No symptoms may be present other than elevated BP readings
- Clinical symptoms rarely occur until damage is done, may include:
    - Headache — may occur early in the morning and improve as day progresses
    - Visual disturbances (due to retinal changes)
    - Dizziness (due to transient cerebral ischemia)
    - Flushing of the face
    - Fatigue

- Nose bleeds (due to vascular disease)
- Nervousness
- Angina pectoris (cardiac failure)
- Shortness of breath (cardiac failure)

Components of initial examination for hypertension

- *Complete medical history to include:*
  - Assessment for risk factors for essential hypertension
  - Personal history of hypertension, including previous and current treatment
  - Patient's understanding of diagnoses and treatment
  - Patient's willingness to make lifestyle changes
  - Personal or family history of diabetes, renal diseases, adrenal dysfunction, pheochromocytoma and hyperparathyroidism
  - Assessment of current medications, the following may exacerbate hypertension: corticosteroids, nonsteroidal anti-inflammatory agents, antihistamines, sympathomimetics, appetite suppressants, phenothiazines, tricyclic antidepressants, and monoamine oxidase inhibitors
- *Physical examination to include:*
  - General appearance
  - Height and weight (to assess for obesity and fluid retention)
  - Blood pressure measurement, sitting and standing in both upper extremities
    A rise in diastolic pressure when standing is consistent with essential hypertension
  - Assessment of peripheral pulses
  - Fundoscopic examination (to detect retinopathy)
  - Auscultation of the heart (Abnormalities of rate, rhythm, abnormal heart sounds)
  - Auscultation of the lungs for rales (pulmonary edema)
  - Palpation of abdomen (detect aneurysm and/or enlarged kidneys)
  - Examination of extremities for edema
  - Neurologic examination (rule out previous stroke)
- *Laboratory and diagnostic testing*
  May be basic or extensive
  - Basic or routine examinations include:
  - Urine for protein, blood and glucose (assess renal status)

- Hematocrit
- Serum potassium (establish baseline)
- Serum creatinine and/or blood urea nitrogen (renal status)
- Electrocardiogram (assess cardiac status)
- Usually included in addition to basic examination
- Microscopic urinalysis
- White blood cell count
- Blood glucose (rule out diabetes and establish baseline)
- Cholesterol to include HDL cholesterol (risk factor)
- Triglycerides (predisposes to hypertension)
- Serum calcium, phosphate, and uric acid
- Chest X-ray (heart size and R/O aortic coarctation)
- Extensive studies for secondary hypertension (not routine)
  - Echocardiogram (Cardiac hypertrophy or anomalies)
  - Intravenous pyelogram (rule out renovascular hypertension)
  - Digital subtraction angiogram (renovascular hypertension)
  - Captopril-induced renogram (renovascular hypertension)
  - Renal arteriogram (renovascular hypertension)
  - Bilateral renal vein catheterization for measurement of plasma renin activity (rule out aldosteronism)
  - 24hr urine for catecholamines (rule out pheochromocytoma)
  - 24hr urine sodium excretion (aldosteronism)

Treatment of hypertension

- Goal of treatment is to reduce cardiovascular morbidity, a lifelong process; there is no "cure"
- Weight loss if overweight (closely related to reduction in BP)
- Low sodium diet (less than 100 mEq/day); sodium related to fluid retention and increased blood pressure
- Reduction of dietary saturated fat and cholesterol
- Dietary calcium and potassium supplementation (recent studies show some patients given supplements have lower BP)
- Alcohol restriction to 1oz of ethanol daily which is 2oz of 100 proof liquor or 4 oz of wine or 24 oz of beer
- Regular exercise for 20-30 minutes three times a week
- Stress reduction
- If smoker, cessation or reduction in smoking

- Caffeine may temporarily increase blood pressure; tolerance develops quickly, however, so usually no restriction is needed
- Medications to control hypertension
- Regular blood pressure check-ups and consultation

Medications for hypertension

- Goal of drug therapy is to return BP to normal with minimal side effects
- A single medication is effective for BP control in over 50% of patients
- All over the counter medications should be cleared with primary care provider before use for possible interactions
- Five classes of drugs are used: diuretics, antiadrenergic agents, vasodilators, calcium entry blockers and angiotensin-converting enzyme (ACE) inhibitors
- Traditionally a stepped-care protocol was used in treatment; New research and new medications have led to new choices for initial therapy and now one of four classes of medications may be selected
  - Low-dose ACE inhibitor
  - Calcium entry blocker
  - Diuretic
  - Beta-blocker
- See Section VII for specific medication information
- Regular follow-up is required with care provider to determine the effect on BP and need for medication or lifestyle changes
- Home BP checks are often helpful in maintaining compliance

Consequences of untreated BP

- Premature death, the most common cause being heart disease
- Cardiac disorders to include:
  - Enlargement of the left ventricle of the heart
  - Angina pectoris
  - Myocardial infarction
  - Heart failure (see also in this section)
- Renal (kidney) disorders due to vascular damage
  - Renal vascular lesions and decreased function
  - Renal failure

- Neurologic disorders due to vascular damage
    - Retinal damage leading to vision changes and possible blindness
    - Headaches, usually in morning
    - Increased risk of cerebral vascular accident (stroke)
    - Hypertensive encephalopathy

Heart Failure (HF)

Definition
- Inability of the heart to pump and adequate amount of blood to meet the needs of the body
- There are several different descriptions of HF to include: acute, chronic, left heart failure, right heart failure, and congestive heart failure

Prevalence
- Now the most common DRG in the USA for patient's over age 65
- Incidence of CHF has increased as the population has aged

Etiology
- May be *acute or chronic* in duration
    - Acute or abrupt HF may occur after myocardial infarction (MI) or other sudden cardiac emergency, acute HF may progress to chronic HF
    - Chronic HF may be begin with progressive narrowing of coronary arteries with only subtle symptoms and gradually progress
- May be *left or right* depending on which ventricle fails first
  In left heart failure, the left ventricle fails first
  In right heart failure, the right ventricle fails first
- Left ventricle HF is more common than right ventricle HF
- Left ventricle HF is the most common cause of right ventricle HF
- Right ventricle HF is uncommon in adults
- Right ventricle HF is an uncommon cause of left ventricle HF
- When both the left and right ventricle fail and there is pulmonary and systemic venous hypertension it is known as *"congestive heart failure"*

Signs and symptoms of heart failure
- *Left sided heart failure* (See also chart)
    - Breathlessness (dyspnea)

- Orthopnea (dyspnea when lying flat)
- Nocturia (urination at night)
- Paroxysmal nocturnal dyspnea (awakes with severe dyspnea)
- Acute pulmonary edema (non-productive cough, dyspnea, tachypnea and wheezing)
- Hemoptysis
- Cheyne-Stokes respirations (late sign)
  Periodic breathing with alternating apnea and tachypnea

Pathophysiology of Left Ventricular Heart Failure

- *Right sided heart failure*
  - Peripheral edema (most dominant sign)
    Related to systemic venous congestion
    Develops over course of day and disappears by morning
  - Weight gain related to edema
  - Enlarged liver (hepatomegaly)
  - Cyanosis
  - Neck vein distension
  - Deep vein thrombosis and pulmonary embolism may occur
  - Heart murmur heard on the lower left border of the sternum (tricuspid valve insufficiency)
  - Possible enlarged and tender spleen
  - Ascites (fluid in abdominal cavity) is a late sign
  - Anasarca (fluid accumulation throughout body) a late sign that often precedes death
- *Congestive heart failure* (biventricular failure)
  - Dyspnea, tachypnea and rales
  - Pleural effusion
  - Edema
  - Pericardial effusion
  - Oliguria (decreased urine output)
  - Proteinuria
  - Weakness
  - Gradual loss of tissue mass
  - Anxiety
  - Anorexia, nausea and vomiting from GI reflux or drugs
  - Headache
  - Insomnia

- Irritability, restlessness, and limited attention span in severe congestive heart failure
- Stupor and coma may occur when cardiac output is severely limited

Components of initial examination for heart failure

- *Complete medical history to include:*
  - Personal or family history of hypertension or heart disease including previous and current treatments and lifestyle changes

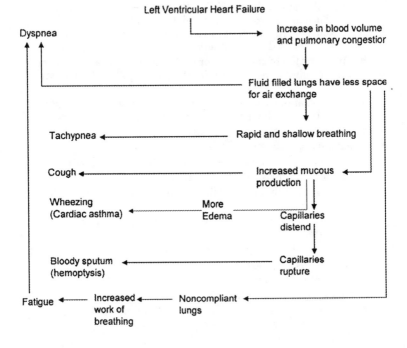

- Patient's understanding of diagnoses and treatment
- Patient's willingness to make lifestyle changes
- History of recent weight gain or loss (fluid shifts)
- Assessment of complaints of signs and symptoms of HF
- *Physical examination to include:*
  - General appearance (in severe HF, patient is pale, sweating, cyanotic and gasping for breath)
  - Weight
  - Respiratory rate and rhythm and blood pressure measurement
  - Auscultation of the lungs for wheezing, rales or rhonchi
    Wheezing from mucous production in lungs
    Rales as fluid accumulates at lung bases
    Rhonchi as fluid accumulation progresses upward in lung
  - Auscultation of the heart for abnormalities in rate, rhythm and for murmurs or extra heart sounds (gallop rhythm with S3)
  - Peripheral pulse assessment for alternating weak and strong pulse (pulsus alternans) usually signifies advanced HF
  - Examination of the extremities for edema
- *Laboratory and diagnostic testing*
  - Urine for protein, blood and glucose (assess renal status)
  - Hematocrit or complete blood count
  - Serum electrolytes (establish baseline or monitor effect from diuretics)
  - Serum creatinine and blood urea nitrogen (BUN) for renal status
  - Cholesterol and triglycerides
  - Arterial blood gases
  - Electrocardiogram
  - Chest X-ray (heart size)
  - Echocardiogram and Doppler study (R/O cardiac disease, valve disorders, congenital heart disorders)
  - Cardiac catheterization (if patient is candidate for surgery)
  - Pulmonary function tests

Treatment of heart failure

- Goal of treatment is threefold
  - Remove the underlying cause of heart failure (may include surgical intervention)

- Remove the current cause for the exacerbation of HF
  Exacerbation of symptoms may be related to:
    Physical or emotional stressors
    Dietary sodium intake
    Obesity
- Treatment of clinical signs and symptoms of HF
- Restriction of physical activity as condition requires
- Activity should be limited to limit dyspnea and fatigue
- Decrease salt in the diet, initially may limit heavily salted foods only and use of table salt if needed a low sodium diet
- Weight loss if indicated
- Reduction in levels of emotional stress
- Oxygen therapy for patients with hypoxia usually via nasal cannula at 4-6 L/min
- Medications to treat signs and symptoms of HF
- Placement of central venous pressure monitoring devices in acute heart failure of acute pulmonary edema
  Also allows for assessment of arterial blood gases
- Thoracentesis or paracentesis to remove fluid from pleural or abdominal cavity (not usually done due to diuretic therapy)
- Surgical intervention — depends on findings of diagnostic tests
- Regular follow-up with careprovider to assess effectiveness of treatment

Medications for heart failure

- Patients with mild HF can be treated with single class of drugs
- A common first line drug treatment is thiazide or a low-dose loop diuretic; in many cases this alone will alleviate symptoms
- Potassium supplements depending upon diuretic choice
- Other first line drug choices include a vasodilator such as an angiotensin converting enzyme inhibitor or a cardiac glycoside
- Combination drug therapy usually involves three classes of drugs
- Diuretics, vasodilators such as hydralazine and isosorbide dinitrate, and digitalis are used at dose level as low as possible. Vasodilators such as an ACE inhibitor like captopril or enalapril and a diuretic are another common combination therapy, used if systemic hypertension is present and there is no evidence of renal impairment

- If symptoms remain despite combination drug therapy intravenous sympathomimetic agents (nitroprusside) may be considered

Myocardial Infarction

Definition
- Heart attack, coronary or MI
- Death of an area of tissue in the heart muscle which results from an inadequate blood supply

Prevalence
- Heart disease is the leading cause of death in USA, most of the deaths due to heart disease are related to MI
- 200 deaths per 100,000 population in USA from MI alone
- 750,000 hospital admissions in USA annually for MI

Etiology
- Risk factors for MI
    - Usually coronary atherosclerosis is present (may have been present for many years prior to MI); this narrows coronary vessels
    - All of the risk factors for hypertension — see Hypertension, this chapter
    - Diabetes mellitus
- Possible acute myocardial infarction etiologies
    - Sudden occlusion of narrowed coronary vessel from thrombus often immediately precedes MI by severly decreasing or stopping blood flow to an area of heart muscle
    - Coronary emboli (infection, fat, neoplasm)
    - Trauma (laceration or contussion of heart)
    - Coronary vasospasm (cocaine or amphetamine abuse, nitrate withdrawal) with "normal coronary arteries"
    - Congenital anomaly of coronary arteries

Symptoms of myocardial infarction
Depending upon the severity and area of the heart damaged, MI may have no clinical symptoms and be diagnosed only upon review of ECG, or patient may experience cardiac death. In general, S&S include:

- Fatigue, chest discomfort, and general feelings of poor health may occur several days prior to onset of MI

- MI usually occurs in early morning hours and is not associated with exertion
- General appearance — pale, sweating (diaphoreis), and restlessness
- Intense, severe, crushing or squeezing chest pain
  Pain is located behind the sternum
  Continous pain which may radiate to left arm, neck, teeth or jaw
- Weakness
- Nausea and vomiting
- Heart palpitations
- Expressions of feelings of impending doom
- Mental confusion, fainting

Components of initial examination for myocardial infarction

- First priority when MI is suspected is to stablize the patient and prevent further cardiac damage
- *Physical examination to include:*
- General appearance and level of distress
  - Cyanosis, pallor, diaphoresis of the skin
  - Restlessness
- Level of consciousness
- Airway for patency and adequacy
- Vital signs to assess for shock and establish baseline
  - Heart rate initially increased
  - Blood pressure initially increased, may be decreased
  - Respirations initially increased due to pulmonary congestion
- Assessment of ECG strip for abnormalities in rate, rhythm
  - ST elevation (persists for hours after MI)
  - T-wave inversion (within first few days)
- Auscultation of the heart for abnormalities of rate, rhythm and abnormal heart sounds
- Ausculation of the lungs for rales (pulmonary edema)
- Pulse oxyimeter readings of oxygen saturation levels
- Fundoscopic examination to detect hemorrhage and/or retinal changes consistent with hypertension
- *Complete medical history to include:*

Due to patient's condition it may not be possible to obtain a complete health history from patient; history may be obtained from medical records or significant other, if present

- Assessment for risk factors for hypertension
- History of hypertension or heart failure to include previous and current treatments
- All current medications
- Any allergies known
- *Laboratory and diagnostic testing*
  - Complete blood count
    - Platelets for possible tx with thrombolytic drugs
    - White blood cells — normal initially increases within two hours and peaks in 2-4 days post MI
    - Erythrocyte sedimentation rate (ESR) — elevated within 48 hrs
    - Serum creatinine and/or blood urea nitrogen
    - Arterial blood gases to evaluate hypoxemia
    - Chest X-ray

Shock

Definition:

- Not a disease; shock is a clinical syndrome
- Circulating blood volume and peripheral blood flow are not adequate to return enough blood to the heart for adequate oxygenation of body tissues and organs

Etiology

- Results from a critical impairment of blood flow to vital organs, may occur for many different reasons
- Shock is classified according to etiology
- Classifications based on etiology include
  - *Hypovolemic*
  - *Cardiogenic*
  - *Septic*
  - *Neurogenic*
- *Hypovolemic* shock results from an inadequate amount of blood volume, usually from a fluid loss from the body, causes include:
  - Blood loss from trauma (eg. accident, gunshot wound)
  - Blood loss from GI bleeding or childbirth
  - Fluid loss from diarrhea, vomiting, or burns
  - Fluid loss from excessive urination

- *Cardiogenic* shock, blood volume is normal, however the heart is unable to pump enough blood, causes include:
  - Acute myocardial infarction (heart attack)
  - Valvular heart disease (aortic or mitral stenosis)
  - Cardiac thrombus, cardiac tamponade or cardiomyopathy
  - Dysrhythmias
- *Septic* shock, blood volume normal, heart normal, however, vasodilatation occurs that the heart is unable to compensate for
  - Usually hospital-acquired not community based
  - Caused by an infection usually a gram-negative organism
  - Common gram-negative bacterial agents include Escherichia coli, Klebsiella, and Pseudomonas
  - Gram-positive bacterial agents include Staphylococcus and Streptococcus
- *Neurogenic* fluid volume is normal, function of heart is normal however, arterial resistance is decreased leading to vasodilation, causes include:
  - cerebral or spinal impairment

Signs and symptoms of shock

- Hypovolemic, see Chart

MAJOR SIGNS AND SYMPTOMS OF HYPOVOLEMIC SHOCK

SIGN/SYMPTON	CAUSE
Blood pressure changes: Initial increase in diastolic BP	Compensatory mechanism due to sympathadrenal stimulation, cannot continue indefinitely Once a rapid loss of 1-1.5 liters of fluid occurs, a rapid fall in BP results in decrease in CVP
Decrease in systolic BP	Due to the loss of circulating blood volume, systolic BP less than 80-90mmHg, CVP below 5cm H_2O
Pulse pressure decreases	Due to the systolic BP decreasing more rapidly than diastolic BP therefore pulse pressure decreases
No measurable BP	Due to the drop in circulating blood volume, low stroke volume and/or severe vasoconstriction
Pulse: Increased, weak and thready	To compensate for the decreasing fluid volume, the heart rate increases
Respiration: Hyperventilation	Initial cause may be anxiety related to trauma or illness; late cause of hyperventilation is acid-base imbalance, body uses hyperventilation to compensate for acidosis
Apnea	Late event occurs when respiratory center fails due to inadequate cerebral perfusion

SIGN/SYMPTON	CAUSE

Acid-base imbalances:
Initial problem
   Respiratory
   alkalosis
	Hyperventilation of patient leads to a loss of carbon dioxide (CO_2), therefore initial blood gases may show low PCO_2, normal bicarbonate (HCO_3), and an increase in the alkalinity of the blood (pH)

Metabolic acidosis	As the BP decreases, the amount of tissue perfusion is also decreased leading to decreased pH and HCO_3
Mixed metabolic and respiratory acidosis	As shock progresses, respiratory acidosis occurs due to severe damage to the lungs leading to the inability to blow off CO_2 (increase in blood PCO_2); at the same time, there remains a continued deterioration of the systems of the body with metabolis acidosis (low pH and HCO_3)
Skin changes: Pale, cool skin	In an effort to compensate for fluid vlume loss, vasoconstriction of blood vessels occurs, blood is decreased to skin and increased to vital organs
Moist skin	Perspiration increases due to epinephrine release by adrenal medulla (sympathetic response)
Thirst occurs	Thirst center in hypothalamus is stimulated by low blood volume in an effort to stimulate fluid intake

Mental function:
   Anxiety,
   restlessness
	Due to stimulation of cerebral cortex by circulating catecholamines

Confusion, lethargy, coma	Due to decreased cerebral tissue perfusion, as shock progresses further, decreased circulating blood volume to the brain occurs with deterioration in mental function and finally somnolence and coma

- Cardiogenic shock
  - Increased heartrate and decreased cardiac output
  - Weak, rapid and thready pulse
  - Cardiac dysrthythmias may occur
  - Decreased urinary output
  - Decreased blood pressure
  - If uncorrected relative hypovolemic shock will occur due to inadequate perfusion of vital organs
- Neurogenic and Septic shock
  Both have vasogenic responses see chart next page

Classification of shock by severity
- Shock is a progressive condition
- **Early reversible shock**
  Vasoconstriction due to sympathetic response

Poor venous return with decrease in blood pressure
Reversible with IV fluids and/or blood

- **Late reversible shock** — Above findings plus:
  Sluggish capillary blood flow
  Acidosis
  Still reversible with fluids

- **Refractory shock**
  Stagnation of blood flow
  Coagulation alterations
  Major end-organ dysfunction
  Difficult to reverse, treatment must be aggressive

- **Irreversible shock**
  Multiple organ failure
  Coma
  Resuscitation unlikely
  Usually fatal

Major Signs And Symptoms Present in Initial Vasogenic Shocks

SIGN/SYMPTON	CAUSE
Blood pressure changes: Normal BP	Early in septic shock, the body is able to compensate for the vasodilation by increasing the heart rate which allows for a normal BP and normal CVP
Decreased BP	Heart is able to compensate for the vasodilation for only a limited time before the BP and CVP will fall
BP may fall and rise	Relative hypovolemic shock will occur if uncorrected
Pulse: Increased	Heart rate increases to compensate for dilation of blood vessels, therefore increasing the pulse and the cardiac output (CO)

Respiration:
  Tachypnea
  Hyperventilation
	Initially may be caused by anxiety, septic reaction to organisms

Apnea	Late event, if relative hypovolemic shock occurs
Temperature: Elevated	Fever if septic vasogenic shock, chills usually will precede the fever Rapid rise in temperature may occur
Hypothermia	Later stages, hypothermia is a common finding
Urinary function: Decreased	Urinary function is decreased despite high cardiac output

SIGN/SYMPTON	CAUSE

Skin changes:
  Warm, flushed,
  dry skin
	Vasodilation causes an increased blood flow to the peripheral areas of the body; skin temperature may be warm to hot due to fever from infection (septic shock)

Cold, moist skin	If uncorrected, relative hypovolemic shock will occur
Mental function: Confusion	Confusion may be the first sign and may precede blood pressure changes by as much as 24 hours Confusion due to cerebral changes in neurogenic shock Confusion due to elevated temperature and infection in septic shock
Coma	If uncorrected, relative hypovolemic shock will occur

Examination for shock

- Assess for type of shock and etiology as soon as possible
- First priority is to stop the progression of shock to prevent serious complications or death
- *Physical examination to include:*
  - General appearance, includes assessment for obvious signs of fluid loss such as bleeding or burns, and signs of trauma
  - Level of consciousness
  - Airway for patency and adequacy
  - Blood pressure (Assess degree of shock and establish baseline)
  - Respiratory rate and rhythm
  - Pulse rate and rhythm
  - Assessment of ECG strip for abnormalities
  - Temperature (R/O elevation from septic shock)
  - Pulse oximeter readings of oxygen saturation level
  - Vital signs should be monitored continuously until recovery
  - Compare VS with patient's previous VS baseline if known
  - Assessment of urinary output in ml/hour
- *Laboratory and diagnostic testing*
  - Complete blood count
  - Serum electrolytes (sodium, potassium, calcium and magnesium)
  - Blood urea nitrogen (BUN) and creatinine
  - Arterial blood gasses
  - Electrocardiogram
  - Chest X-ray
  - Arterial central pressure monitoring (eg. Swan-Gantz)

- Lactic acid
- Blood cultures if sepsis is suspected
- Toxicology screen if etiology of shock is unknown
- Cardiac enzyme panels if cardiogenic shock is suspected
- Echocardiogram with Doppler study for unexplained shock
- Ventilation-perfusion lung scan to R/O pulmonary emboli
- Computed tomography (CAT) to R/O stroke, aortic dissection
- Cardiac catheterization if cardiogenic shock is suspected
- *Complete medical history*
  - Due to patient's condition it may not be possible to obtain a complete health history from patient
  - If possible obtain previous medical records
  - When possible and patient's condition permits obtain health history from significant other
  - Health history may provide clues to etiology of shock if unknown
  - Any present or recent illness should be explored as well as previous conditions of the heart, lungs, kidneys, liver or brain
  - All current medications
  - Any allergies known

Treatment of shock

- Primary goals are to determine and correct the cause of shock, maintain the vital organs, and prevent complications
- Due to the life-threatening nature of shock a critical care team is required, interventions are often carried out simultaneously
- Establishment and maintaince of an adequate airway
  - Endotracheal intubation may be required
  - Mechanical ventilation may be required
- For suspected or known trauma, immobilization of the head and back until critical injuries to these areas have been ruled out
- Reverse trendelenburg positioning unless contraindicated by head or chest injuries
- Supplemental oxygen for suspected or confirmed hypoxemia
- Establishment and maintaince of at least two intravenous lines
  - Large bore catheters (16-18 gauge) for fluids or blood
  - Fluid replacement is determined by pulmonary capillary wedge pressure (PCWP) measurements, blood pressure and urine flow

- Isotonic solutions such as normal saline or Ringers lactate are used initially
- Blood product replacement as indicated; whole blood, plasma, plasmanate, 5% human serum albumin or fresh frozen plasma may be ordered
- Plasma substitites such as dextran or hydroxyethyl starch (Hetastarch) which is newer and has less side effects than dextran
- Urinary catheter to determine renal perfusion
  - Monitor for oliguria (less than 30 ml/hour)
- Hemodynamic monitoring and arterial line insertion
  - Measurement of pulmonary artery pressure, PCWP, and cardiac output
- Nasogastric tube to provide gastric decompression
- Cardioversion or temporary cardiac pacing may be necessary when arrhythmias occur (usually fluid replacement and treatment with vasopressors are adequate to reverse arrhythmias)

Medications for shock

- Inotropic and vasopressor agents to reverse profound hypotension
  - Drug selection and dosage is individualized to maintan adequate blood pressure
  - Norepinephrine (4 mg/1000 ml D5W) continuous IV infusion at 1-4 ml/minute (0.050-1.0 ug/kilo/minute to:
    Increase cardiac output
    Direct blood flow from extremities to heart and brain
    Increase arterial blood pressure
    Lack of response to norepinephrine indicates severe heart muscle damage
  - Dopamine continuous IV infusion at 1-10 ug/kilo/minute to:
    Increased cardiac output
    Decreased peripheral resistance
  - Epinephrine at 0.005-0.02ug/kilo/minute
    Increases cardiac output, produces peripheral vasodilation
    Increases heart rate
  - Dobutamine continuous IV infusion at 2-15 ug/kilo/minute
    Improve cardiac output
    Reported to have a lower incidence of arrhythmias than dopamine

- Isoproterenol (not recommended for cardiogenic or septic shock)
  Increases heart rate, contractility and cardiac output
- Amrinone intial dose of 0.75mg/kilo/over 3-5 minutes followed by continous IV infusion of 5-10 ug/kilo/minute
  Reduces systemic vascular resistance, vasodilator
- Vasodilators for microcirculatory vasodilation
  - Sodium nitroprusside 50 mg in 250-1,000 ml of D5W (wrap bag in aluminum foil to prevent deterioration from light) 10 ug/min initial rate via continuous IV infusion
    Causes relaxation of both arteries and veins
- Sodium bicarbonate titrated to maintain pH of 7.30 or greater for the correction of acidosis
- Morphine for ischemic chest pain and acute pulmonary edema, 2-5 mg every 5-30 minutes IV slow push
- Medications for the treatment of arrhythmias, may include:
  - Lidocaine, bretylium and procainamide for ventricular tachycardia
  - Digitalis glycosides, calcium channel blockers and/or beta-adrenergic blockers for supraventricular tachycardias
  - Atropine for sinus bradycardia
- Parenteral antibiodics are administered once blood cultures and other appropriate cultures based on assessment are completed if septic shock is suspected. When etiology of septic shock is unknown, the following may be given:
  - Gentamicin or tobramycin IV or IM plus Nafcillin
  - Carbenicillin or ticarcillin if *Pseudomonas* is suspected
- Adrenal corticosteroids to support peripheral resistance and limit cellular injury from endotoxins-Methylprednisolone 30 mg/kg, repeated at 6-12 hour intervals for 24-48 hours; use is controversial
- Heparin if disseminated intravascular coagulation is present
- Diuretics, furosemide if patient has oliguria

Section VI — DIETS

- Diet is important in the treatment of cardiovascular disease
- Some individuals with hypertension may achieve blood pressure levels within the standards with dietary management alone
- Dietary management is the primary treatment for hyperlipidemia
- Diet may be comprised by one or all of the following components:
    - Weight reduction if patient is overweight
        - Overweight is defined here as patient who is more than 110% of ideal body weight
        - Obesity and blood pressure are closely related
        - Weight loss in patients with hypertension has been shown to decrease blood pressure
        - Research suggests that those with fat deposits in the abdomen may also have a higher risk of hypertension
        - Diet may be ordered as low calorie with specific number of calories included (1200, 1500)
    - Restriction of sodium to less than 100 mEq/day or less than 2.3 grams of sodium, used for almost all types of cardiovascular diseases
        - Estimates of sodium intake in typical American diet range from 175-265 mEq or 4-6 grams sodium per day
        - Minimum requirement for sodium is 0.5 grams/day
        - In sodium-sensitive individuals moderate sodium restriction has been shown to reduce blood pressure
        - It is estimated that about 50% of individuals with high blood pressure are sodium-sensitive
        - Moderate sodium restriction allows 70-100 mEq/day
        - For patients on diuretic therapy sodium restriction lessens the risk of hypokalemia
        - Dietary sources of sodium include:
            Table salt (1 tsp contains 87 mEq of sodium)
            Foods to which sodium is added in preparation
            Foods that contain sodium naturally
            Bottled, tap or softened water that contains sodium
            Medications (antacids, laxatives, cough medicines)

- Diet may be ordered as NES or no extra salt (no added salt) limits foods high in salt, restriction of added salt in cooking and table salt
- Restriction of alcohol intake
  - Restriction to 1oz of ethanol/day for hypertension and/or serum triglycerides greater than 250 mg/dl
  - Abstinence from alcohol if triglycerides greater than 500mg/dl
  - An association between amount of alcohol consumed and blood pressure has been established
  - 1 oz of ethanol is equal to 24oz beer, 8oz wine, or 2oz of 100 proof whiskey
  - Diet may be ordered as no or low alcohol
- Adequate dietary potassium, calcium, and magnesium has been noted to be important in the treatment of hypertension
  - Potassium supplements may be prescribed for patients treated with diuretics
- Reduce dietary saturated fat and cholesterol intake
  - Decreasing total fat intake to 30% of total calories
  - Decreasing saturated fat intake to less than 7-10%
  - Using unsaturated fats in recommended amounts
  - Decreasing cholesterol intake to 200-300 mg/day
  - Diet may be ordered as low fat and/or low cholesterol
- Decreasing sugar and sugar-containing foods may be helpful for patients with high triglycerides
  - Some patients with high triglycerides are sensitive to simple sugars, this may be related to an exaggerated insulin response
  - Sucrose intake should be less than 5% of total calories
  - Beneficial effect may be greater for men than women
  - Diet may be ordered as low simple sugar
- Fluid restriction
  - May be necessary for patients with congestive heart failure if decreased sodium in blood occurs (hyponatremia)
  - Restriction to 1.5-2 liters per day is common
  - A patient in acute or severe failure may be restricted to 1 liter per day

- Level of fluid restriction should be specified
- Small frequent meals
  - May be helpful following cardiac surgery, myocardial infarction or in heart failure
  - Usually better tolerated than a large meal
  - Ingestion of food increases heart rate, blood pressure, and cardiac output
  - Large feedings increase myocardial oxygen demand
  - Small meals decrease cardiac workload
- Limiting caffeine-containing beverages
  - May be limited in hypertension or congestive heart failure
  - Totally restricted in intensive care units post-myocardial infarction
  - Lowers the risk of increased heart rate or dysrhythmias
  - Caffeine-containing beverages are limited to no more than 3 cups per day
  - Level of caffeine restriction if any should be included in diet order

NO EXTRA SALT (NES) DIET

General description	Contains 70-150 mEq of sodium and is a moderate sodium restricted diet (2-3 grams) Primary purpose is to limit foods high in sodium and to avoid added table salt and salt in food preparation
Indications	For sodium-sensitive individuals who have known cardiovascular disorders and/or renal disorders to include hypertension, cardiac failure, fluid retention, kidney failure or myocardial infarct
Allowable items	Foods that are low in sodium — check labels Federal regulations have been formulated for food labels by the Food & Drug Administration *Sodium-free* means less than 5mg or 0.2mEq/serving *Very low sodium* is 35mg or 1.5mEq/serving *Low sodium* is 140mg or 6mEq/serving or less *Reduced sodium* means food has been altered to reduce usual level of sodium by at least 25% *Without added salt, Unsalted,* and *No salt added* means that food was once processed with salt and is now processed without salt — check the amount of sodium on label *Lite* and *Light* means product may be reduced in calories, fat or sodium — check the label *Light in sodium* means the sodium content has been reduced by 50% Examples of foods allowed include: unsalted meats, cottage cheese, eggs, milk, puffed cereals, low sodium breads, unsalted cooked pasta, rice and potatoes, unsalted vegetables, fruits, fruit juices, creams, oils, unsalted margarines/butter, beer, coffee, carbonated drinks, tea, cooked puddings, ice cream, angel food cake
Restricted items	Salt is limited to 1/2 tsp/day for cooking and table use combined Limiting of high sodium foods; check food labels for ingredients such as sodium benzoate, sodium citrate or other sodium additives used in food processing or preservation Examples of foods restricted include: canned soup, canned meats, hot dogs, salted crackers, baking soda, canned vegetables, baking powder, soy sauce, shellfish — Check all food labels
Nutritional value	Diet, if well balanced, should provide all of the needed nutrients; caloric intake will vary
Other comments	Toothpaste and mouthwash may be high in sodium; rinse after use Medications high in sodium include aspirin, cough medicine, laxatives and antacids; check all drugs with primary health care provider; There are low-sodium salt substitutes available; these should be used in moderation; check label for sodium and potassium content

LOW FAT DIET

General description	Diet contains less than 30% of its total caloric intake from fats with saturated fats making less than 7-10% of total dietary intake 2,000 kcal diet should have less than 600 kcal from fat or no more than 65 grams of fat total with no more than 200 kcal or 20-22 grams of fat from saturated fat sources
Indications	Cardiovascular disease or hyperlipidemia Recommended for all individuals to promote a healthy lifestyle
Allowable items	Foods low in fat; check label for grams of fat *Low-fat* on label means 3 grams/serving or less *No-fat* or *fat-free* means 0-0.5 grams/serving Examples of allowable foods include: skim or 1% milk, nonfat yogurt, non-fat or fat-free cheese, low-fat cottage cheese, lean meats, fish, poultry without skin, water-packed tuna, salmon, low-fat hot dogs, low-fat cold cuts, dried beans, whole-grain bread, cereals, muffins, bagels, pasta, rice, potatoes, low-fat crackers, angel food cake, plain popcorn, pretzels, fig bars, fresh or frozen fruits and vegetables, polyunsaturated oils to include safflower, corn, sunflower, soybean, sesame or cottonseed, monounsaturated oils to include olive, canola or peanut oil, no-fat or fat-free spreads, dressings, cream cheeses or sour cream
Restricted items	High fat foods; check label Examples of high fat foods include: whole milk, ice cream, organ meats, fatty and marbled meats, cold cuts, hot dogs, sausage, bacon, canned meats, pies, cakes, cookies, donuts, pastries, chips, saturated fats to include butter, lard, bacon drippings, hydrogenated margarine and shortening, coconut oil, cocoa butter, palm oil, nondairy creamers, gravies, cream sauces, half-and-half, coconut, most dips and crackers
Nutritional value	A well-balanced diet will provide all of the required nutrients; caloric intake will vary
Other comments	Reducing overall fat intake may lead to loss of weight and overall improvement in cardiovascular health

LOW SIMPLE SUGAR

General description	Sucrose is limited to 5% of total caloric intake
Indications	For patients with high triglycerides that are sensitive to simple sugars
Allowable items	Foods low in sugars For patients who desire sweet tastes: unsweetened fruit juices, sugar free carbonated beverages, fresh fruits, frozen or canned unsweetened fruits, sugar-free cocoa, sugar-free gelatins or puddings All unsweetened foods such as meats, vegetables, pastas, unsweetened cereals, crackers, muffins, bread sticks, pretzels
Restricted items	All sweetened products to include: regular carbonated beverages, lemonage, sweetened fruit drinks and juices, products containing corn syrup or corn sweeteners, cakes, pies, donuts, pastries, ice cream, sherbert, sweetened gelatins or pudding, sweetened cereals, candy, chocolate, jams, jelly, honey, sugar
Nutritional value	Decreasing simple sugars within a well-balanced diet will not affect nutrition.

Section VI — DRUGS

The tables supply only general information, a drug handbook or the physicians desk reference (PDR) should be consulted for details. Each classification includes detailed information about the example drug, this drug is representative of the other drugs in the classification and can be used as a model.

Every effort has been made to include the major classes of drugs used in the treatment of cardiovascular diseases, other classes include:

Diuretics — see Renal System

ANGIOTENSIN-CONVERTING ENZYME (ACE) INHIBITORS
Action: Prevents Angiotensin I from conversion to Angiotensin II, reduces peripheral vascular resistance and lowers blood pressure. Preserves blood circulation to the heart and brain.
Indications: Hypertension and congestive heart failure.
Example: Captopril (*Capoten*)
Route: PO
Pharmacokinetics: Onset 15 min, Peak 1-2 hrs, Duration 6-12 hrs
Contraindications: Pregnancy
Common adverse effects: Maculopapular rash, cough
Life-threatening adverse effects: Agranulocytosis, angioedema
Other adverse effects: Headache, dizziness, paresthesias, insomnia, heart rate increase, fatigue, fainting, nausea, vomiting, abdominal pain, dry mouth, constipation, diarrhea, appetite loss, taste percepion alteration, weight loss, hyperkalemia, neutropenia, pancytopenia, arthralgia, azotemia impaired renal function, nephrotic syndrome, urticaria, pruritus, positive ANA titer, photosensitivity
Interventions:
Administer 1 hour before meals (food reduces absorption)
Hypotension may occur within 1-3 hours of first dose so bedrest and BP assessment are recommended until 3 hours after first dose is given
Proteinuria occurs in 1-2% of patients, baseline urinary protein level should be done before first dose
WBC with differential count is recommended before first dose
BUN, serum creatinine levels should be monitored for increases
Serum K+ should be monitored for hyperkalemia
May decrease fasting blood sugar levels

Assess for agranulocytosis — unexplained fever, unusual fatigue, sore mouth, easy bruising or bleeding, report to primary care provider ASAP

Assess for angioedema — swelling of face, tongue or lips and difficulty breathing, contact primary care provider ASAP

Instruct patient to use over the counter medications only after checking with primary care provider

Examples of other drugs in this classification:

Benazepril hydrochloride (*Lotensin*), Oral, headache common side effect

Enalaprilat (*Vasotec I.V.*), IV, Common side effects include: headache, dizziness & postural hypotension, slow IV push 1.25 mg/5 min, compatible with D5W or NS, may be diluted with up to 50 cc of same, Report hematuria, oliguria, or dysuria

Enalapril maleate (*Vasotec*), PO, see also enalaprilat

Fosinopril (*Monopril*), PO, Assess BP before administration

Lisinopril (*Prinivil, Zestril*), PO, Assess BP before administration, monitor sodium level

Quinapril hydrochloride (*Accupril*), PO, Taking with high fat meal may decrease absorption

Ramipril (*Altace*), PO

ANTIARRHYTHMICS

Action: Depresses the excitability of the heart to electrical stimulation and thereby reduces electrical irregularities and corrects dysrhythmias

Indications: Abnormal electrical pattern on ECG, possible irregular pulse, complaints of palpitations, weakness, dizziness. Symptoms may occur when stimulants (caffeine, cigarettes, medications) are taken, or they may occur spontaneously. There may be no obvious symptoms

Divided into four different classes:

       IA and IB — sodium channel blockers

       II — beta-adrenergic antagonists

       III — drugs from other classes that prolong action potential

       IV — calcium channel blockers

Example: Procainamide HCL (*Procan, Pronestyl, Pronestyl SR*) Class IA

       IM 0.5-1 gram q4-6hr until able to tolerate oral

       IV 100 mg q5min at rate of 25-50 mg/min until arrthymia controlled or 1 gram then 2-6 mg/min

Route: PO, IM, IV
Pharmacokinetics: Peak 15-60 min IM, 30-60 min PO, Duration 3hr, 8hr SR
Contraindications: Myasthenia gravis, hypersensitivity to procainamide or or procaine, blood dyscrasias, complete AV block, second and third degree AV block unassisted by pacemaker
Common adverse effects: Prolonged use SLE like syndrome, polyarthralgia, pleuritic pain, pleural effusion, erythema, skin rash, myalgia, fever
Life-threatening adverse effects: Ventricular fibrillation, with repeated use, agranulocytosis
Other adverse effects: Dizziness, mental depression, psychosis, AV block, hypotension, pericarditis, tachycardia, flushing, bitter taste, nausea, vomiting, diarrhea, anorexia, thrombocytopenia, fever, muscle and joint pain, angioneurotic edema, maculopapular rash, pruritus, eosinophilia
Interventions:
Administer before meals (take on empty stomach) or 2 hrs after meals
Administer with full glass of water (enhances absorption)
If gastric distress occurrs may administer with food
Do not crush sustained release (SR) tablets
First oral dose is given at least 4 hours after last IV dose
During IV administration monitor therapuetic drug levels, 3-10 µg/ml is normal, 8-16 µg/ml is potentially toxic with levels >16 µg/ml toxic
IV infusion requires an infusion pump
Keep patient supine during IV infusion, assess for signs of too rapid administration irregular pulse, tightness in chest, flushed face, headache loss of consciousness, shock and cardiac arrest
Check apical pulse before each dose during periods of dose adjustment
Monitor ECG and BP continuously during IV administration
Stop drug if arrthymia is interrupted, toxic effects are noted, QRS widens greater than 50%, PR interval is prolonged or if BP drops 15 mmHg or more
Notify primary care provider if above occurs and obtain rhythm strip
Report ASAP chest pain, dyspnea and increasing anxiety
Report S&S of kidney dysfunction to include changes in I&O, body weight, and edema
Record episodes of fibrillation
Laboratory tests that may elevate include alkaline phosphatase, bilirubin, lactic dehydrogenase and AST

Incompatibile with bretylium and ethacrynate
Examples of other drugs in this classification:
Acebutolol hydrochloride (*Monitan, Sectral*) Class II, See
   Beta-adrenergic antagonist

Adenosine (*Adenocard*), Rapid IV push over 1-2 seconds, follow by
   rapid saline flush, transient facial flushing is common, solution
   must be clear. Monitor heart rate sinus bradycardia or
   tachycardia may occur for a few seconds and resolve without
   intervention

Amiodarone hydrochloride (*Cordarone*), PO, Common side effects
   include: muscle weakness, fatigue, dizziness, corneal
   microdeposits, anorexia, nausea, vomiting, constipation,
   photosensitivity, Administer with food or milk, auscultate chest
   frequently, elevation of liver enzymes occurs frequently,
   supervision during ambulation is needed if muscle weakness is
   noted, monitor for S&S of thyroid dysfunction, pulse below 60
   should be reported

Bretylium tosylate (*Bretylate, Bretylol*), Rapid IV push or continuous
   IV infusion, IM, Common side effects include hypotension,
   nausea, vomiting. No more than 5 ml in any one IM site, keep a
   record of IM injection sites. Anticipate vomiting

Deslanoside (*Cedilanid-D, Cedilanid*), Class III, see Cardiac
   glycoside

Digoxin (*Lanoxicaps, Lanoxin*) Class III, see Cardiac glycoside

Diltiazem (*Cardizem, Dilacor XL*), Class IV see Calcium channel
   blockers

Disopyramide phospate (*Napamide, Norpace, Norpace CR,
   Rythmodan*), PO, common side effects include hypotension,
   blurred vision, dry mouth, constipation, urinary hesitancy and
   retention, hypokalemia, no alcoholic beverages with drug

Esmolol hydrochloride (*Brevibloc*) Class II see Beta-adrenergic
   antagonist

Flecainide (*Tambacor*), PO, Common side effects include dizziness,
   blurred vision, difficulty in focusing and nausea, plasma level
   monitoring of drug is recommended 0.7-1 ug/ml for trough, report
   visual disturbances

Lidocaine hydrochloride (*Anestacon, Dilocaine, L-Caine,
   Lida-Mantle, Lidoject-1, LidoPen Auto Injector, Nervocaine,
   Octocaine, Xylocaine*), IV, IM or direct to vein, Deltoid muscle is
   recommended for IM — avoid inadvertant IV administration,
   assess for signs of cardiac depression, auscultate the lungs for

rales, theraputic blood levels 1.5-6 ug/ml, levels greater than 7 are toxic

Mexiletine (*Mexitil*), PO, Common side effects include dizziness, tremor, nervousness, incoordination, nausea, vomiting and heartburn. Effective serum concentration is 0.5-2 ug/ml, supervise ambulation

Moricizine (*Ethmozine*), PO, Common side effects include dizziness, anxiety headache, euphoria, perioral numbness and lightheadedness

Nifedipine (*Adalat, Procardia*), Class IV, see calcium channel blockers

Phenytoin (*Dilantin*), Class III, see Anticonvulsants

Propafanone (*Rhthmol*), PO, Common side effects include dizziness, blurred vision and taste alterations

Quinidine (*Apo-Quinidine, Quinidex extentabs, Quinora, Duraquin*) PO. Common side effects include nausea, vomiting, diarrhea and abdominal pain. Take with full glass of water on empty stomach

Sotalol (*Betapace*), Class II, see Beta-adrenergic antagonist

Tocainide hydrochloride (*Tonocard*), PO, Common side effects include: tremors, dizziness, lightheadedness, visual disturbances, vertigo and tinnitus. Administer with food, effective serum concentration is 3.5-10 ug per ml, onset of tremors indicates maximum dose is being approached, CBC should be monitored for blood dyscrasia

Verapamil hydrochloride (*Calan, Isoptin, Veralens*) Class II, see Calcium Channel Blockers

ANTILIPEMIC — BILE ACID SEQUESTRANT

Action: Increases loss of bile acids in the stool which leads to lowered total serum cholesterol

Indications: Hypercholesterolemia

Example: Cholestyramine Resin (*Cholybar, Questran, Questran Light*)

Route: PO

Contraindications: Complete biliary obstruction, hypersensitivity to bile acid sequestrants

Common adverse effects: Constipation

Life-threatening adverse effects: none

Other adverse effects: Uveitis, fecal impaction, hemorrhoids, abdominal pain, abdominal distention, flatulence, bloating sensations, belching, nausea, vomiting, heartburn, anorexia, diarrhea, steatorrhea, urticaria, dermatitis, asthma, shortness of

breath, weight loss or gain, increased livido, iron, calcium, vitamin A, D, and K deficiencies, rash, irritations of skin, tongue and perianal areas, hypoprothrombinemia
Interventions:
Place 1 pkg in 4-6 ozs of water or preferred liquid, allow to stand for 1-2 minutes without stirring, then stir until uniform
Administer before meals, always dissolve powder before drinking
Report any abnormal bleeding, petechiae, ecchymoses or tarry stools
Supplemental vitamins may be ordered
Serum cholesterol levels are reduced within 24-48 hours of therapy
High bulk diet with increased fluid intake is recommended for constipation

Examples of other drugs in this classification:
Colestipol hydrochloride (*Colestid*), PO, Give other medications 1 hr before or 4 hours after colestipol, monitor Na+ and K+ levels, check with primary care provider regarding alcohol use

ANTILIPEMICS — LIPID LOWERING AGENTS
Action: Act directly on the formation of cholesterol to produce lower cholesterol levels
Indications: High serum cholesterol levels that have not responded to dietary interventions
Example: Lovastatin (*Mevacor, Mevinolin*)
Route: PO
Pharmacokinetics: Onset 2 weeks, Peak 4-6 weeks
Contraindications: Active liver disease, unexplained elevations of serum transaminases
Common adverse effects: Drug is generally well tolerated
Life-threatening adverse effects: None
Other adverse effects: Dizziness, mild headache, insomnia, fatigue, nausea, blurred vision, dyspepsia, dysgeusia, heartburn, constipation, diarrhea, flatus, abdominal pain, rash, pruritis
Interventions:
Monitor liver function tests for increase in serum transaminases
Report any muscle tenderness or pain
Low-fat diet should be continued

Examples of other drugs in this classification:
Clofibrate (*Atromid-S*), PO, Nausea is a common side effect, laboratory monitoring to include CBC, renal function tests, urine steroid levels, serum electrolytes and blood sugar is recommened, agranulocytosis is a possible life-threatening side effect, give with meals

Dextrothyroxine sodium (*Choloxin*), PO, Patients with cardiac disease need close monitoring, report any change in cardiac condition, MI is a possible life-threatening adverse effect

Gemfibrozil (*Lopid*), PO, not for use in patients with gallbladder disease, kidney or liver dysfunction, common side effects include abdominal or epigastric pain, cholelithiasis, Administer 30 minutes before meals, monitor cholesterol, triglycerides, CBC, and blood glucose levels, report any unexplained bleeding

Niacin (*Vitamin B3, Niac, Nicobid, Nico-400, Nicolar, Nicotinex*) PO, SC, IM, Common side effects include: Transient headache, tingling of extremities, generalized flushing, sensations of warmth, jaundice, bloating, flatulence nausea, pruritus, Administer with meals and cold water, Patient should avoid sudden postural changes, alcohol should be limited

Pravastatin (*Pravachol*), PO, Should be given in evening

Probucol (*Lorelco*), PO, Common side effect is diarrhea, Administer with meals, monitor pulse during initial treatment, ventricular arrhythmias may occur, periodic ECG's may be ordered during treatment, Any unexplained bleeding should be reported, Alcohol intake may be limited or prohibited, Swelling on face, hands should be reported

Simvastatin (*Zocar*), PO, Administer in evening, report unexplained muscle pain

BETA ADRENERGIC ANTAGONIST
Action: Decrease heart-rate and cardiac output
Indications: Cardiac arrhythmias, myocardial infarction, hypertension and angina
Example: Propranolol hydrocholoride (*Inderal, Inderal LA*)
Route: Oral (PO), IV
Pharmacokinetics: PO, Peak 60-90 minutes, IV 5 minutes
Contraindications: Greater than 1st degree heart block, congestive heart failure, sinus bradycardia, cardiogenic shock, mitral valve disease, bronchial asthma or bronchospasm, severe chronic airway disease (COPD), allergic rhinitis, patients on MAO inhibitors
Common adverse effects: Confusion, fatigue, drowsiness, bradycardia
Life-threatening adverse effects: Agranulocytosis, laryngospasm, cardiac arrest
Other adverse effects: Erythematous, pruritus, fever, pharyngitis, vertigo, respiratory distress, psychosis, sleep problems, depression, agitation, giddiness, lightheadedness, syncope, weakness, insomnia, hallucinations, delusions, palpitations, AV heart block, hypotension,

angina, acute CHF, tachyarrhythmia, paresthesia of hands, dry eyes, visual disturbances, conjunctivitis, tinnitus, hearing loss, nasal stuffiness, dry mouth, nausea, vomiting, heartburn, diarrhea, constipation, flatus, abdominal cramping, transient eosinophilia, thrombocytopenic purpura, hypoglycemia, hyperglycemia, hypocalcemia, dyspnea, bronchospasm, alopecia, pancreatitis, weight gain, impotence, decreased libido, arthralgia

Interventions:

Administer before meals and at bedtime, tablet may be crushed

Take pulse and blood pressure before administration, withhold if pulse is below 60 or systolic BP is below 90

IV administration requires monitoring of ECG, BP and pulmonary wedge pressure

Monitor I&O and daily weights to assess for fluid retention and CHF

Assess for signs of hypoglycemia in diabetic or fasting patients

Examples of other drugs in this classification:

Acebutol hydrochloride (*Sectral*), PO, Other common side effects include: diarrhea and constipation

   Atenolol (*Tenormin*), PO, IV over 5 minutes or in solution over 15-30 mins

Betaxolol hydrochloride (*Betoptic, Betoptic-S, Kerlone*) Topical for open-angle glaucoma, PO for hypertension

Carteolol hydrochloride (*Cartrol*), Opthalmic for glaucoma, PO for high blood pressure, Do not crush tablet, if pulse is below 50 withhold drug

Esmolol hydrochloride (*Brevibloc*), IV for supraventricular tachyarrhythmia and used to control heart rate in MI, Administer via infusion pump, use of butterfly needles is not recommended, for short-term use only, monitor BP, pulse and ECG during infusion, burning, redness at IV site may occur temporarily, stop infusion if bradycardia, dizziness, drowsiness, dyspnea, cyanosis or seizures occur

Metoprolol tartrate (*Lopressor*), PO for angina or hypertension, IV push in MI at rate of 5 mg over 60 seconds, monitor BP, pulse and ECG with IV push, Assess for depression, report to primary care provider if noted, usual pulse increase after exercise may not occur, provide frequent oral care, Patient should wear medical identification bracelet

Nadolol (*Corgard*), PO, Prophylactic angina pectoris or hypertension

Penbutolol (*Levatol*), PO, Patient should avoid excesses of alcohol

Pindolol (*Visken*), PO

Sotalol (*Betapace*), PO, Administer on empty stomach, Do not
   administer with milk or milk products, Initial dosing should be
   monitored with ECG

Timolol Maleate (*Blocadren, Timoptic*), Ophthalmic solution for
   glaucoma, PO for hypertension, Tablets may be crushed

CALCIUM CHANNEL BLOCKERS
Action: Inhibit the passage of calcium into the cell decreasing the
cells contractability, this reduces blood pressure by causing
peripheral blood vessel dilitation
Indications: High blood pressure
Example: Nifedipine (*Adalat, Adalat CC, Procardia, Procardia XL*)
<u>Route:</u> PO, SL
<u>Pharmacokinetics:</u> Onset 10-30 minutes, Peak 30 minutes
<u>Contraindications:</u> Known sensitivity to Nifedipine
<u>Common adverse effects:</u> Dizziness, lightheadedness, headache,
facial flush, heat sensations, peripheral edema and diarrhea
<u>Life-threatening adverse effects:</u> Myocardial infarction
<u>Other adverse effects:</u> Nervousness, mood changes, weakness,
jitteriness, sleep disturbances, blurred vision, retinal ischemia,
balance problems, hypotension, palpitations, nausea, heartburn,
constipation, cramps, flatus, joint stiffness, muscle cramps, sore
throat, weakness, dermatitis, fever, pruritus, urticaria, gingival
hyperplasia, sweating, chills, congestion
<u>Interventions:</u>
May be given sublingual in an emergency situation, puncture
capsule and express contents out under tongue
Monitor blood pressure before administration, hold if BP <90
Monitor blood sugar in diabetic patients
Assess for gingival hyperplasia, report if noted, provide oral/dental
care
Assess for any increase in angina and report
Smoking decreases the effectiveness of this medication
Examples of other drugs in this classification:
Amlodipine (*Norvasc*), PO, Common adverse effects include
   peripheral and facial edema, dose-related palpitations may occur
Diltiazem (*Cardizem, Cardizem CD, Cardizem IV, Cardizem SR,
   Dilacor XL*), PO, IV for atrial fibrillation, may increase digoxin
   levels, incompatible with furosemide in solution, Administer
   before meals and at bedtime
Felodipine (*Plendil*), PO, Common side effects include palpitations,
   edema, and fatigue, Do not crush tablets, report tachycardia,
   may increase levels of digoxin

Isradipine (*Dynacirc*), PO, Assess for signs of increasing heart failure, monitor ambulation

Nicardipine hydrochloride (*Cardene, Cardene SR*), PO, Common side effects include fatigue, peripheral edema, diaphoresis, increased angina, and hypotension, Administer on empty stomach, Measure BP 1-2 hours after dose for peak effect and 8 hours after dose for trough effect, instruct patient to make postural changes slowly, notify physician of irregular heartbeat, shortness of breath, or drop in BP

Verapamil hydrochloride (*Calan, Calan SR, Isoptin, Isoptin SR, Veralens*), PO, IV for supraventricular tachycardia, Incompatable in IV form with aminophylline, amphotericin B, cotrimazole, hydralazine, ampicillin, mezlocillin, nafcillin, oxacillin, and sodium bicarbonate, Administer oral with food, Monitor for AV block if given with digitalis, monitor I&O, ECG monitoring is required for IV use, Take pulse before administration report irregular pulse or slowed pulse

CARDIAC GLYCOSIDES

Action: Increase the force of cardiac contraction, increasing cardiac output, blood pressure is decreased, and the heart rate is slowed

Indications: Congestive heart failure and arrhythmias

Example: Digoxin (*Lanoxicaps, Lanoxin*)

Route: IV, PO

Pharmacokinetics: PO, Onset 1-2 hrs, Peak 6-8 hrs, Duration 3-4 days; IV, Onset 5-30 min, Peak 1-5 hrs, Duration 3-4 days

Contraindications: Digitalis hypersensitivity, ventricular fibrillation, ventricular tachycardia unless due to CHF

Common adverse effects: Nausea

Life-threatening adverse effects: AV block

Other adverse effects: Fatigue, muscle weakness, headache, paresthesias, facial neuralgia, mental depression, hallucinations, confusion, agitation, drowsiness, dizziness, arrhythmias, hypotension, visual disturbances, anorexia, vomiting, diarrhea, diaphoresis, dysphagia

Interventions:

Tablet may be crushed and mixed with food and fluid

Assess radial pulse 1 full minute prior to administration, hold if pulse is below 60, unless other parameters are noted, know patients baseline VS any change in pulse rate or rhythm is a sign of digitalis intoxication

Assess baseline levels of serum electrolytes, creatinine clearance, level of serum digoxin, magnesium and calcium, notify primary care provider if abnormal levels are found

Assess for anorexia, nausea, vomiting, diarrhea, visual disturbances are possible indicators of digitalis toxicity

Therapeutic range of digoxin is 0.8-2 ng/ml, with toxic levels 2ng/ml

Digoxin levels should be drawn 5-6 hrs after dose and just before the next scheduled dose

Monitor I&O during digitalization, assess for edema and ausculatate lungs for rales

Examples of other drugs in this classification:

Deslanoside (*Cedilanid-D, Cedilanid*), IV at rate of 0.2 mg /min,
Used for rapid digitalizing in emergency situation, monitor for hypercalcemia

CENTRAL-ACTING ANTIHYPERTENSIVES

Action: Stimulate the adrenergic nervous system to decrease blood pressure

Indications: High blood pressure

Example: Methyldopa (*Aldomet*)

Route: PO, IV

Pharmacokinetics: Peak 4-6 hrs, Duration 24 hours on oral, 10-16 hrs IV

Contraindications: Active liver disease, blood dyscrasias

Common adverse effects: Fever, sedation, drowsiness, decreased mental acuity, sodium and water retention, nasal stuffiness, decreased libido, impotence

Life-threatening adverse effects: Granulocytopenia, agranulocytosis, hepatic necrosis

Other adverse effects: Skin eruptions, ulcerations of feet, flulike symptoms, lymphadenopathy, eosinophilia, sluggishness, headache, weakness, fatigue, dizziness, vertigo, inability to concentrate, mild psychoses, depression, nightmares, orthostatic hypotension, syncope, bradycardia, myocarditis, edema, sodium and water retention, diarrhea, constipation, abdominal distension, nausea, vomiting, dry mouth, sore tongue, black tongue, sialadenitis, jaundice, hepatitis, gynecomastia, lactation and hypothermia

Interventions:

During IV infusion monitor VS and observe for adequate urinary output

Take BP in lying, sitting and standing on at least one occasion to obtain baselines

Supervise ambulation and position changes until patients response to drug is known

Monitor I&O, report decrease in urine output, weigh patient daily

Monitor CBC and liver function tests
Assess mental status and report any changes to primary care provider
Provide for patients safety during showers as hot water may enhance orthostatic hypotension

Examples of other drugs in this classification:

Clonidine hydrochloride (*Catapres, Catapres-TTS*) PO, Transdermal patch, Common adverse effects include: dry mouth and constipation, Assess patient with history of depression for excerbation of depression, Patient should carry medical alert card, Report any rash or irritation under transdermal patch, patch should not be cut or trimmed in any manner

Guanabenz acetate (*Wytensin*), PO, Dry mouth is another common adverse effect, Administered usually at bedtime, Additional laboratory tests to be monitored include urinalysis for protein and sugar, and blood chemistry, Offer frequent oral care if dry mouth is a problem

Guanfacine hydrochloride (*Tenex*), PO, Common adverse effects also include: fatigue, dry mouth and constipation, Administered at bedtime, frequent oral care to prevent dry mouth, Alcohol use or other CNS depressents may increase drowsiness and should be avoided

Mecamylamine hydrochloride (*Inversine*), PO, Common adverse effects also include: orthostatic hypotension, blurred vision, dry mouth, anorexia, nausea, vomiting, constipation, diarrhea and urinary retention, Assess for signs of paralytic ileus (abdominal distention, decreased bowel sounds — report ASAP), Instruct patient to lie down if dizziness or lightheadedness is felt, Smaller doses may be required in the summer, frequent oral care should be given

NITRATE VASODILATORS

Action: Dilation of large veins promotes decrease in blood pressure
Indications: Angina pectoris, high blood pressure
Example: Nitroglycerin (*Deponit, Minitran, Nitro-Bid, Nitro-Bid IV, Nitrocap, Nitrodisc, Nitro-Dur, Nitrogard, Nitrogard-SR, Nitroglyn, Nitrol, Nitrolingual, Nitrong, Nitrong SR, Nitrospan, Nitrostat, Nitrostat IV, Nitro-T.D., Transderm-Nitro, Tridil*)
<u>Route:</u> SL, PO, IV, Topical
<u>Pharmacokinetics:</u> SL Onset 2 minutes, Duration 30 minutes
PO, Onset 3 minutes, Duration 3-5 hours
Ointment, Onset 30 minutes, Duration 3-6 hours
<u>Contraindications:</u> Hypersensitivity to nitrates, severe anemia, head

trauma, increased intracrainial pressure, glaucoma, hypovolemia, pericarditis, pericardial tamponade

<u>Common adverse effects:</u> Headache and postural hypotension

<u>Life-threatening adverse effects:</u> Circulatory collapse and anaphylactic reaction

<u>Other adverse effects:</u> Apprehension, blurred vision, weakness, vertigo, dizziness, faintness, palpitations, tachycardia, increased angina, syncope, nausea, vomiting, abdominal pain, dry mouth, methemogloboinemia, vasodilation with flushing, rash, dermatitis, muscle twitching, pallor, perspiration, and cold sweat

<u>Interventions:</u>

Aministration of SL medication: place under tongue at onset of angina, have patient sit or lie down, instruct patient to not swallow tablet but to let it dissolve slowly, if pain is not relieved additional tablet may be administered after 5 minutes (no more than 3 tablets in 15 minutes)

Administration of extended release buccal tablets: Placed between lip and and gum or cheek and gum, dissolve slowly over 3-5 hours

Administration of PO tablets or capsule: Take on empty stomach with one full glass of water, do not crush or chew

Administration of ointment: Express out ordered amount of ointment into applicator and spread in a thin layer on non-hairy skin surface, cover transparent wrap and tape, rotate sites

Administration of IV form: Use infusion pump, manufacture suggested tubing and IV glass bottle, Titrate as ordered, monitor for signs of ethanol toxicity to inlcude vomiting, lethargy, coma, alcohol smelling breath

Remain with patients during angina attacks, assess effectiveness of drugs, notify physician if drug is not effective, remove SL med when angina gone

Assess baseline vital signs and take VS as ordered during administration

Overdose S&S include hypotension, tachycardia, warmed flushed skin, headache, palpitations, confusion, nausea, vomiting, fever, paralysis, coma, convulsions and heart failure report to physician ASAP

Record all angina attacks, use of nitroglycerin and its effectiveness

Postural hypotension may occur, supervise ambulation and position changes until response to medication is known

Examples of other drugs in this classification:

Amyl Nitrite, Inhalation agent in glass ampule, ampule is crushed
   between fingers and vapors inhaled, gauze should be used to hold

ampule during crushing, patient should sit during administration to prevent fainting

Erythrityl Tetranitrate (*Cardilate*), PO, SL, Monitor apical pulse for 1 full minute tachycardia is a common side effect

Isosorbide Dinitrate (*Dilatrate-SR, Iso-Bid, Isordil, Isotrate, Sorbitrate, Novosorbide, Sorbitrate SA*) PO, Chewable tablet should be chewed totally before swallowing, Do not chew sustained release forms

Pentaerythritol Tetranitrate (*Duotrate, Pentylan, Peritrate, PETN*), PO, Not for relief of acute angina attacks

NON-NITRATE VASODILATORS

Action: Reduces blood pressure by relaxing the smooth muscle inside the blood vessels to cause vasodilatation

Indications: High blood pressure, congestive heart failure

Example: Hydralazine hydrochloride (*Alazine, Apresoline*)

Route: PO, IM, IV

Pharmacokinetics: Onset 20-30 mins, Peak 2 hrs, Duration 2-6 hrs

Contraindications: Coronary artery disease, mitral value disease, MI, tachycardia, systematic lupus erthymatoeous

Common adverse effects: Headache, palpitations and tachycardia

Life-threatening adverse effects: Shock

Other adverse effects: Dizziness, tremors, depression, anxiety, angina, disorientation, flushing, orthostatic hypotension, arrhythmias, anorexia, nausea, vomiting, diarrhea, constipation, abdominal pain, paralytic ileus, lacrimation, conjunctivitis, dysuria, glomerulonephritis, rash, uticaria, pruritus, fever, chills, arthralgia, eosinophilia, cholangitis, hepatitis, jaundice, nasal congestion, muscle cramps, rheumatoid and edema

Interventions:

IV drug may be given 10mg over 1 minute IV push, monitor pulse and BP

Monitor BUN, creatinine clearance, uric acid, serum K+, blood glucose, LE cell preparation, antinuclear antibody titer and ECG during therapy

Monitor I&O during IM and IV therapy

Monitor weight, assess for edema daily

Assist patient with ambulation until response to drug is known, postural hypotension may occur, have patient lie or sit down if dizziness occurs

Examples of drugs in this classification:

Cyclandelate (*Cyclan, Cyclospasmol*), PO, Relatively few side effects, take with food or milk

Dipyridamole (*Persantine, Pyridamole, IV Persantine*) PO, IV, Take on empty stomach

Ethaverine hydrochloride (*Ethaquin, Ethatab, Ethavex-100, Isovex*), PO, Monitor pulse for 1 minute and take blood pressure before administration, withold drug if significant changes from baseline have occurred, notify primary care provider, drug may cause arrhythmias and depression of respirations, monitor liver function studies, assess for jaundice

Minoxidil (*Loniten, Rogaine*) PO, Take pulse and BP before administration, report pulse increase of 20 bpm or greater above baseline, monitor I&O and auscultate for rales daily, report shortness of breath, lightheadedness, fainting, chest pain, weight gain of 2 pounds or more in 24 hours, assess for hypertrichosis (increased pigmentation of body hair with long thick hairs may occur on face, arms and backs), this medication is also used to treat baldness in topical form

Nitroprusside sodium (*Nipride, Nitropress*), IV, Used for hypertensive crisis, solutions must be used within 4 hours of preparation, no other drugs can be added to nitroprusside solution, solution will have faint brownish tint, wrap solution in aluminum foil to protect drug from the light, monitor BP continously during administration, titrate drug to BP response

Papaverine hydrochloride (*Cerespan, Genabid, Pavabid, Pavased, Pavatyme, Paverolan*), PO, IM, IV, Used primarily for MI with arrhythmias, cerebral and peripheral ischemia associated with arterial spasm, IV drug is not compatible with Lactated Ringers

RAUWOLFA ALKALOID

Action: Blocks sympathetic neurons (blocks the release or storage of norepinephrine) and therefore decreases blood pressure
Indications: High blood pressure
Example: Reserpine (*Serpalan, Sk-Reserpine*)
Route: PO
Pharmacokinetics: Peak 2 hours
Contraindications: Hypersensitivity to Rauwolfa alkaloids, patients with depression, peptic ulcer, ulcerative colitis, electroconvulsive therapy, use of MAO inhibitors within 1-2 weeks
Common adverse effects: Drowsiness, lethargy, edema, and nasal congestion
Life-threatening adverse effects: Respiratory depression
Other adverse effects: Depression, nervousness, anxiety, nightmares, headache, appetite increases, tremors, muscle rigidity, convulsions, hypothermia, bradycardia, orthostatic hypotension,

arrhythmias, epistaxis, lacrimation, blurred vision, miosis, ptosis, dry mouth or excess saliva, nausea, vomiting, abdominal cramping, diarrhea, heartburn, purpura, rash, anemia, thrombocytopenia, pruritus, asthma, menstrual irregularities, breast engorgement, galactorrhea, gynecomastia, feminization in males, impaired sexual function, impotence, muscle aches, dysuria

Interventions:

Administer with meals or milk, monitor VS, monitor I&O, assess for mental depression, assess for drowsiness and need for assistance in ambulation

Report dizziness or lightheadedness, assist patient with showers or baths

Assess for weight gain and edema, monitor blood glucose in diabetics

Section VIII — GLOSSARY OF TERMS

Aneurysm	Abnormal dilation of a vessel due to weakness in the vessel wall, may be congenital
Angialgia	Pain in vessel
Angina pectoris	Severe chest pain lasting seconds to minutes, related to insufficient blood supply to cardiac tissues, may radiate to shoulder and left arm
Angiogram	X-ray of blood vessels using contrast dye
Aortitis	Inflammation of the aorta
Apex of heart	Bottom tip of the heart
Arrhythmia	Abnormal rhythm of the heart detectable on ECG monitoring or noted on auscultation
Atherosclerosis	Build-up of fatty deposits in the blood vessels
Atrioventricular node (AV)	Part of the heart's electrical conduction system
Atria	The two upper chambers of the heart that receive blood
Atrioventricular valves (AV)	The valves located between the atria and ventricular chambers of the heart
Bicuspid valve (mitral value)	Separates the left atrium and left ventricle, one of the AV valves
Blood pressure (BP)	Amount of pressure exerted on the inside walls of a blood vessel
Bradycardia	Heart rate below 60 beats per minute (adult)
Bundle of His	Part of the electrical conduction system of the heart which conducts electrical stimulation from the AV node to the medial surfaces of the ventricles
Cardiac	Pertaining to the heart
Cardiac catheterization	A diagnostic procedure where a radiopaque catheter is inserted into the heart via a vein in arm or leg and threaded into the vena cava, right atrium, or right ventricle; catheter may

	also be threaded into an artery to assess the aorta, left atrium and left ventricle
Cardiac output (CO)	The amount of blood the left ventricle ejects into the aorta per minute, calculated by SV x HR
Code	Code arrest, an emergency involving arrest of breathing (respiratory arrest) or heartbeat (cardiac arrest)
Crash cart	Slang term for a resuscitation cart used in code emergencies
Defibrillation	Stopping the fibrillation of the heart with drugs or electrical means; electrical defibrillation applies a countershock to the heart via electrodes on the chest
Diastole	The period of relaxation in the heart cycle when the ventricles fill with blood
ECG	Abbreviation for electrocardiogram
Echocardiogram	Ultrasound examination of the heart non-invasive procedure where a transducer is moved over the chest, and sound waves are bounced off the structures of the heart, able to detect an enlargement of the heart
Electro-cardiogram	ECG/EKG: A diagnostic test that records the electrical activity of the heart, used to diagnose abnormal cardiac rhythms
Embolism	Obstruction of vessel caused by a clot or foreign substance in circulating blood
Endocarditis	Inflammation of the endocardium
Endocardium	Thin layer of endothelium lining the inner aspect of the heart
Epicardium	Transparent outer layer of the heart wall
Extracorporeal circulation	Procedure to circulate blood during cardiac surgery while bypassing the heart and lungs
Fibrillation	Quivering or contraction of individual cardiac muscle fibers, may be atrial or ventricular

Hyperkalemia	Serum potassium above level of 3.8-5.0 mmol/L
Hypertension	High blood pressure
Hypokalemia	Serum potassium is below level of 3.8-5.0 mmol/L
Intravenous	A system to deliver fluids through the veins (IV) consisting of a catheter placed in the vein, and a flexible tubing connected to a solution bag
Mitral valve (Bicuspid valve)	Separates the left atrium from the left ventricle
Myocardial infarction (MI)	Death of an area of tissue in the myocardium of the heart (coronary, heart attack)
Myocardium	Cardiac muscle tissue
Palpitation	A sudden throbbing or flutter in the heart
Pericardial sac	Serous membrane that encloses the heart
Pericarditis	Inflammation of the pericardium
Phlebitus	Inflammation of a vein
Purkinje fibers	Part of the electrical conduction system of the heart
Semilunar valves	Two valves located between ventricles and arteries that prevent blood from flowing back into the heart
Sinoatrial node	The pacemaker of the heart, initiates the cardiac cycle
Stroke volume	The amount of blood the heart ejects during contraction (systole) from the ventricle (average 70 cc/beat)
Systole	The period of ventricular contraction in the heart cycle
Tachycardia	Heart rate above 100 beats per minute in an adult

Tricuspid valve   Separates the right atrium and right ventricle, so called because it contains 3 flaps; one of the two atrioventricular valves

Ventricles   The two lower heart chambers

Vital signs   Temperature, pulse, respirations and blood pressure

Respiratory System

RESPIRATORY SYSTEM

Table of Contents

Section I — THE OVERVIEW

Primary Functions

- Respiration: the exchange of oxygen and CO_2 between the atmosphere and the blood, may be external or internal
- External respiration, exchange of gases between the external environment (air) and internal environment (lungs)
- Internal respiration, exchange of gases at the cellular level between the alveoli and the blood
- Filtering, warming, and humidification of incoming air through the nose
- Formation of the sounds known as speech

Components (Figure 2A)

Contains components used in external respiration

> Nose, pharynx, larynx (voice box), trachea (windpipe), bronchi, and lungs and internal respiration
>
> Alveoli and capillaries

Nose

- Made of cartilage and bone, divided by the septum into two chambers
- Primary entry point for air entering the body
- Filtering center for incoming air: lined with tiny hairs called cilia which filter dust and particles out and then trap them in mucous to prevent them from entering the sterile environment of the lungs
- Warming and humidification of incoming air begins here as it passes over the network of tiny blood vessels within the nose

Pharynx (The back portion of the nose and mouth)

- A 5 inch muscular tube extending from the base of the skull to the level of the 6th vertebra
- Contains 3 parts, the nasopharynx, the oropharynx, and the laryngopharynx
- On one end of the pharynx is the nose on the other end it communicates with the esophagus and the larynx
- Air continues to be humidified and warmed in the pharynx
- Pharynx also provides the passageway for food from the mouth into the esophagus and then the stomach

Components Used in External Respiration

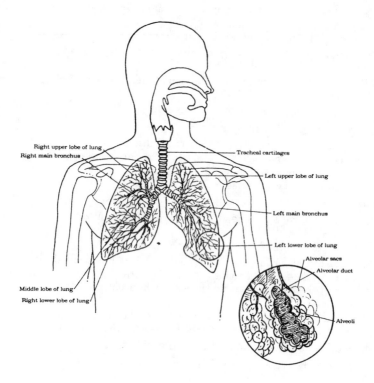

Figure 2A

Larynx (voice box or Adam's apple)

- Link between the pharynx and the trachea consisting of nine cartilages bound together by an elastic membrane and muscle
- Approximately 36mm long in females and 44mm in males
- The epiglottis covers the entrance to the larynx during swallowing to prevent food or drink from entering the lungs
- Interior of the larynx contains the ventricular folds (false vocal cords) and the vocal folds (true vocal cords)
- Also coated with mucous to filter incoming air

Trachea (windpipe)

- Large 4½ inch tube made up of bands of C-shaped cartilage
- Located between the larynx and the bronchial tubes
- Beginning at the sixth cervical vertebrae extending to the fifth thoracic vertebra
- Divides into two bronchi; the right and the left, the point of division is known as the carina tracheae
- Mucous lined passage for air movement into and out of the lungs

Bronchi (bronchus = singular)

- Located inside the lungs
- The right bronchus is shorter, wider and more vertical than the left; for this reason a foreign object is more likely to become lodged in the right bronchus than the left
- Both bronchi branch out like a tree; there are five smaller bronchi which lead into the five lobes of the lungs, these further divide into about 50-80 terminal bronchioles in each lobe
- Each of terminal bronchioles further divide into two respiratory bronchioles, each of which divide further into 2-11 alveolar ducts which give rise to alveolar sacs and alveoli (about 300 million in the lungs)
- Internal respiration or gas exchange takes place in alveoli

Lungs

- Lungs are connected to the trachea by the right and left bronchi
- Right lung is thicker and broader and has three lobes
- Left lung has two lobes and an indentation for the heart known as the cardiac depression
- Function is to bring air and blood into close proximity so O2 and CO_2 can be exchanged (internal respiration)

Concepts
Respiration
- Average adult at rest breathes 14-20 times/minute
- About 500ml of air is inspired per breath, maximum amount of air that can be inhaled is about 3000 ml (*inspiratory reserve*)
- Maximum amount of air that can be exhaled after a normal breath is about 1200 ml (*expiratory reserve*)
- The amount of air that can be exhaled forcibly after inhaling the largest breath possible is about 4700ml (*vital capacity*).
- The amount of air left in the lungs that you are not able to exhale even forcibly is about 1200 ml (*residual volume*)

Internal Respiration
- Unoxygenated blood enters the lungs lobes through the pulmonary arteries leaving the heart
- Pulmonary arteries are large and then progressively branch and narrow, until they become capillaries
- Capillaries, like the alveoli, are located throughout the lungs
- In the capillaries blood is exposed to oxygen on all sides as it passes through the alveolar wall
- Each individual blood cell contains millions of hemoglobin molecules which are each able to bind four molecules of oxygen
- While the hemoglobin molecule is picking up oxygen; it is releasing carbon dioxide molecules
- This exchange of gas molecules is termed internal respiration

Control for respiration
- The respiratory regulatory center is located in the lower portion of the brain stem (medulla oblongata)
- Breathing is not usually a conscious act, the respiratory center sends the message to the diaphragm and intercostal muscles
- We can consciously alter our breathing, we can breathe faster or slower at will
- The respiratory center receives constant feedback from the body which it uses to adjust the rate or depth of breathing and thereby control the amount of oxygen the body receives and the amount of carbon dioxide the body loses
- The respiratory center has chemoreceptors that monitor carbon dioxide levels in the blood

- When the carbon dioxide is elevated, neurons in the respiratory center increase the rate of respiration, so more carbon dioxide is blown out of the body and more oxygen enters restoring the proper blood levels
- Carbon dioxide levels in the normal healthy body will always provide the stimulus for respiration (in persons with chronic lung disease who have elevated levels of carbon dioxide, this is not the case)

The mechanics of breathing

- The mechanics of breathing (movement of air into and out of the chest) is a response to changing pressures
- Between respirations, the pressure outside the body and the pressure inside the body are equal
- To start respirations, the respiratory center in the brain sends a signal to the diaphragm and the intercostal muscles to contract
- With contraction the lungs increase in depth and circumference, increasing lung volume and causing the lung pressure to drop below atmospheric pressure
- When the pressure drops, air moves into the lungs (inspiration); the pressure in the lungs is again equal to the air pressure outside the body
- A message is then sent for the diaphragm and intercostal muscles to relax, this reduces lung volume and forces air out of the lungs into the atmosphere (expiration) See Figure 2B

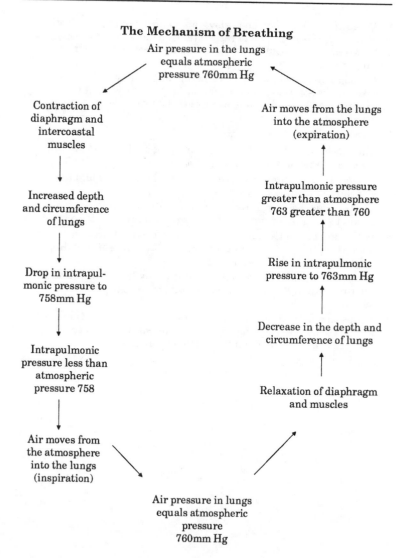

The Mechanism of Breathing

Air pressure in the lungs equals atmospheric pressure 760mm Hg

Contraction of diaphragm and intercoastal muscles

Increased depth and circumference of lungs

Drop in intrapulmonic pressure to 758mm Hg

Intrapulmonic pressure less than atmospheric pressure 758

Air moves from the atmosphere into the lungs (inspiration)

Air moves from the lungs into the atmosphere (expiration)

Intrapulmonic pressure greater than atmosphere 763 greater than 760

Rise in intrapulmonic pressure to 763mm Hg

Decrease in the depth and circumference of lungs

Relaxation of diaphragm and muscles

Air pressure in lungs equals atmospheric pressure 760mm Hg

Figure 2B

Section II — ASSESSMENT

HEALTH HISTORY

Chief complaint

- Common chief complaints for this system include:
    Cough, productive or nonproductive
    Dyspnea (difficulty breathing)
    Chest pain
    Wheeze
    Hemoptysis (blood in sputum)
    Shortness of breath

Family and personal history

- Obtain specific diagnoses and age at diagnosis when known
- Obtain ages and causes of death in immediate family members
- Assess for presence and past treatment of the following:
    Tuberculosis
    Lung cancer
    Chronic airway diseases (COPD); i.e., emphysema, bronchitis
    Asthma
- If personal or family history of tuberculosis note date of last TB test or chest x-ray and results
- If above condition exists assess for required life style changes and current treatment of condition to include medications

Shortness of breath

- Assess if activity related
- Frequency and duration of attacks

Cough

- Onset
- Factors that aggravate the cough (temperature, talking, position, drinking, eating, time of day)
- Productive (with sputum) or non-productive in nature
- If productive, amount, color and character of sputum (eg. viscous, thin)
- Presence of pain with cough

Chest pain

- Assess location, severity, duration and if pain radiates
- Pain that is sharp and well localized may be pleurisy, pneumothorax, rib fracture or non-pulmonic in nature

- Pleuritic pain and pain from rib fracture is made worse by deep breathing or coughing and improves with immbolization of chest (holding side or splinting a pillow against chest)
- See also chest pain under cardiovascular system

Respiratory system testing

- Assess for tests completed or ordered and patient's knowledge and understanding of any test procedures or results

RESPIRATORY SYSTEM ASSESSMENT FORM

Chief Complaint

Complaint_____ Onset_____ Symptoms_____

Frequency_____ Duration_____ Other areas affected_____

Have you had this before?_____ When_____

What have you done for this?_____

What do you think caused this to happen?_____

What changes have you had to make in your life?_____

Personal and Family History

	Patient date	Family member		Patient Only Now	In Past
Tuberculosis	____	____	Shortness of Breath	____	____
Lung Cancer	____	____	Wheezing	____	____
Pneumonia	____	____	Bloody sputum	____	____
COPD	____	____	Pain in chest	____	____
Asthma	____	____	Where_____	When_____	
Emphysema	____	____	URI	____	____

Do you have a cough?_____ Productive_____ Color of Sputum_____

Respiratory System Testing

Chest X-rays_____ Pulmonary function studies_____

Bronchoscopy_____ Lung biopsy_____ CT scan_____ Mediastinoscopy_____

Other_____

Current Treatments/Medications

Name_____ Dose_____ Frequency_____ Route_____

Cigarettes/day____/____/____yrs   Alcoholic drinks____/____/____yrs

What is your usual weight?_____ Have you lost/gained?_____

PHYSICAL ASSESSMENT

- Respiratory assessment is done in the following order:
  1. Inspection
  2. Palpation
  3. Percussion
  4. Auscultation
- Patient is generally undressed to the waist for this exam

INSPECTION

General appearance

- Assess patient's chosen positioning — Patient who is short of breath may position themselves in high fowlers position
- A patient in respiratory distress may not tolerate the supine position or other position changes
- Appearance — Patients with chronic airway diseases may appear cachexic secondary to increased effort required for respirations which leads to fatigue and a greater caloric need

Skin

- Color — Assess for cyanosis (gray or blue color) of the lips, mouth, under tongue, and nailbeds
- Cyanosis can be caused by decreased oxygen due to pulmonary or heart disease or it can be caused by the patient being cold
- Clubbing of fingers and curvature of nails on fingers/toes is abnormal and is usually related to chronic lung or heart disease

Respirations

- Assess rhythm, rate and effort
- Breathing should be regular, rate of 10-20 times per minute and unlabored
- Chest should be symmetrical during inspiration and expiration
- Expiratory phase of breathing is normally longer than the inspiratory phase in the adult at rest

Abnormal respiratory effort

- If the expiratory phase is excessively long, assess for use of abdominal muscles aiding in respiration
- Labored, rattling breaths, wheezing or shallow respirations are abnormal for the adult at rest
- If labored breathing is noted assess for mouth breathing, pursed lips, flared nostrils, use of accessory muscles, and/or retractions in chest, any of these findings are abnormal in the adult at rest

- Pursed lip breathing is associated with chronic airway diseases
- Flaring nostrils may be present in asthma attack or respiratory distress
- Accessory muscle use may include the trapezius (shoulder), scalenus, sternomastoid (neck) during inspiration, as well as the abdominal muscles during expiration

Apneic Episodes

- Apnea is a temporary stop in breathing
- May occur from low levels of carbon dioxide in the blood, damage to the brain or even be voluntary (breath holding)
- If present assess duration (seconds), frequency of episodes
- If patient is on respiratory monitoring (apnea monitor or cardiac monitor) assess alarm limits

Cough

- Note if cough is productive
- Assess sputum for amount (scant, moderate, or copious), consistency (thick or thin), color (white, yellow, green, blood-tinged), odor

Chest

- Inspect for shape
- Barrel chest — Rounded appearance with ribs more horizontal than normal, sternum is prominent, seen in infants and the elderly or those with pulmonary disease
- Funnel chest — Part or all of the sternum is depressed, if the depression is severe enough it can interfere with respirations
- Pigeon chest — Sternum protrudes anteriorly and the chest resembles the thorax of a fowl

PALPATION

- Warm hands to avoid starting patient
- Palpate any areas where masses appear, document location, size, and tenderness if present

Respiratory excursion

- Procedure:
  Place thumbs on either side of the spinal cord at the level of the 10th rib with palms flat on the posterior chest
  Ask the patient to inhale, assess expansion of patients lungs by estimation or measurement
- Normal results are symmetrical expansion

- A lack of symmetry may mean underlying disease

PERCUSSION

- Percuss over chest wall for solid, fluid, or air filled spaces
- Resonance — Hollow sound heard over most of the normal lung
- Hyperresonance — Low pitched, booming sound, abnormal; heard when lung is overinflated as in chronic airway diseases
- Tympany — Loud high pitch sound (drum like); abnormal over chest, normal on stomach
- Dullness — Soft, high pitched dull sound; heard over heart or solid surface such as in consolidated lungs

AUSCULTATION

- Use the diaphragm of the stethoscope for lung sounds
- Have patient breathe deeply through his/her mouth
- Listen for one full breath at each location
- Monitor patient for dizziness from hyperventilation

Breath sounds

- *Bronchial breath sounds* — Loud, high pitched blowing sounds
  Inspiratory time less than expiratory time
    Normal over the trachea
    Abnormal over other areas of the chest
- *Bronchovesicular breath sounds* — Medium intensity sounds
  Inspiratory and expiratory time are equal
    Normal over both of the bronchi
- *Vesicular sounds* — Soft, light breath
  Inspiratory time is greater than expiratory time
    Normal over lung surfaces
- *Crackles* — Crackling, popping sound that may be fine, medium or coarse in intensity which results from fluid in airways or from small atelectatic areas that expand with deep breathing
    Always abnormal
- *Gurgles* — Loud, coarse, low pitched sounds, (snoring sound), that result from thick secretions in the larger airways   Usually heard on expiration
    Always abnormal
- *Wheezes* — High pitched, musical, whistling sound resulting from a narrowed airway (as in asthma)
  Heard on expiration, may be heard on inspiration if severe

Always abnormal
- *Plural friction rub* — A rough grating sound resulting from the visceral and plural linings of the lung rubbing together
    Always abnormal

RESPIRATORY SYSTEM ASSESSMENT FORM

INSPECTION

General appearance / Posture_____

General skin color_____ Mucous membranes_____ Nails_____ Clubbing_____

Breathing: Regular_____ Irregular_____ Rate_____ _ U nlabored_____

Symmetrical movement of chest_____ Expirations >Inspirations_____

Labored_____ Rattling_____ Wheezing_____ Shallow_____ Ot her_____

Mouth breathing/Pursed lips_____ Flaring nostrils_____ Retractions_____

Where_____ Use of accessory muscles: neck____ shoulder____ abdomen____

Apneic episodes_____ How long_____ How Many____/____ Monitor on/off_____

Cough_____ Sputum_____ Amount_____ Consistency_____ Color_____ Odor___

Shape of Chest: _____ Symmetrical_____

PALPATION

Respiratory excursion: Symmetrical_____ Inspiration/cm's_____

Pain on palpation_____ Masses_____ Location_____

PERCUSSION

Resonance_____ Tympany_____ Dullness_____ So und symmetry_____

AUSCULTATION

Symmetrical Breath Sounds: Anterior_____ Posterior_____ Absent_____

Bronchial (Trachea/I<E)*: _____ Bronchovesicular (Bronchi/I=E)*:_____

Vesicular (Peripheral areas/I>E)*: _____ Decreased_____

Crackles_____ Gurgles_____ Wheezes_____ R ubs_____

Assessment Notes_____

_____

_____

_____

*I=Inspiration   E=Expiration

Section III — LABORATORY AND DIAGNOSTIC TESTS

In the following section traditional laboratory values and SI units are given, it is important to recognize that "normal" values vary from laboratory to laboratory. Check the normal values at the agency or institution where the test is performed. Most labs print their normal values on the laboratory reporting slip or page.

Table of Common Laboratory Tests

Test Name	Indications	Comments
Acid-fast bacilli (AFB) Sputum test **Normal:** No mycobacterium tuberculi bacili found	Tuberculosis Mycobacterial lung disease	**Regarding collection:** Hold antibiotics until collection Early morning sputum recommended Use sterile sputum container Have pt rinse mouth with water before collection At least 1 tsp of sputum required Wear gloves for collection **Results:** May take up to 3 weeks for results
Alphal-antitrypsin test (AlAT, ATT) Blood test **Normal:** over 250 mg/dl Genetic typing MM	Emphysema Family history of emphysema	**Regarding collection:** Collect 5-10 ml **Results:** Genetic typing of ZZ or SS have blood levels <50 mg/dl and develop emphysema in 3rd or 4th decade Genetic typing of MZ or MS have levels between 50-250 mg/dl and are at risk to develop emphsema

Arterial blood gases (ABGs) Arterial Blood
 	
Normal:
pH 7.35-7.45
PCO_2 35-45mmHg
HCO_3 24-28mEq/L
PO_2 80-100 mmHg
O_2 sat 90-100%
 	
See also Arterial blood gas determination later in this chapter
	Respiratory or metabolic disease Trauma Cardiac failure Drug overdose Life threatening emergencies	**Regarding collection:**
		Use heparinized needle and syringe
		collect 1-5 ml of arterial blood
		Allow no air in syringe or tube
		Apply pressure to site for 2-5 min
		Record oxygen rate and oximeter reading on lab slip as indicated
		Place on ice, send to lab ASAP
		Results:
		Respiratory acidosis
		  pH PCO_2 HCO_3 normal
		Respiratory alkalosis
		  pH PCO_2 HCO_3 normal
		Metabolic acidosis
		  pH PCO_2 normal HCO_3
		Metabolic alkalosis
		  pH PCO_2 normal HCO_3

Test Name	Indications	Comments
Carboxyhemoglo-bin (COHb) Blood test **Normal:** <3% Smoker <12%	Carbon monoxide poisoning	**Regarding collection:** Use lavender- or green-top tube Collect 5-10 ml Assess pt for confusion, dizziness **Results:** Critical value >20% Death occurs values >60%
Legionnaire's dis-ease antibody test Blood test **Normal:** No Legionella anti-body titer	Legionnaire's disease	**Regarding collection:** Use red-top tube, collect 5-7 ml **Results:** Titer of 1:256 or greater indicates active Legionnaire's Two blood samplings at 1 & 3 weeks after onset of symptoms may be used to assess for rise in titer
Sputum culture & sensitivity (C&S) Sputum test **Normal:** Usual cells, no infec-tions present	Respirtory infection Pneumonia	**Regarding collection:** Hold antibiotics until collection Early morning sputum recommended Use sterile sputum container Have patient rinse mouth with water before collection At least 1 tsp of sputum required Wear gloves for collection **Results:** Preliiminary report available in 24 hrs, cultures require 48 hrs
Sputum cytology Sputum test **Normal:** Usual cells, no tumor cells	Lung carcinoma	**Regarding collection:** Early morning sputum recommended Use sterile sputum container Have patient rinse mouth with water before collection At least 1 tsp of sputum required Wear gloves for collection Usually collected on 3 separate days **Results:** Positive test indicates malignancy
Tuberculin test (PPD skin test) **Normal:** Negative reaction or reaction <5mm	Tuberculosis	**Regarding testing:** Routine screening test Assess for previous positive PPD, history of TB or BCG immunization PPD is injected intradermally to form wheal on forearm **Results:** Assess area in 48-27 hrs, measure any area of hardening (millimeters) Notify physician of positive PPD

Test Name	Indications	Comments
Tuberculosis culture (BACTEC) Sputum, urine, spinal fluid, or biopsy tissue **Normal:** No mycobacterium tuberculi found	Tuberculosis Atypical mycobacterial nontuberculosis disease	**Regarding collection:** Check for type of blood fluid Sputum – use early morning sputum Urine – use early morning specimen Wear gloves for collection **Results:** Faster than AFB testing, results available in 24 hrs If positive drug-susceptibility testing is completed

Table of Common Diagnostic Tests

Test Name	Indications	Comments
Bronchogram X-ray with contrast dye **Normal** structure of larynx, trachea and bronchi	Tracheobronchial obstruction or tumor Bronchiectasis Tracheobronchial malformation Done less often now with development of flexible fiberoptic bronchscope	**Pre-procedure:** Signed consent form is required Expectorants and postural drainage may be ordered 2-3 days before test to remove mucus and secretions NPO 6-8 hrs before test Assess for allergy to iodine, seafood or contrast dyes Explain procedure Catheter or bronchoscope wll be passed into trachea and dye injected Administer meds as ordered **Post-procedure:** Assess for complications: laryngeal edema, bronchspasm or bleeding NPO for 2 hrs or until gag reflex is present Encourage coughing to clear out dye Monitor VS frequenty Assess lung sounds for rhonchi Postural drainage may be ordered
Bronchoscopy Endoscopy May be flexible fiberoptic bronchoscope or rigid bronchoscope **Normal** structure of larynx, trachea and bronchi	Unexplained cough Hemoptysis Tracheobronchial tumor or lesion Foreign body Procedures which may be done: Bronchogram Biopsy of lesions Encobronchial radiation therapy Laster therapy Aspiration of deep sputum for C&S	**Pre-procedure:** Explain procedure Flexible or rigid tube will be used to visually examine the tracheobronchial tree Signed consent form is required NPO for 4-8 hrs before test Record baseline vital signs Have pt rinse mouth with water Pre-procedure drugs may be ordered Procedure takes about 1 hr **Post-procedure:** NPO 2 hrs or until good gag reflex Assess for bleeding, pneumothorax, laryngospasm or signs of shock Fever may develop within 24 hrs

Test Name	Indications	Comments
Chest X-ray X-ray **Normal** lungs and surrounding structures	Lung inflammation Lung tumor Trauma to chest Pleural effusion Pneumothorax	**Pre-procedure:** Remove all metal objects Assess for pregnancy in females **Post-procedure:** No activity restructions
Computed tomography of the chest (CT scan) X-ray **Normal** structure	Tumors, nodules Abscess, cysts, Pleural effusion Enlarged lymph nodes	**Pre-procedure:** Signed consent form may be required Assess for allergy to iodine Procedure takes 30-45 mins NPO for 4 hrs of contrast dye **Post-procedure:** If contrast dye, encourage fluids No activity restrictions
Lung biopsy Microscopic exam of tissues **Normal** tissue, no pathology Thoracentesis	Lung disease Lung carcinoma Sarcoidosis Lung infection	**Pre-procedure:** Signed consent form is required Biopsy may be obtained via needle aspiration, thoracotomy or by bronchscope NPO for 8-12 hrs Pre-medication will be given **Post-procedure:** Monitor VS frequently Assess for shortness of breath Obtain chest X-ray as ordered to assess for pneumothorax
Lung scan **Ventilation/ perfusion scanning** (VPS, V/Q scan) **Normal** uptake of nuclear material by the lung	Defects in blood perfusion within the lungs Pulmonary embolism Tuberculosis Emphysems, COPD Pneumonia, tumors Atelectasis	**Pre-procedure:** Signed consent form may be required Assess for recent chest X-ray Remove jewelry or metal from chest Tracer doses of radioactive isotope will be given via IV **Post-procedure:** No activity restrictions are needed No radiation precautions are needed
Mediastinoscopy Endoscopy **Normal** mediastinal lymph node tissue	Lung metastasis Lung carcinoma Lumph node biopsy Lymphoma Sarcoidosis	**Pre-procedure:** Signed onsent form is required Obtain type and screen for blood as ordered Complete pre-operative checklist NPO for 8-12 hrs Pre-medication will be given Mediastinoscope will be inserted into sternal notch surgically **Post-procedure:** Usual post-operative procedures Assess breath sounds carefully

Test Name	Indications	Comments
Oximetry Photodiagnostic **Normal** >95%	Assessment during peri-operative or post-operative period Mechanical ventilation	**Pre-procedure:** Place sensor probe on earlobe or fingertip as indicated Record percentage as ordered **Post-procedure:** No activity restrictions required
Pulmonary angiography X-ray with contrast dye **Normal** pulmonary vessels	Pulmonary embolism Lesions of pulmonary vessels Pulmonary tumors	**Pre-procedure:** Signed consent form is required Assess for allergies to iodine Assess for history of arrhythmias, esp. ventricular; report if found NPO for 8-12 hrs Pre-medication will be given Procedure takes about 1 hr **Post-procedure:** Assess catheter insertion site for bleeding, inflammation or hematoma Assess pulse on affected extremity Monitor VS, bedrest for 12-24 hrs
Pulmonary function testing Airflow testing **Normal** airflow for age, sex, height, & weight See also pulmonary function studies later in this chapter	Pre-operative test COPD, asthma Pulmonary tumor Chest wall trauma Scleroderma Pneumonia Interstitial fibrosis	**Pre-procedure:** Discuss need for cooperation No smoking 6-8 hrs before testing No bronchodilators within 6-8 hrs Obtain pt's weight & height List all medications on lab slip **Post-procedure:** Pt with lung disease may need rest after procedure
Thoracentesis Fluid analysis **Normal** pleural fluid	Pulmonary infection or infarction Lung carcinoma Pleural hemorrhage Tuberculosis effusion Trauma	**Pre-procedure:** Explain procedure to pt Pleural fluid is aspirated using a needle inserted through the chest Signed consent form is required A local anesthetic will be given **Post-procedure:** Assess for bleeding, pneumothorax, trauma to liver or spleen Turn patient to affected side for 1 hr Label specimens and send to lab Obtain chest X-ray Monitor VS, assess lung sounds Normal activity after 1 hr

ARTERIAL BLOOD GASES (ABGs)

- Ordered for a variety conditions to gain information on
  - How well the patient is oxygenated (PO_2)
  - Acid base status of the patient (pH)
  - Ability of the lungs to eliminate carbon dioxide (PCO_2)

Helpful definitions

pH The degree of acidity or alkalinity, ranges from 0-14
Neutral pH is 7, it is neither acidic or alkaline
A pH below 7 is considered to be acidic
A pH above 7 is considered to be alkaline
Normal blood pH is slightly alkaline, between 7.35-7.45
A blood pH below 6.8 or above 7.8 is incompatible with life

Acid A substance that liberates hydrogen ions (H+) in a solution
An acid can neutralize a base and has a pH less than 7.0

Base A substance that accepts hydrogen ions (H+) in a solution
A base can neutralize an acid and has a pH greater than 7.0
A base is considered to be alkaline

PCO$_2$ Represents the partial pressure of carbon dioxide (CO_2)
The normal blood value is 35-45 mm Hg
CO_2 is eliminated by the lungs, therefore, if respiration
increases or decreases the acid/base balance changes
The PCO$_2$ reflects the RESPIRATORY component of acid base

HCO$_3$ Represents the bicarbonate content
The normal blood value is 22-26 mEq/L
HCO$_3$- levels are regulated by the kidneys
The HCO$_3$- reflects the METABOLIC component of acid base

PO$_2$ Represents the partial pressure of oxygen
A PO$_2$ of less than 50 mmHg requires supplemental oxygen

B.E. Represents the base
− sign means a deficit
+ sign means an excess

Normal arterial blood gas values

Measurement	Value
pH	7.35-7.45
PCO$_2$	35-45 mm Hg
HCO$_3$-	22-26 mEq/L
PO$_2$	80-100 mm Hg
O$_2$ Sat	95% or >
B.E.	−2 — +2

Analyzing ABG's

• Four major classifications of acid-base abnormalities:
Respiratory acidosis
Metabolic acidosis

Respiratory alkalosis
Metabolic alkalosis

Acid-base abnormality	pH	PCO$_2$	HCO$_3$-
Respiratory acidosis	Decreased below 7.35	Increased above 45	In normal range
Metabolic acidosis	Decreased below 7.35	In normal range	Decreased below 22
Respiratory alkalosis	Increased above 7.45	Decreased below 35	In normal range
Metabolic alkalosis	Increased above 7.45	In normal range	Increased above 26

Consult the chart and observe:

- When the pH is decreased below 7.35 the condition is *ACIDOSIS*
- When the pH is increased above 7.45 the condition is *ALKALOSIS*
- When the PCO$_2$ is affected, the condition is *RESPIRATORY*
- When the condition is *RESPIRATORY*, the HCO$_3$- is in normal range
- When the HCO$_3$- is affected, the condition is *METABOLIC*
- When the condition is *METABOLIC*, PCO$_2$ is in normal range

The words and numbers can be replaced with arrows

- Arrows in the same direction are with *METABOLIC* conditions
- Arrows in opposite directions are with *RESPIRATORY* conditions

Acid-base Abnormality	pH	PCO$_2$	HCO$_3$-	Direction of arrows
Respiratory acidosis	↓	↓	WNL	Different
Metabolic acidosis	↓	WNL	↓	Same
Respiratory alkalosis	↑	↓	WNL	Different
Metabolic alkalosis	↑	WNL	↑	Same

When analyzing ABG's using arrows may be helpful

Abnormal arterial blood gases

- Respiratory and renal systems are responsible for maintaining the body's acid base balance between 7.35 and 7.45

INCREASED pH VALUES (ALKALOSIS)

Body must either lose acids or increase bicarbonate

- **Respiratory causes for lost acid**
  Acid is lost when excess CO_2 is blown off by the lungs as when breathing is too fast (hyperventilation)
  - Can occur during anxiety or pain
  - When ventilator settings deliver too many breaths/minute
- **Metabolic causes for lost acid**
  Acid can be lost from the GI tract during illness
  - During vomiting (acid lost from stomach)
  - When bile is lost (acid lost from lower GI tract)
  - During gastric suctioning/lavage
- **Metabolic causes for gaining bicarbonate**
  - Ingestion of baking soda or other alkaline substances

DECREASED pH VALUES (ACIDOSIS)

Body must either gain acid or lose bicarbonate

- **Metabolic causes for losing bicarbonate**
  - Ileostomy causes body to lose HCO_3-
  - Intestinal fistulas
- **Respiratory causes for gaining acid**
  Acid is retained when too little CO_2 is blown off as when breathing is too slow (hypoventilation)
  - Emphysema or pneumonia where gas exchange is impaired
  - Airway obstruction where no gas exchange can take place
- **Metabolic causes for gaining acid**
  - Uncontrolled diabetes with fat breakdown and metabolism (ketoacidosis)
  - Starvation diets (breakdown/metabolism of fatty acids)
  - Poor renal function (Increase in BUN and creatine)
  - Cardiac disorders (poor circulation /hypoxia)
  - Overdose of salicylates (Aspirin)

COMPENSATION

- When imbalances occur the body must try to compensate

- **The role of the lungs in compensation**
  Retain or blow off CO_2 by changing respiratory rate and depth
  Retain CO_2 by breathing less frequently (decrease pH)
  Blow off CO_2 by breathing more rapidly (increase pH)
  Lungs can compensate for pH changes faster than the kidneys
- **The role of the kidneys in compensation**
  Retain or excrete bicarbonate (HCO_3-)
  Retaining bicarbonate (increase pH)
  Excreting bicarbonate (decrease pH)

HOW THE BODY COMPENSATES FOR ACID/BASE IMBALANCES

Respiratory acidosis Cause	Signs & Symptoms	Compensation
Hypoventilation Pneumonia Emphysema Asthma COPD Drug overdose Head injury Reyes syndrome CHF	Hypoventilation Confusion Weakness Disorientation Drowsines Hea dache Blurred vision Coma	Lungs Hyperventilation Kidneys Retain HCO_3- Secrete H+ ions CNS

Metabolic acidosis Cause	Signs & Symptoms	Compensation
Diabetes Starvation diets Poor renal function Systemic infections Tissue anoxia	Weakness Confusion Stupor Kussmal breathing Unconsciousness Cardiac arrhythmias Hypokalemia Increased pulse Decreased BP	Lungs Hyperventilation Kidneys Excrete HCO_3- Secrete H+ ions Retain K+ (potassium Retain NA+ (sodium)

Respiratory alkalosis Cause	Signs & Symptoms	Compensation
Hyperventilation Anxiety Pulmonary emboli Fever Salicylate overdose	Hyperventilation Hypoventilation (late) Numbness/tingling in extremities Convulsions (late) Tetany	Lungs Hypoventilation Kidneys Excrete HCO_3- Retain H+ ions

Metabolic alkalosis Cause	Signs & Symptoms	Compensation
Vomiting Irritability Cushing's disease Corticosteriod tx Gastric suctioning	Hypoventilation Confusion Tetany (late)	Lungs Hypoventilation Kidneys Excrete K+ Excrete Na+ Excrete HCO_3- Retain H+ ions

Arterial blood gas values in compensation

* During compensation for an acid-base imbalance it may be difficult to detect the original problem
* The pH may be near normal or within the normal range
  pH 7.36 PCO_2 50 HCO_3- 29
* When a normal pH is noted along with an abnormal PCO_2 or HCO_3-, the body is compensating for an acid base imbalance
* Check which end the pH is nearest, acidosis or alkalosis 7.36 is low normal, acidosis was the primary problem
* Check for increase or decrease in the other values
  PCO_2 was increased to 50 HCO_3- was increased to 29
* Check which type of acidosis has an increased value in PCO_2 or HCO_3-

  Out of two types of acidosis, only one has an increased PCO_2, respiratory acidosis
  Metabolic acidosis does not have an increased HCO_3-, therefore, the body must be trying to compensate for the respiratory acidosis by retaining more HCO_3-
* Another example of acid base compensation:
  pH 7.36 PCO_2 26 HCO_3- 12
* Check which end the pH is nearest, acidosis or alkalosis acidosis
* Check for increase or decrease in other values
  PCO_2 decreased to 26, HCO_3- decreased to 12
* Check which type of acidosis has a decreased value in PCO_2 or HCO_3-

  Out of the two types of acidosis, neither one has a decreased PCO_2
  Metabolic acidosis has a decreased HCO_3-, therefore, the original imbalance was metabolic acidosis
  The body must be trying to compensate for the metabolic acidosis by increasing the rate of respirations which would blow off CO_2 resulting in a decreased PCO_2

Acid base imbalance problems for practice

pH	PCO2	HCO3-	Answer
7.20	65	24	Respiratory Acidosis
7.20	45	18	Metabolic Acidosis
7.60	25	23	Respiratory Alkalosis
7.33	49	24	Respiratory Acidosis
7.30	40	15	Metabolic Acidosis
7.36	52	30	Respiratory Acidosis, compensated
7.43	49	32	Metabolic Alkalosis, compensated

Interventions for acid base disorders

Disorder	Intervention	Rationale
Respiratory acidosis	Bronchodilators	To open the airway
	Oxygen	Increase O_2 concentration
	Frequent vital signs	Respiratory depression may occur
	Turn cough and deep breathe	To promote lung expansion
	Force fluids	To thin secretions
	Assess level of consciousness	Decreased LOC may occur
	Administer narcotics, sedatives & hypnotics with care	To prevent further CNS depression
Metabolic acidosis	Assess for dehydration	Due to hypovolemia
	Frequent vital signs	
	Strict input & output	Assess for hypovolemia
	Seizure precautions	To protect patient
	Neurological checks	To assess for change in neurological status
	Kayexalate for hypokalemia	Hypokalemia may occur
	Monitor ECG	
		Cardiac arrhythmias may occur due to hypokalemia
Respiratory alkalosis	Rebreathing mask if due to hyperventilation	CO_2 will be inhaled; paper bag will work if mask if not available
	Assess for cause	Pain, anxiety, head injury
	Administer pain meds prior to intense pain	To reduce pain, promote relaxation
	Provide back rubs	To reduce anxiety and to promote relaxation
	Assess for hypokalemia	Hypokalemia may occur
	Assess for headache, paraesthesia, tetany	Due to vasoconstriction
Metabolic alkalosis	Assess vital signs	Decreased respirations may occur
	Administer Diamox as ordered	Help kidney excrete HCO_3-
	Administer Chloride or K+ and Cl- or KCL as ordered	Help kidney excrete HCO_3- Serum K+ may be decreased
	Assess for tetany	Late possible sign of metabolic alkalosis

PULMONARY FUNCTION TESTS

- Used as an aid in the diagnosis of respiratory disorders
- Primary purpose to establish baseline functioning of the lung
- Normal values vary with age (decreased in advancing age) and sex (women have generally lower values by as much as 25%). Race and body weight may also affect values.

PULMONARY FUNCTION EXPECTED TEST RESULTS

Name of test	Normal Results Definition
Tidal volume (TV, Vt)	500 ml. Amount of air inhaled and exhaled in a single breath at rest. A spirometer may be used for 1 min and total divided by number of breaths taken in the min.
Inspiratory reserve volume (IRV)	3000-3100 ml. Maximum amount of air that can be inhaled after a normal inspiration.
Inspiratory capacity (IC)	3500-3600 ml. The total amount of air that can be inhaled in one breath. IC = TV + IRV 3600 = 500 + 3100 3600 = 3600
Functional residual capacity (FRC)	2300-2400 ml. The amount of air left in the lung at the end of a normal exhalation.
Expiratory reserve volume (ERV)	1100-1200 ml. The total amount of air that can be exhaled after a normal exhalation.
Residual volume (RV)	1200-1300 ml. The amount of air left in the lungs that you cannot exhale; this air keeps the alveoli slightly inflated. Increased RV may result from emphysema where the lungs contain an abnormally large amount of air even after maximum exhalation. RV = FRC - ERV 1200 = 2400 - 1200 FRC = ERV + RV 2400 = 1200 + 1200
Vital capacity	4600-4800 ml. Amount of air exhaled slowly and totally, after inhaling the largest breath possible. A decreased VC may result from pulmonary edema, pneumonia, collapsed lung tissue, or any disorder that inhibits full lung expansion. VC = ERV + TV + IRV 4800 = 1200 + 500 + 3100 4800 = 4800

Name of test	Normal Results Definition
Total lung capacity (TLC)	5800-6000 ml. The total volume of air in the lung after a maximum inhalation, this must be calculated. A decreased TLC may result from pulmonary edema, collapsed areas of lung, tumors, pneumonia or any condition that inhibits lung expansion. An increased TLC may result from emphysema where the lung hyperinflates. TLC = RV + ERV + TV + IRV 6000 = 1200 + 1200 + 500 + 3100 6000 = 6000
Forced vital capacity (FVC)	4600-4800 ml. The amount of air that can be forcefully exhaled quickly, after maximum inhalation, FVC usually equals VC. The measurement of FVC can be further broken down into forced expiratory volume timed.
Forced expiratory volume timed (FEVt)	Measured during the FVC, the amount of air the patient can exhale in seconds is recorded. Example: FEVt 0.5 would be the amount of air expired in one-half a second.

Section IV — PROCEDURES

Oxygen Administration

- Room air is approximately 21% oxygen, exhaled air is about 16% . Oxygen is administered as a drug to treat hypoxemia
- Hypoxemia is a deficiency of oxygen in the blood
- Hypoxemia may result from trauma, cardiac or pulmonary conditions, anemia, shock or surgical interventions
- The most reliable indicator of hypoxemia is PaO_2 (see ABG's)
- Normal PaO_2 is 80-100 mmHg
- A patient with a PaO_2 below 50 mmHg always requires oxygen
- A decreased PaO_2 may occur long before the signs and symptoms of hypoxemia are present
- The signs & symptoms of hypoxemia include:
  - Dyspnea (Shortness of breath, difficulty breathing)
  - Cyanosis (bluish tinge to lips, mouth, or nailbeds)
  - Anxiety, feelings of impending doom, restlessness
  - Confusion
  - Tachycardia with elevated blood pressure
  - Pale, cool extremities (due to vasoconstriction)

Prior to administration of oxygen:

- Assess patient's current respiratory condition to include:
  - Respiratory rate, rhythm and effort
  - Presence of cyanosis of mucous membranes or nailbeds
  - Results of arterial blood gases if available
- Record baseline vital signs
- Assess order for method and rate of oxygen administration

Cannula nasal	Consists of tubing with curved nasal prongs
	Delivers 24% oxygen at 2 L/minute
	Flow rates greater than 5 L dry nasal membranes
	Patient should breathe through the nose to prevent a loss of oxygen
	Lubricating nares will prevent cannula irritation
Mask	Face mask needs to cover both the mouth and nose and fit tightly enough to prevent dilution of oxygen with room air
	Flow rate of 8-15 L/minute delivers 40-60% oxygen concentration

- Obtain equipment
    Wall oxygen unit or portable oxygen bottle
    Mask, cannula or other oxygen setup with tubing
    Distilled water and humidifier unit for oxygen set-up
- Remove any fire hazards from area
    Remove unneeded electrical equipment
    Oils should not be used on or near the patient
- Oxygen must always be humidified prior to use to prevent drying of the mucous membranes (Distilled water or normal saline)

Oxygen and the patient with chronic carbon dioxide retention:

- Patients with chronic pulmonary diseases (COPD) have become conditioned to higher carbon dioxide (CO_2) levels
- The respiratory regulatory center is no longer using the level of blood CO_2 as an indicator of a need for more oxygen
- The respiratory center has become dependent upon hypoxemia
- If the oxygen level is suddenly increased it will depress the stimulus to breathe and decrease respirations
- Persons with chronic CO_2 retention need a lower concentration of oxygen than other patients and must be carefully monitored
- Monitor ABGs before and during oxygen administration

Complications of oxygen administration

- Oxygen is a drug and can be toxic if too much is administered
- The following are symptoms of oxygen toxicity:
    Nausea
    Restlessness
    Pallor
- Oxygen toxicity can lead to permanent brain and lung damage
- Premature neonates exposed to high concentrations of oxygen may develop visual impairment or blindness

CHEST TUBES
Used to remove fluid, blood and/or air from the pleural cavity

The pleural cavity
* Normally contains no air or blood and is located between two layers of tissue, the visceral pleura, and the parietal pleura
* Has a thin layer of lubricant that allows the two pleura to slide and move with each other
* Works like a vacuum, holds the pleura together during and between respirations
* During inspiration the diaphragm contracts and moves down creating more lung space, the pleura then expand together
* During expiration when the diaphragm relaxes the pleura prevent the elastic lung tissue from collapsing
* Any separation of the two pleura destroys the vacuum and prevents the two layers from moving as a unit
* When the vacuum is destroyed, the lungs will collapse and the air available for gas exchange will decrease

Pleural cavity abnormalities
* Pneumothorax — Air in the pleural cavity
* Hemopneumothorax — Blood and air in the pleural cavity
* Hemothorax — Blood in the pleural cavity
* Hydrothorax — Fluid in the pleural cavity
* Hydropneumothorax — Fluid and air in the pleural cavity
* Pyothorax — Pus in the pleural cavity
* Abnormalities may be "open or closed"

Closed:
* Visceral pleura (pleura closest to the lungs) is damaged and air and/or fluid/blood enters the pleural cavity but cannot exit
* The vacuum is destroyed and the lung begins to collapse
* During inspiration air moves into the pleural cavity, during expiration, not all of the air moves out, some is trapped
* During the next respiratory cycles, the lung cannot expand fully due to trapped air, eventually a portion or all of the lung collapses
* A closed pneumothorax can result from:
  > Rupture of an abscess or bleb on lung surface
  > Internal puncture by fractured rib
  > Ruptured bronchus or perforated esophagus
  > Pulmonary barotrauma from mechanical ventilation

Open:

- The chest wall, parietal pleura, and visceral pleura are entered from an external source (trauma or incision)
- Air entering the lungs can escape into the atmosphere and air from the atmosphere can enter the lungs
- An open pneumothorax also destroys the vacuum

How chest tubes work

- Purpose is to restore the normal lung pressure, and/or to drain air or fluid from the pleural cavity
- When these goals are met, the lung can rexpand
- One end of the chest tube is inserted into the chest wall, the other is connected to a chest drainage system
- The most commonly used chest drainage system is the disposable three compartment system

1st Compartment — The Collection chamber

- Collects any fluid leaving the lung

2nd Compartment — The Water seal chamber

- Prevents any air from the atmosphere from entering the lung through the chest tube
- Has water in it; the water allows air from the pleural cavity traveling via the chest tube to pass out of the pleural cavity and prevents air from the atmosphere from entering the pleural cavity
- To understand this concept, think of a straw. A straw allows you to blow air through it but the end of the straw is underwater and no air can enter this end until all of the water is gone

3rd Compartment — Suction control chamber

- This compartment contains water, which determines the degree of suction, suction is needed to remove the unwanted air and/or fluid from the pleural cavity
- The amount of suction can be changed by changing the volume of water in this compartment
- Although the chest drainage system connects to a suction control unit, the amount of suction depends on the level of water in this compartment

Assisting with chest tube insertion

- Prior to the procedure
  - Assess reason for chest tube insertion

- Obtain and record respiratory rate, rhythm and breath sounds, decreased or absent breath sounds may be present when air or fluid is trapped in the pleural cavity
- Check orders for any premedication or special instructions
- Signed informed consent is needed
- Gather equipment
  Sterile chest tube insertion tray with antiseptic, sterile chest tube, chest drainage system unit, sterile petrolatum gauze, covered hemostat
  Sterile water or normal saline to keep at bedside
  Local anesthetic (usually lidocaine)
  Covered hemostat to keep at bedside (booted hemostat)
- Set up the chest drainage system as ordered, maintain sterility of system, follow directions on system package
- During insertion
  - Maintain strict sterile conditions to prevent infection
  - Patient should be in the high Fowler's position
  - Incision will be made by primary care provider on
    Midclavicular line high on chest if only air is to be removed
    Midaxillary line low on chest if blood, fluid alone, or blood and fluid with air is to be removed
    Patient should be instructed not to cough
  - Pain will be present as the pleura are difficult to anesthetize
  - Once chest tube has been inserted then it is connected to the drainage system using a barrel connector
  - The chest tube is sutured to the chest wall, and the petrolatum gauze is placed around insertion site
- Post-procedure
  - Assess respiratory rate, rhythm, and breath sounds for any change
  - Observe for gentle bubbling in the suction control chamber
  - Observe for gentle bubbling in the water seal chamber; this should be present if the purpose is to remove air the pleural cavity (pneumothorax)
  - Assess drainage collection chamber for type and amount of drainage, if bloody drainage assess amount and report any sudden increase
  - Tape all connections tightly to prevent accidental disconnection

- Assess dressing for drainage and airtight seal
- It is important to note here that not all systems are connected to suction, some drain by gravity

Problem solving with chest drainage systems

There are five major areas where problems arise when working with chest tube drainage systems, these are:

- Suction control chamber
- Water seal chamber
- Collection chamber
- Tubing
- Respiratory distress in the patient

Problems with suction control chamber:

- If any of these are noted on assessment there is a problem with the suction control chamber
  - No bubbling in suction control chamber
  - Vigorous bubbling in suction control chamber
  - Decreased suction in unit

Problem: No bubbling in suction control chamber

1. Is suction source turned on?
   If not, turn on suction until bubbling appears
2. Check and tighten all connections
3. Check for obstructed tubing from suction source to water collection chamber — remove any kinks
4. Replace suction unit if unit is still not bubbling
5. Report problem to primary care provider

Problem: Loud vigorous bubbling

1. Turn down suction until bubbling is gentle

Problem: Decreased suction in unit

1. Check water level, is it at ordered suction level?
   If not, follow manufacture's instructions to add sterile water or saline to unit (see unit back)

Problems with the water seal chamber:

- If any of these are noted on assessment there is a problem with the water seal chamber
  - Fluctuation of water level in chamber
  - Sudden stop of bubbling of water in chamber
  - Bubbling in water seal chamber

Problem: Fluctuation of water in chamber
1.   No problem, the pressure within the pleural cavity is restored to normal, the pneumothorax is resolved

Problem: Sudden stop in bubbling in water seal chamber
1.   Check for kink in tubing — release if found
2.   Check for obstruction of tubing — remove obstruction
3.   Assess patient for respiratory distress — if found, report to primary care provider STAT

Problem: Bubbling in water seal chamber
1.   Bubbling is normal for patient with a pneumothorax
     Air is being removed from the pleural cavity
2.   If patient does not have a pneumothorax then there is a air leak within the system — tighten all connections
3.   If bubbling continues then use booted hemostat to clamp tubing momentarily at chest dressing. If bubbling stops proceed to 4. If bubbling does not stop proceed to 5
4.   Unclamp the tubing and remove the chest tube dressing, is the chest tube out? If so, cover wound with petroleum gauze and report to the primary health care provider STAT. If chest tube remains in, replace dressing and see if the bubbling stops; if bubbling still occurs report STAT, the air leak is in the chest
5.   Unclamp the hemostat and move it down about 12 inches from patients chest and reclamp on tubing, if the bubbling stops when clamped then you know the leak is in the tubing between the hemostat and chest. Locate the leak and tape. If the bubbling continues, relocate the clamp down the tubing another 12 inches, repeat this until the leak is located or chest unit is reached.
6.   If the bubbling continues and no leak is found in the tubing, replace the chest drainage unit.

Problems with the collection chamber:
• If any of these are noted on assessment there is a problem with the collection chamber
   • No drainage in collection chamber
   • Sudden increase in drainage
Problem: No drainage in collection chamber
1.   If patient has pneumothorax no drainage is expected

2. If patient has a hemopneumothorax or hemothorax, check previous shift report, was it draining earlier?
3. Check tubing for kinks or dependent loops, lower the chest drainage system and reassess for drainage in chamber
4. Assess patients breath sounds, if decreased breath sounds then fluid remains in lungs
5. If fresh bleeding was noted on previous shift, gently milk tubing according to agency policy
6. If tubing still is not draining on patient with decreased breath sounds report interventions and findings to primary care provider

Problem: Sudden increase in drainage
1. Take patient's vital signs, assess for increased pulse and decrease in blood pressure. If present, notify primary care provider STAT
2. Assess for recent position change. If present, monitor amount of drainage, drainage will return to normal level if increase was due to position change. If increase in drainage does not return to previous level notify primary care provider STAT

Problems with the tubing:
*   If any of these are noted on assessment there is a problem with the tubing
    *   Disconnection of tubing between unit and chest
    *   Kink or loop in tubing
    *   Pressure on tubing

Problem: Disconnection of tubing
1. Assess whether tubing touched floor or other surface. If tubing did not contact any surface, reconnect and tape connection securely
2. If tubing contacted surface change tubing, reconnect and tape

Problem: Kink in tubing or dependent loop in tubing
1. Remove kinks or loops, system may need to be lowered to prevent reoccurrence

Problem: Pressure on tubing
1. Check to see if patient is lying on tubing. If so, reposition patient

2.   Assess for any equipment on tubing or pressing against tubing and remove or reposition as appropriate

Problems with respiratory distress
- If any or all of these are noted on assessment the patient is having respiratory distress
  - Increase in dyspnea and/or shortness of breath
  - Tachypnea
  - Tachycardia
  - Anxiety and/or restlessness

Problem: Respiratory distress is present
1.   Place patient in high-Fowler's position
2.   Assess vital signs — report abnormal vital signs STAT
3.   Continue to monitor vital signs regularly until respiratory distress is resolved
4.   Is the chest tube drainage system below the level of the chest? If not reposition unit to below chest level
5.   Check for tubing obstruction (kinks, loops, clot). If present, remove the obstruction
6.   Check for any air leaks in system, tighten and tape all connections
7.   Check for any increase in chest tube drainage
8.   Report any unusual findings STAT — respiratory distress may indicate an increased accumulation of air or fluid in the pleural cavity
9.   Assess for tension pneumothorax. This is the most serious complication of chest tubes. It occurs when air is trapped in the lungs and cannot escape so with each increasing breath, the space is under more pressure. Eventually, the heart and great vessels are pushed to the opposite side by the increasing pressure and the ability of heart to receive and pump blood is compromised.

Signs and symptoms of tension pneumothorax:
Severe dyspnea (difficulty breathing)
Pain: Sudden sharp chest pain
  Pain may be referred to shoulder or abdomen
Diminished to absent motion and breath sounds on affected side
Affected side will appear inflated with air, but does not fall on expiration

Tympany on percussion of chest; diminished or absent
tactile fremitus
Heartbeat displaced secondary to mediastinum shift
Trachea is displaced to the unaffected side
Onset of shock
Decreased blood pressure
Pulse thready and fast
Hypoxemia
X-ray of chest confirms pneumothorax

RESPIRATORY ISOLATION

- Used to stop the transmission of pathogens from the respiratory tract of an infected person to an uninfected person
- Transmission of pathogens can occur by direct contact or by the airborne route
- Direct contact may occur from soiled linen or tissue
- Airborne route may include droplets coughed, sneezed, or breathed

Diseases where respiratory isolation would be required:

- Epiglottis with *Hemophilus influenzae*
- Erythema infectiosum
- Measles (rubeola)
- Meningitis with *Meningococcal H. Influenzae* or bacterial meningitis of unknown etiology
- Mumps
- Pertussis (whopping cough)
- Meningoccemia
- Pneumonia with *Hemophilus influenzae* in children

Measures taken in respiratory isolation

- Private room, unless two patients are infected with same pathogen
- Door to the room is kept closed
- Hands are washed before entering the room
- Masks should be worn by health care workers to enter the patient's room and while providing care
- Patient should be instructed to cover the mouth and nose when coughing or sneezing

- Patient should wear a mask when leaving the hospital room and carry tissues and a bag for their disposal
- Gloves/gowns are needed for direct contact with infected sputum or body secretions (not needed for mumps)
- Gowns and gloves are not needed by visitors unless they plan to contact secretions, all visitors should wear masks
- Contaminated materials such as tissues or linen are placed in plastic bag, sealed and placed in another bag for contaminated materials as per agency policy prior to removal from room
- Articles directly contaminated with secretions must be disinfected upon leaving the room
- Hands are washed upon exiting the room

Isolation recommendations for tuberculosis (AFB or TB isolation)

- Tuberculosis has it's own isolation recommendations due to the appearance of *Mycobacterium tuberculosis* or MTB and isoniazid (INH) resistant
- MTB is an acid-fast, aerobic bacterium (AFB) that is found in droplet nuclei that are released when an infected person coughs, sneezes, speaks or sings. The AFB can then be inhaled by a susceptible host
- Those most susceptible to MTB include:
  - Children (underdeveloped immune systems)
  - Elderly individuals (immune systems are diminished)
  - Undernourished or malnourished individuals
  - Those living in overcrowded living quarters
  - Immunodeficient individuals (HIV positive)
- Immunodeficient persons with HIV and a low CD4 cell count may not have a positive tuberculin skin test due to their inability to mount an immune response this complicates detection of MTB.

Measures taken in addition to respiratory isolation for TB

- Private room with negative pressure ventilation
  Rooms draws air into itself and thus reduces the potential for movement of AFB outward. The ventilation system of the room can not empty into the general ventilation system. Air from the room should be exhausted directly to the outside of the building away from intake vents, people and animals. The CDC recommends that isolation rooms undergo six total air changes per hour, including at least two outside air changes per hour.

- Tightly fitted masks or particulate respirator masks must be worn by staff who will share air space with the patient. The MTB organism is small (1-5 microns) therefore mask must not have any gaps, it should fit snugly on the face.
- Patient must wear a tightly fitted mask or valveless particulate respirator at all times when leaving their room
- Food trays and utensils are handled and washed the same way they are for other patients. Environmental surfaces are rarely associated with transmission of infection. AFB generally must be inhaled for infection to occur.

MECHANICAL VENTILATION

- Invasive medical procedure used to provide life support when the patient is unable to breathe or cannot breathe effectively
- The goal is to achieve optimal gas exchange
- Delivers a combination of air and oxygen to the patient by literally blowing it into the lungs
- Effectiveness is assessed by arterial blood gas results
- Does not provide a cure for respiratory problems; it will simply provide respiratory support until the cause of the respiratory problem can be resolved (if possible)

Indications for mechanical ventilation

1. Apnea (lack of spontaneous breathing)
2. Clinical respiratory distress with poor respiratory effort
3. PaO_2 of less than 50-60 mm Hg despite oxygen therapy
4. Elevated PCO_2 greater than 55-60 mm Hg
5. pH below 7.25-7.35
6. General anesthesia

Types of mechanical ventilation

- Pressure-cycled
- Volume-cycled

Pressure-cycled ventilators

- Flow into the lungs stops when a pre-determined pressure within the lungs is reached
- An advantage of a pressure-cycled ventilator is that good control is maintained over respiratory pressure
- Used more often in neonates and children than volume-cycled ventilation

- Disadvantages are that tidal volume is poorly controlled, and the system does not respond to changes in lung compliance

Volume-cycled ventilators
- Flow into the lungs stops when the pre-determined volume has been reached (regardless of pressure)
- The same volume of air and oxygen is delivered even if the airway resistance or the compliance of the lungs changes
- A safety feature that will stop the flow if excessive peak airway pressure occurs (usually set for 10 cm H20 pressure above the peak inspiratory pressure setting)
- Used when prolonged ventilation is required, rarely used on newborns

Terms used in mechanical ventilation
- *Respiratory Rate* — Rate of breaths that the ventilator will deliver, not always the same as patients respiratory rate Patient may have some unassisted breaths
- *FIO2* — Percentage of oxygen delivered, initially may be 100% changed according to the arterial blood gas results or the pulse oximeter readings
- Mean airway pressure (MAP) — Average pressure that is required to deliver the gas to the patients lungs
- *High pressure alarm* — Sounds if the preset pressure point is exceeded during the tidal volume delivery
- *Tidal volume* — Actual volume of gas the ventilator will deliver, usually set at 10-12 ml of gas per kilogram of weight Tidal volume is closely regulated in volume-cycled ventilators and poorly regulated in pressure-cycled ventilators
- *Respiratory mode* — When the ventilator is delivering all breaths the patient takes it is in the control mode
- *Peak or inspiratory flow rate* — Rate at which the tidal volume of air is delivered, usually between 50-80 liters per minute
- *Positive end-expiratory pressure (PEEP)* — Independently controlled with pressure-limited, time cycled ventilators, allows for regularized respiration
- *Inspiratory time (IT)* — a pre-set amount of time in which the gas will be delivered
- *Peak inspiratory pressure (PIP)*

Preparing for mechanical ventilation
- An adequate airway is always needed for effective ventilation

- Intubation can be achieved by either an oral or nasal endotracheal tube or by tracheostomy
- Once intubated, the tube is taped securely in place to prevent accidental extubation, taping an ET tube requires two persons — one tapes, the other maintains tube position
- Mark the entry level of the tube and record, the level should be assessed at least once per shift or if respiratory distress occurs
- Chest x-ray is done to confirm placement
- Lungs should be auscultated with equal breath sounds on both sides, if not equal notify the primary care provider
- Assess patients consciousness and agitation level, use restraints only if other means fail to reduce agitation and patient may extubate themselves. Remember agitation may be related to pain, hypoxemia, increased respiratory secretions, fear or anxiety. Obtain order for restraint use.
- Administer sedatives or muscle relaxation agents as ordered to prevent or decrease agitation and potential extubation

Assessment during mechanical ventilation

- Assess actual respiratory rate, rhythm and effort
- Auscultate breath sounds in all lung lobes, decreased breath sounds may indicate pneumothorax, rhonchi may indicate need for suctioning
- Assess for equal bilateral lung expansion.
- Check all ventilator settings against orders every 1-4 hours depending on patients condition and agency policy
- Record rate, PEEP, PIP (abrupt rise in PIP may indicate a pneumothorax with volume-cycled ventilation), IT, MAP, FIO2 and temperature setting (should be between 32-36 degrees)
- If at any time you must change the FIO2 chart the time, change and reason
- Check all alarm settings, alarms should not be disarmed Never leave a patient's bedside with the alarms in the off position
- Check all connections along the ventilator tubing to be sure they are tightly secured
- Assess the color and consistency of sputum for signs of infection
- Monitor patient's temperature and report any elevations

Care of patient during mechanical ventilation

- Explain all procedures to patient to reduce anxiety

- Suction as needed to maintain the patency of the airway Assessment findings that indicate a need for suctioning include an increase in restlessness and the presence of rhonchi
- Pre-oxygenate with a higher concentration of oxygen for 1-2 minutes prior to suctioning, to reduce hypoxia
- Suction for only 15 seconds or less and then provide high concentration of oxygen again, reassess lung sounds and chart
- Obtain regular blood gas testing as ordered (generally 15-20 minutes after any changes in rate, FIO_2 or ventilator pressure
- Reposition patient every 1-2 hours, by rotating position all lobes of the lung will be adequately perfused and skin breakdown will be minimized

Complications of mechanical ventilation

- Equipment malfunction
- Obstruction of the endotracheal tube by thick secretions
- Pneumothorax, pneumomediastinum, and subcutaneous emphysema
- Barotrauma from high pressure, occurs when the alveoli are overdistended and rupture which leads to alveolar necrosis
- Cardiac arrhythmias
- Nosocomial infection of the respiratory tract

Section V — CONDITIONS

Asthma

Definition

- Syndrome with recurring attacks of airway narrowing resulting in shortness of breath, wheezing, and coughing that resolve with treatment or spontaneously
- Attacks last minutes to hours followed by symptom free periods
- Asthma has three components: airway obstruction to airflow, thickening of airway epithelium, and presence of secretions within the airway
- Non-progressive, most asthmatics have less frequent and less severe attacks as they age
- Status asthmaticus is a severe airway obstruction that lasts for days or weeks
- Acute episodes can be fatal (unusual)

Prevalence

- Affects adult men and women equally, in childhood males are affected more than females
- About 4-5% of US population has S&S consistent with asthma
- About 50% of all cases have onset before age 10

Etiology

- Etiology is unknown
- Asthma triggered by physical exertion is known as "exercise-induced asthma"
  - Exercise is one of the most common precipitating factors
  - Exercise in cold whether may be less tolerated
- Asthma triggered by a known allergy is known as "extrinsic asthma or allergic asthma"
  - Frequently seasonal
  - Onset usually in childhood or young adults
  - Exposure to allergen results in immediate symptoms
  - A late reaction 6-10 hrs after initial reaction may occur
- Attacks are also known to be triggered by air pollution, occupational exposure to metal salts, dusts, pharmaceutical agents, industrial chemicals, biologic enzymes, animals, infections or emotional stress

- Asthma that occurs without any known trigger is "intrinsic asthma or idiosyncratic asthma"

Symptoms of asthma attack

- Shortness of breath (dyspnea), wheezing and cough are the three most typical symptoms
    - Wheezing heard on inspiration and expiration
    - Non-productive cough at onset
    - Productive cough with thick stringy mucus at end of attack
- Feeling of tightness in the chest
- Hoarseness
- Tachypnea, respiratory rate often 25-40 breaths per minute
- Use of accessory muscles during inspiration
- Intercostal retractions during inspiration
- Prolonged expiratory phase during breathing
- Tachycardia
- Anxiety

Components of initial examination for asthma

- *Complete medical history to include:*
- Personal history of asthma including previous and current treatment
- Onset time of this episode and date of last previous attack
- Patient's understanding of diagnoses and treatment
- Any factor that patient or family believe triggered current attack (provoking stimulus)
- Family and/or personal history of allergic diseases such as eczema, rhinitis or urticaria (hives)
- History of awakening from sleep with dyspnea and/or wheezing
- *Physical examination to include:*
- General appearance and level of distress (anxious, fearful)
    - Patient's preferred position, may not tolerate supine
- Respiratory rate, rhythm and effort
    - Degree of breathlessness is not closely related to degree of airway obstruction
    - Respirations are often audibly harsh and labored
    - Shallow respirations may occur with severe obstruction
    - Gasping may occur if mucous plug obstructs airway

- Assessment of chest for hyperinflation, retractions, use of accessory muscles to aid in respiration
- Pulse rate and rhythm
  - Usually tachycardiac
  - Pulsus paradoxus, fall in pulse at close of each full inspiration, correlates with severe attacks
- Blood pressure measurement, mild systolic hypertension is common
- Auscultation of the lungs for
  - Wheezing
  - Rhonchi if secretions are present in airway
  - Rales indicating localized infection
  - Symmetrical breath sounds, atelectasis or even spontaneous pneumothorax may occur (rare)
  - Decreased or absent breath sounds indicate severe obstruction
- Assessment of lips and nailbeds for cyanosis
- Sputum, often clear or opaque may be yellow or green-tinged (color does not always indicate infection)
- *Laboratory and diagnostic testing:*
The diagnosis of asthma is based on establishing that airway obstruction is intermittent and reversible, no specific tests
- Pulmonary function testing
- Arterial blood gases (only done if severe or prolonged)
- Skin testing for various suspected allergens
- Serum IgE levels (helpful, not specific for asthma)
- Sputum and blood eosinophilia (not specific for asthma)
- Chest X-ray (often normal, may show hyperinflation)

Treatment of asthma

- Goals of treatment are to:
  - Remove known or suspected allergens from environment
  - Obtain a symptom free state with minimum amount of medications
  - Achievement of best pulmonary function possible
- Desensitization therapy for suspected allergens
- Medications in aerosol form for treatment of acute symptoms (beta-adrenergic agonists)

Medications for asthma
- Beta-adrenergic agonists produce airway dilatation, used for acute episodes of asthma in aerosolized forms and include catecholamines such as epinephrine, isoproterenol and isoetharine; resorcinols such as metaproterenol, terbutaline and fenoterol, and saligenins such as albuterol and salbutamol
- Methylxanthines for bronchodilatation such as theophylline for patients with asthma complaints at night
- Glucocorticoids to reduce airway inflammation such as hydrocortisone and methylprednisolone for persistent symptoms
- Mast cell stabilizing agents such as cromolyn sodium and nedocromil sodium for patients with persistent symptoms and unstable lung function
- Anticholinergics to produce bronchodilation such as atropine methyl nitrate and ipratropium bromide

Chronic Airway Diseases
Definition
- Also known as chronic obstructive lung diseases (COLD) or chronic obstructive pulmonary disease (COPD)
- Includes chronic bronchitis, chronic obstructive bronchitis, and emphysema
- Grouped together in one category because patients will have characteristics predominant of bronchitis or emphysema and also have some characteristics of the other disorder as well
- *Bronchitis* is an inflammation of the mucous membrane of the bronchial tubes that causes a productive cough from stimulation of mucous secretions, impaired mucus clearance due to interference with ciliary activity and impaired resistance to bronchial infection
- *Chronic bronchitis* must have occurred for at least 3 months out of the year for more than 2 consecutive years
- *Chronic obstructive bronchitis* is a severe disabling condition with an irreversible narrowing of the bronchioles and small bronchi, also known as small airways disease
- *Emphysema* is an abnormal, permanent enlargement of the air spaces distal to the terminal bronchioles with destructive changes in the alveolar walls

Prevalence
- Males are affected more frequently than females, however with recent increases in female smokers this may change
- More common in persons over age 50 than in younger adults
- *Chronic bronchitis* may affect up to 20% of adult males
- *Emphysema* is found in varying degrees at autopsy of most adults

Etiology
The following are contributory factors:
- Cigarette smoking is the single most important causative factor
- Air pollution, higher incidence in heavily industrialized areas
- Occupations that involve organic dusts or noxious gases
- Infections are known to contribute to exacerbations
- Family factors, children of smokers have increased exposure to carbon monoxide and smoke and an increased risk
- Genetic factors, studies of twins have shown a genetic predisposition may be present independent of environment

Symptoms of chronic airway diseases
Most patients have some characteristics of both syndromes although they may show predominance for one or the other

Bronchitis — Mild early disease
- Cough, upon arising after the first cigarette is smoked
  - Productive cough
  - Occurs most often in winter months
  - Increased cigarette use or respiratory infection increases cough and sputum production
  - If patient stops smoking symptoms usually disappear

Bronchitis — Progressive obstructive disease
- Shortness of breath with severe disease
- Impairment of ability to do physical work
- Severe disability may occur with chronic respiratory failure
- Cough, throughout the day and throughout the year
  - Increased sputum production often purulent
  - Episodes of severe coughing occur
  - Wheezing may occur at end of coughing spell (bronchospasm)
  - Wheezing may occur when lying down (secondary to sputum)
- Frequent bronchial infections
- Swelling of lower extremities

Emphysema
- Severe shortness of breath
- Cough
  - Scant amount of sputum
- Weight loss

Components of examination for airway disease
Most patients have some characteristics of both syndromes
- *Complete medical history to include:*
- Personal history of airway disease including diagnosis, previous and current treatments
- Patient's understanding of diagnosis, treatment and life-style changes required
- Cigarette use, type (low or high tar) number of years and packs per day
- History of respiratory infections to include frequency
  - *Bronchitis* — Frequent bronchial infections
  - *Emphysema* — Infrequent bronchial infections
- History of cough, assess for productivity, frequency
  - *Bronchitis* — Persistent cough with copious sputum for many years, starts before shortness of breath
  - *Emphysema* — Minimal cough with only small amount sputum, onset of cough follows shortness of breath
- Shortness of breath and effect on activities of daily living
  - *Bronchitis* — Mild with exertion
  - *Emphysema* — Severe, often limits activity
- History of weight changes
  - *Bronchitis* — Weight gain related to water retention
  - *Emphysema* — Weight loss related to increased work of breathing
- *Physical examination to include:*
- General appearance — *Bronchitis,* sometimes referred to as "blue bloaters"
  - Frequently overweight
  - No apparent respiratory distress at rest
  - Lying down may lead to wheezing from retained secretions
  - Productive cough, episodes of severe coughing
  - Cyanosis may be present due to heart failure
  - Peripheral edema may be present due to heart failure

- General appearance — *Emphysema,* sometimes referred to as "pink puffers"
  - Stooped posture
  - Evidence of weight loss
  - Apparent respiratory distress
- Respiratory rate, rhythm and effort — *Bronchitis*
  - Rate is normal or slightly increased
  - No use of accessory muscles
- Respiratory rate, rhythm and effort — *Emphysema*
  - Obvious increased work of breathing, labored
  - Patient leans forward when sitting, extending arms to brace themselves
  - Obvious use of accessory muscles to aid in respiration — lift of sternum and intercostal retractions with each inspiration, neck vein distention is noted during expiration
  - Pursed lip breathing
  - Grunting sound may be heard at beginning of expiration
- Respiratory percussion and auscultation — *Bronchitis*
  - Normal chest percussion
  - Auscultation with coarse rhonchi & wheezes which change in location and intensity after a deep cough (productive)
- Respiratory percussion and auscultation — *Emphysema*
  - Chest percussion is hyperresonant
  - Breath sounds are diminished
  - Faint high-pitched rhonchi may be heart during end of expiration
  - Prolonged period of expiration

It is important to again note that most patients develop a mixture of symptoms from both bronchitis and emphysema

- *Laboratory and diagnostic testing:*
- Chest X-ray, normal in early disease
- Complete blood count (CBC) with differential study
- Sputum examination for suspected infections
- Pulmonary function tests to assess lung function
- Arterial blood gasses to assess for hypoxemia
- Ventilation-perfusion lung scans
- Electrocardiogram

Treatment of chronic airway diseases

The goals of treatment are to relieve airway obstruction symptoms, limit further disease, control cough and sputum production, prevent infections, decrease hospitalizations and interference with daily activities of living, and to control or prevent cardiovascular complications

- Cessation of smoking to slow or limit advancement
- Avoidance of known respiratory irritants such as air pollution, aerosol sprays (deodorants, hair sprays, insecticides)
- Yearly influenza vaccine against common or expected strains
- Pneumococcal polysaccharide vaccine (once in lifetime)
- Bronchial hygiene methods such as postural drainage for patients with hypersecretion
- Exercise as tolerated (daily walking) to improve exercise tolerance and improve well-being
- Oral dietary supplements if malnutrition is noted
- Avoidance of high altitudes
- Home oxygen therapy for severe exertional hypoxemia
- Phlebotomy if hematocrit is above 60%
- Avoidance of narcotics, sedatives and tranquilizers for patients with chronic hypercapnia
- Vocational rehabilitation and occupational therapy to encourage active lifestyle
- Lung transplantation for severe disease
- Bilateral carotid body resection and periodic use of negative pressure ventilation are two controversial treatments

Medications for chronic airway diseases

- Bronchodilators such as theophylline or aminophylline, albuterol and metaproterenol
- Antibiotics if purulent mucus is present
- Diuretics if pedal edema or heart failure is present
- Corticosteroids such as prednisone if bronchodilators and bronchopulmonary drainage measures have been tried without success
- Digitalis for heart failure

PULMONARY EMBOLISM (PE)

Definition
- An emboli within the pulmonary artery or one of it's branches that leads to the partial or complete obstruction of arterial blood flow to the lung tissue fed by that artery
- The emboli is usually a thrombus or blood clot that has traveled to the lungs via the blood stream
- a sudden onset life-threatening condition, death due to pulmonary embolism can occur within 1-2 hours, often before a treatment plan can be begun

Prevalence
- Occurs in 1-2% of general surgical patients over the age of 40, with higher incidence in orthopedic surgical patients, the elderly, obese, or those with previous venous disease, post-operative infection or prolonged bed rest
- Annual incidence in US from 500,000-600,000 cases
- Directly responsible for more than 50,000 deaths in the US annually, prognosis is excellent if detected early

Etiology
- 95% of pulmonary emboli arise from deep vein thrombi (blood clots) in lower extremities
- Fat droplets, tumor cells, air bubbles, pieces of intravenous catheters, or other materials are rare causes of PE

Symptoms of pulmonary emboli
- Range from no symptoms to sudden death, symptoms depend upon the degree of blockage and whether pulmonary infarction occurs
- Sudden and unexplained onset of shortness of breath may be the only symptom
- Sudden feelings of apprehension occurs in about 50% of cases
- Pleuritic chest pain may be present if pulmonary infarction has occurred occurs in about 74% of patients

Components of initial examination for pulmonary emboli
- *Complete medical history to include:*
- Presence of sudden pain in the chest
- History of current or previous thrombosis in lower extremities or pre-existing venous disease

- Recent history of immbolization, general or orthopedic surgery, postoperative infection or any other condition that contributes to prolonged bed rest (risk factor for thrombi formation)
- Recent history of trauma (may be surgical) with blood vessel damage, particularly in lower extremities or pelvis
- Cancer of the lung, breast, or abdominal viscera (strong association with venous thromboembolism)
- Personal history of increased blood coagulability
- Family history of venous thrombosis or hereditary abnormality of anticoagulant factor
- Pregnancy, post-partum period
- *Physical examination to include:*
- Findings may be normal, diagnostic testing is required for diagnosis
- The extent of the obstruction from the emboli will determine how pronounced the symptoms are
- General appearance and level of distress
  - Patient is short of breath
  - Substernal or pleuritic chest pain only if pulmonary infarction has occurred
  - Patient may be anxious or have feelings of doom
- Respiratory rate, rhythm and effort
  - Rate usually increased
  - Breathing may be labored
  - Hemoptysis (sputum with frothy bright red blood) may occur
- Pulse, rate is elevated, often above 100
- Temperature may be elevated if infection or infarction is present
- Auscultation of the lungs for
  - Air exchange within all lung areas
  - Rales may be heard related to atelectatic areas
  - Wheezes may be heard (rare)
  - Pleural friction rub will not be present unless infarction has occurred
- Assessment of lower extremities for deep vein thrombosis (seldom clinically apparent), cold, pale, bluish extremity with loss of pulse below the obstruction
- *Laboratory and diagnostic testing:*
- Pulmonary arteriography, the definitive test for diagnosis of PE

- Ventilation-Perfusion lung scans to assess regional pulmonary blood flow
- Computed tomography and magnetic resonance imaging
- Arterial blood gases to determine level of hypoxemia
- Electrocardiogram to rule out myocardial infarction
- Chest X-ray
- Thoracentesis, pleural effusions are common in PE
- Clotting times, partial thromboplastin times (PTT) to monitor heparin therapy

Treatment of pulmonary embolism
Goal of treatment is threefold
- Limit the size of the embolus
- Conclusion of the pulmonary embolus
- Prevent any reoccurrence
- Medication therapy (heparin) is the number one treatment
- Surgical intervention (pulmonary embolectomy or vena caval interruption) is rarely considered and is used for patients unable to have heparin therapy

Medications for pulmonary embolism
- Heparin administration is the initial therapy because the effect is immediate and is begun even before diagnostic confirmation is made, routes include:
  - Continuous intravenous infusion delivered by infusion pump
  - Intermittent intravenous infusion
  - Intermittent subcutaneous injection
- Thrombolytic agents such as streptokinase, urokinase, and tissue plasminogen activator, tPA to hasten resolution of venous thrombi
- Oral anticoagulation with warfarin may be begun 1-2 days after heparin therapy

Section VI — DIETS

- No diets specific for this system
- Patients with chronic respiratory conditions may benefit from inclusion of the following dietary components
- Increased caloric diet if patient is underweight
  - Underweight here is defined as less than 85% of ideal body weight
  - Anorexia may occur related to dyspnea, weakness, and fatigue from a variety of respiratory disorders to include chronic airway diseases and lung neoplasms
  - Oral dietary supplements may be ordered for improved muscle strength and less fatigability which may decrease breathlessness
- Pancreatic enzymes
  - In cystic fibrosis obstruction of large and small intestines may occur with loss of appetite, emesis and pain
  - In cystic fibrosis insufficient pancreatic enzyme release yields to protein and fat malabsorption
- Use of antiemetics to improve nutritional intake
  - Nausea may occur related to viscous respiratory secretions

Section VII — DRUGS

The tables supply only general information; a drug handbook or the Physicians Desk Reference (PDR) should be consulted prior to administering any unfamiliar drug. Each classification includes detailed information about the example drug, this drug is representative of the other drugs in the classification and can be used as a model.

Every effort has been made to include the major classes of drugs used in the treatment of respiratory diseases.

ANTITUSSIVES
Action: Inhibit the cough reflex
Indications: Used for patients with a dry, non-productive cough
Example: Benzonatate (*Tessalon*)
Route: PO
Pharmacokinetics: Onset 15-20 minutes, Duration 3-8 hours
Common adverse effects: Low incidence of adverse effects
Life-threatening adverse effects: None
Other adverse effects: Drowsiness, headache, mild dizziness, constipation, nausea, skin rash, and pruritus
Interventions: Must be swallowed whole, Assess for productive cough, color, quantity of sputum
Examples of other drugs in this classification:
Dextromethorphan (*Benylin DM, Cremacoat 1, Delsym, DM Cough, Hold, Mediquell, Ornex DM, Pedia Care, Pertussin 8 hour Cough formula, Robitussin DM, Romilar CF, Romilar Childrens Cough, Sucrets Cough Control*), Contraindicated in asthma, productive cough, chronic cough, and liver impairment, can be purchased over the counter

BRONCHODILATORS
Action: Relaxes the smooth muscle of the bronchi and pulmonary vessels, stimulates the respiratory center to increase the vital capacity of the lungs
Indications: Bronchial asthma, bronchospasm, chronic bronchitis, emphysema
Example: Theophylline (*Bronkodyl, Elixophyllin, Lanophyllin, Respbid, PMS theophylline, Quilbron-T, Slo-Bid, Slo-Phyllin, Somophyllin, Theo-Dur, Theo-24, Theolair, Theospan and Uniphyl*)
Route: PO, IV
Pharmacokinetics: PO, uncoated tablet, Peak 1 hr, Duration 4-8 hrs

PO, sustained release, Peak 4-6 hours, Duration 4-8 hrs
IV, Peak 30 minutes

<u>Contraindications</u>: Hypersensitivity to xanthines, coronary artery disease, angina pectoris if stimulation might be harmful

<u>Common adverse effects</u>: Tachycardia and nausea

<u>Life-threatening adverse effects:</u> Drug-induced seizures, circulatory failure and respiratory arrest

<u>Other adverse effects:</u> Irritability, restlessness, insomnia, dizziness, headache, tremor, hyperexcitability, muscle twitching, palpitations, extrasystoles, flushing, hypotension, vomiting, anorexia, epigastric pain, diarrhea, irritation of peptic ulcer, urinary frequency, kidney irritation, tachypnea, fever and dehydration

<u>Interventions</u>:

Administer with a full glass of water, coated tablets or sustained release forms should be swallowed whole, chewable tablets must be chewed/crushed thoroughly, sprinkles can be mixed with applesauce
IV rate should not exceed 20 mg/minute
Therapeutic range is 10-20 µg/ml, levels greater than 20 µg/ml are toxic
Cigarette smokers may require an increase in dosage levels
Monitor for dizziness and assist with ambulation as needed
Monitor vital signs and input and output as ordered, encourage fluids
Assess for signs of toxicity anorexia, nausea, vomiting, dizziness, shakiness, restlessness, abdominal pain, irritability, palpitations, increased pulse, hypotension, and seizures
Check with pharmacist for drug incompatibilities if patient is on other medications

Examples of other drugs in this classification:

Aminophylline(*Theophylline ethylenediamine*) Monitor IV infusion carefully

Dyphylline (*Dilor, Dylline, Lufylin, Neothylline, Thylline*)
Therapeutic drug level is 12ug/ml, theophylline levels cannot be used to monitor this medication, Avoid alcohol and large amounts of xanthine beverages to include cocoa, colas, and teas

Oxtriphylline (*Choledyl, Choledyl-SA, Choline Theophyllinate*), 64% of this drug is theophylline

Example: Isoproterenol Hydrochloride (*Dispos-a-Med, Isoproterenol, Isuprel*)

<u>Route:</u> Inhaler, IPPB, IV

<u>Pharmacokinetics</u>: Onset immediate, Duration inhalation 1 hour, SC 2 hours

<u>Contraindications</u>: Cardiac arrhythmias, cariogenic shock, simultaneous administration with epinephrine

<u>Common adverse effects</u>: Ventricular arrhythmias and tachycardia

<u>Life-threatening adverse effects:</u> None

<u>Other adverse effects:</u> Mild tremors, nervousness, anxiety, lightheadedness, vertigo, insomnia, excitement, fatigue, flushing, palpitations, unstable blood pressure, anginal pain, nausea, vomiting and sweating

<u>Interventions</u>:

Infusion pump must be used for IV use, Monitor vital signs for titration rate of solution per orders, Continuous ECG monitoring is required, Check orders and agency protocol for parameters, Generally infusion is decreased or stopped if heart rate is greater than 110 bpm, heart rate, ECG pattern, BP and central venous pressure should be recorded

Sublingual tablets may cause flushing, palpitations, and precordial pain

Sublingual tablets may be given rectally as ordered, they should not be swallowed whole

Intermittent Positive-Pressure Breathing (IPPB) inhalation usually takes 15-20 mins, and may be ordered up to 5 times per day, saliva and sputum may be pink after treatment

Observe patient using metered dose inhaler for correct use, check the manufacturer's instructions, monitor patients use for frequency of use

Patient should not use OTC drugs without primary care provider input

Examples of other drugs in this classification:

Albuterol (*Proventil, Proventil Repetabs, Salbutamol, Ventolin, Ventolin Rotocaps*), Available PO or Metered dose Inhaler, most common adverse effect is fine tremor in fingers

Bitolterol Mesylate (*Tornalate*), Inhalation medication, if reaction to drug is not known epinephrine should be available

Isoetharine Hydrochloride (*Arm-a Med Isoetharine, Beta-2, Bronkosol, Dey-Lute, Dispos-a Med Isoetharine*), Nebulizer or metered dose inhaler, Do not administer simultaneously with epinephrine, increase fluids

Terbutaline sulfate (*Brethaire, Brethine, Bricanyl*), PO or SC injection, Inhalation use, Tablet may be crushed and mixed with fluid or taken with food, SC injection is usually into the lateral deltoid area, Check pulse and blood pressure with each dose if baseline is altered significantly, notify primary care provider, No other bronchodilator inhalation should be used with aerosol terbutaline

Example: Epinephrine (*Bronkaid Mist, Epinephrine, EpiPen Auto-Injector, Primatene Mist Suspension, AsthmaHaler, Bronkaid Suspension, Bronitin Mist Suspension, Epitrate, Medihaler-Epi, Epifrin, Glaucon, MicroNefrin*)
Route: SC, IV, Inhalation
Pharmacokinetics: Onset 3-5 minutes, Peak 20 minutes
Contraindications: Hypersensitivity to sympathomimetic amines, glaucoma, cariogenic shock, cardiac dilatation, cerebral arteriosclerosis, coronary insufficiency, arrhythmias, organic brain disease, local anesthesia of fingers, toes, ears, nose and genitalia
Common adverse effects: Burning, stinging, nervousness and tremors
Life-threatening adverse effects: Palpitations, ventricular fibrillation and pulmonary edema
Other adverse effects: Dryness of nasal mucosa, sneezing, rebound, congestion, lacrimation, browache, headache, restlessness, sleeplessness, fear, anxiety, severe headache, cerebrovascular accident, weakness, dizziness, syncope, pallor, nausea, vomiting, sweating, dyspnea, urinary retention, precordial pain, hypertension, tachyarrhythmias, metabolic acidosis, tissue necrosis, blood glucose elevations, altered state of perception and thought
Interventions:
SC injection, use tuberculin syringe, shake vial or ampule thoroughly to disperse particles, protect from light and inject promptly, carefully aspirate before injection to avoid accidental IV injection, for quick absorption massage site, rotate sites to prevent tissue necrosis
IV injection, given 1 mg over 1 minute, may be given more rapidly in cardiac arrest, check concentration and dosage carefully, monitor BP, pulse and respirations, Assess urinary output, if cardiac rhythms occur, withhold drug and notify primary care provider
Inhalation, Pt should be upright during inhalation use, assess pt for effectiveness after use, Pt should rinse mouth and throat with water after inhalation to avoid swallowing residual medication, Report to the primary care provider if symptoms are not relieved within 20 minutes of use, check orders for any respiratory care treatments (postural drainage)
Check orders for fluid intake, encourage adequate intake
Examples of other drugs in this classification:
Ephedrine (*Efedron, Ectasule, Ephedsol, Vatronol*), PO, IM, SC, IV,
     Offer dosage before bedtime to prevent insomnia, Monitor I&O,

Do not take OTC drugs unless cleared by primary care provider, many OTC drugs for colds, coughs, allergies and asthma contain ephedrine

EXPECTORANTS
Action: Decreases the viscosity of phlegm to help in expectoration of sputum, decreases cough as well
Indications: Dry nonproductive cough from colds and/or bronchitis
Example: Guaifenesin (*Amonidrin, Anti-Tuss, Breonesin, Gee-Gee, GG-Cen, Glyceryl Guaiacolate, Glycotuss, Glytuss, Guaituss, Hytuss, Malotuss, Mytussin, Nortussin, Robitussin*)
Route: PO
Common adverse effects: Low incidence of adverse effects
Other adverse effects: Nausea, drowsiness, gastric upset
Interventions: Administer with full glass of water, monitor effectiveness of drug, increase fluid intake to loosen secretions
Examples of other drugs in this classification:
Potassium Iodide (*Pima, SSKI*), PO, Also antithyroid agent and may alter thyroid function testing, Administer with meals, avoid giving with milk, Serum K+ levels should be assessed prior to therapy, report to primary care provider any GI bleeding, abdominal pain, nausea, vomiting or distention, Avoid over the counter drugs that contain iodides

MUCOLYTICS
Action: Decreases the viscosity of sputum
Indications: Abnormally thick mucous secretions, chronic bronchopulmonary diseases, cystic fibrosis, tracheostomy and atelectasis
Example: Acetyl cysteine (*Mucomyst, Mucosol, N-Acetyl cysteine*)
Route: Inhalation, Instillation, PO
Contraindications: Hypersensitivity to Acetyl cysteine, patients at risk for gastric hemorrhage
Adverse effects: Vomiting; Dizziness, drowsiness, nausea, stomatitis, bronchospasm, rhinorrhea, burning sensation in respiratory passage, epistaxis, urticaria
Interventions:
May also be given by injection or into tracheostomy
Encourage patient to cough up secretions
Drug has an unpleasant odor and this may lead to vomiting

Section VIII—GLOSSARY

Alveoli	Small air sacs within the lungs where internal respiration (gas exchange) occurs
Alveolus	One air sac within the lung where gas exchange occurs (singular form of alveoli)
Apnea	Break or period of no breathing
Atelectasis	Collapse of lung tissue
Bronchiectasis	Chronic abnormal state with spasms of coughing, purulent sputum due to chronic dilation of the bronchus
Bronchiolitis	Inflammation of the bronchioles
Bronchitis	Inflammation of the mucous membrane of the bronchi
Bronchoplasty	Repair of the bronchus
Bronchospasm	A spasm of the muscles located around the bronchi
CO_2	Carbon dioxide, the odorless, colorless gas which is a cellular waste product our lungs expel
COPD	Chronic obstructive pulmonary disease, term for obstructive pulmonary disorders such as asthma, emphysema and bronchitis
Diaphragm	Muscle that separates the thoracic and abdominal cavities. The primary muscle used in respiration, when the diaphragm contracts, the lungs expand and inspiration occurs; when it relaxes, expiration occurs
Dyspnea	Difficult breathing
Emphysema	Obstructive lung disease where the alveoli increase in size due to damage or destruction
Epiglottis	The flap-like structure that covers the larynx during swallowing
Epistaxis	Bleeding from the nose, nosebleed

Eupnea	Normal breathing, no distress in breathing
Hemopneumo-thorax	Blood in the pleural cavity
Hemoptysis	Blood in the sputum
Hyperventilation	Rapid breathing which is prolonged and deep
Hypoventilation	Slow, shallow breathing
Larynx	Also called the voice box. Located at the upper end of the trachea, the larynx contains the false and true vocal cords which aid in speech
Laryngitis	Inflammation of the larynx
Nares	Nostrils
O$_2$	Oxygen, an essential element for life
Pertussis	Whooping cough
Pharynx	An upper airway tube that extends from the nasal cavity (and oral cavity) to the larynx, divided into three parts: Nasopharynx — upper portion above the palate Oropharynx — palate to hyoid bone Laryngopharynx — hyoid bone to larynx
Pleural cavity	The space (potential not actual) between the two pleural layers of the lung, the parietal pleura and the visceral pleura
Pleurisy	Inflammation of the pleura
Pneumonia	Congestion and inflammation of the lungs
Pneumohemo-thorax	Air and blood in the pleural cavity
Pneumothorax	Air in the pleural cavity
Pulmonary edema	Fluid in the lung tissues
Rales	Term for crackles, an adventitious lung sound resulting from small atelectatic areas

Respiration   The act of breathing, the exchange of gases
                     between the atmosphere and the lungs

Rhinitis   Inflammation of the nasal membranes

Rhinoplasty   Cosmetic procedure for repair of nose, also
                     known as a "nose job"

Thoracentesis   Drainage of fluid via needle aspiration from
                     the chest wall

Trachea   An airway tube that extends from the larynx
                     to the right and left bronchi, also called the
                     windpipe

Neurologic System

NEUROLOGIC SYSTEM

Table of Contents

Section I — The Overview

Primary functions

- Control and management of most body functions needed for survival
- Receives, decodes, interprets messages from the body to include:
  - Changes in respiration and heart rate
  - Changes in levels of circulating hormones and enzymes
  - Changes in body core temperature
  - Changes in acid base balance of the blood
- Transmits messages to the cells of the body to include:
  - Initiation and continuation of respiration via the stimulation of the intercostal muscles and diaphragm
  - Amount and types of secretions from glands
  - Control of muscular movement, coordination, balance and posture
- Interaction and communication with the external environment by receiving, decoding, and interpreting messages such as:
  - External environment changes to include temperature, level of safety and sensations of movement
  - Sensory stimulation to include olfactory, auditory, tactile, gustatory or visual stimuli
  - Allows for the creation, development, perception, transmission and evaluation of thoughts and ideas
  - Ability to send and receive messages (communication) via speech, gesture, written word, or technological advancement (telephone, telegraph, computer)
  - Ability to learn new concepts and use these concepts to manufacture new idea's, create new products or alter the environment
- Responsible for the individual distinct characteristics such as temperament, feelings, cognition, and personality

Components

- This system contains the central nervous system (CNS), peripheral nervous system (PNS), and the sensory organs
- The CNS contains the brain and the spinal cord

- The PNS contains the cranial nerves, spinal nerves and the autonomic nervous system which contains both the sympathetic nervous system (SNS) and the parasympathetic nervous system
- The sensory organs that are included in this discussion are the eye and the ear

THE CENTRAL NERVOUS SYSTEM (CNS)

- Continuous organ system divided into two principal components; the brain and spinal cord
- The CNS has a protective covering called the meninges composed of three layers; dura mater, pia mater, and the arachnoid membrane
- Cerebral spinal fluid is produced in the ventricles and circulated along the brains surface and around the spinal cord

Brain

- Complex organ with four principal parts of the brain (Figure 3A)
  - Brainstem
  - Cerebellum
  - Diencephalon
  - Cerebrum

Principal Parts of the Brain

I.   Brain stem

Interconnects the spinal cord, cerebellum, diencephalon, and cerebral cortex

Controls basic body functions needed for survival (respiration, eating and movement)

Individual may live with all parts of the brain destroyed except the brainstem

Ten of the twelve pairs of cranial nerves (CN) originate here

Has three components; medulla oblongata, pons, and the mesencephalon

- Medulla oblongata

  Continuation of the spinal cord into the skull, contains vital life-support centers

  Cardiac center: Regulates the rate and contraction force of the heart and diameter of blood vessels

  Respiratory center: Regulates respiratory rhythm

  Control center for basic reflexes: swallowing, gagging, coughing, sneezing hiccupping, vomiting, and salivating

The Brain and Meninges

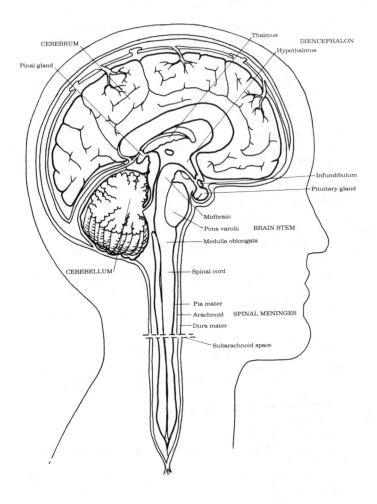

CEREBRUM

Pinal gland

Thalmus

DIENCEPHALON

Hypothalmus

Infundibulum

Pituitary gland

Midbrain

Pons varolii   BRAIN STEM

Medulla oblongata

Spinal cord

CEREBELLUM

Pia mater

Arachnoid   SPINAL MENINGES

Dura mater

Subarachnoid space

Figure 3A

- Innervates the tongue (CN IX and XII), lateral eye movement (CN VI), vagus nerve (CN X) and facial expression (CN VII)
- The pons
  Connection between the upper & lower levels of the CNS
  Innervates the muscles used in chewing and for jaw movement during speech (CN V)
- Mesencephalon or midbrain
  Innervates the muscles used in movements of the eyeballs and raising the eyelids
  Regulates pupillary size and lens shape (CN III)
  Involved in the function of localizing sound sources

II. The cerebellum

Coordinates motor movement with visual, auditory, somesthetic and vestibular information to produce smoothly controlled movements

Needed for coordination, balance, posture, and muscle tone

Studies suggest that rote movements such as touch-typing or finger movements to play an instrument originate here

III. The diencephalon

Composed of the dorsal thalamus, hypothalamus and subthalamus

- Dorsal thalamus (commonly referred to as the thalamus)
  Sensory stimuli (except olfactory) are received here and then relayed to cortical areas
  Makes the sensation of pain, crude touch and temperature possible
- Hypothalamus
  Homeostatic control center: Integrates and maintains blood gas concentration, fluid balance, body temperature, hunger, and the major aspects of hormonal control
- Subthalamus
  Needed for movement control

IV. Cerebrum

Forms the bulk of brain tissue

Contains a right and left cerebral hemisphere interconnected by the corpus callosum

Each cerebral hemisphere contains white matter, gray matter, and basal ganglia

Each hemisphere contains four different lobes; frontal, temporal, parietal and occipital named after bones of the skull

- Frontal lobe
  Site of personality and intellectual functioning
  Area where ideas are developed and plans made
  Area also controls movement and produces speech
- Temporal lobe
  Site of auditory cortex; allows for discrimination of sound frequency and needed to determine the meaning sounds and speech
  Long-term memory recall is stored here
- Parietal lobe
  Primary sensory cortex; allows for discrimination of sensory input such as location, and intensity
  Needed to feel vibration and determine the position or movement of body parts
- Occipital lobe
  Primary visual cortex; interprets visual input

The Spinal Cord
- Link between the brain and the peripheral nerves
- Extends from the foramen magnum at the base of the skull to the conus medullaris located at the first or second lumbar vertebra
- The cord itself is made up of both white and gray matter and housed in the bony vertebral canal

THE PERIPHERAL NERVOUS SYSTEM (PNS)
- All nerve impulses are transmitted to and from the CNS by the PNS
- Composed of the cranial nerves, spinal nerves and the autonomic nervous system

Cranial nerves (CN)
- There are 12 pairs of cranial nerves that are attached to the base of the brain.

CRANIAL NERVES

CN	CN Name	CN Function	Malfunction Indications
I	Olfactory	Perception of smell	Loss or disturbance in perception of smell
II	Optic	Vision	Blindness may be partial or complete depending on lesion location

CN	CN Name	CN Function	Malfunction Indications
III	Oculomotor	Movement of both eyes to center, upper right & upper left position Movement of left eye to side right & to lower left position Movement of right eye to side left & to lower right position Regulates pupillary size Raises eyelid	Deviation of eye outward Double vision Dilatation of pupil Ptosis (drooping eyelid)
IV	Trochlear	Movement of left eye to lower right & left	Deviation of eye upward & outward
V	Trigeminal	Sensory input to face Chewing	Pain or sensation loss in face, forehead, eye or temple Difficulty chewing
VI	Abducens	Movement of right eye to side right Movement of left eye to side left	Deviation of eye outward Double vision
VII	Facial	Facial expression Glandular secretion Taste	Paralysis of one side of face Loss of taste in foods
VIII	Acoustic Vestibulocochlear	Hearing Sense of equilibrium	Ringing in ears Deafness, dizziness Nausea or vomiting
IX	Glossopharyngeal	Taste perception Ability to swallow	Altered taste perception Difficulty in swallowing
X	Vagus	Involuntary muscle & gland control Swallow and speech Taste	Hoarseness Difficulty in swallowing Difficulty with speech
XI	Spinal accessory	Movement of shoulder & head Ability to swallow Speech	Drooping of shoulder Loss of full ROM in head
XII	Hypoglossal	Tongue movement	Deviation of tongue Thick speech Paralysis of one side of tongue

A memory jogger for learning the cranial nerves is:

On Old Olympus Towering Tops A Finn And German Viewed Some Hops

Each letter corresponds to the first letter of the nerves in order from I-XII.

Spinal nerves

- 31 pairs of nerves branch off the spinal cord providing a pathway for feedback to and from the brain
  - 8 pairs of cervical nerves (C1-C8)
  - 12 pairs of thoracic nerves (T1-T12)
  - 5 pairs of lumbar nerves (L1-L5)
  - 5 pairs of sacral nerves (S1-S5)
  - 1 pair of coccygeal nerves
- They alert the brain of sensory changes such as hot/cold temperatures, pressure from touch, and pain
- Figure 3B shows how the spinal nerves innervate the body, the numbers on the regions correspond to the spinal nerve
- Sensory information is transmitted in chemical codes from peripheral nerves to spinal cord receptors and then to the brain for decoding and interpretation
- The ability to detect pain, cold, heat, and pressure depend on specific sensory neurons used for that specific task
- Referred pain occurs when the areas of injury share the same innervation pathway. An example of referred pain is the shoulder and arm pain that may be felt during a heart attack
- Phantom pain (pain felt in an amputated limb) may be due to the stimulation of the remaining nerve pathways in the stump

AUTONOMIC NERVOUS SYSTEM (ANS)

- Controls involuntary bodily functions such as the regulation of smooth muscle, cardiac muscle (heart) and gland function
- Divided into the sympathetic and parasympathetic systems
  - Sympathetic nervous system
    Enables the body to withstand stress, increases the heart rate and blood pressure to prepare for a "flight or fight" response
    Blood is shifted away from organs that are non-vital (skin, bladder, and stomach) to organs that survival may depend on such as skeletal muscle or the brain
  - Parasympathetic nervous system
    A restorative system that can increase glandular activity (such as salivation) to facilitate an organ function (such as digestion)

Nerves of the Body

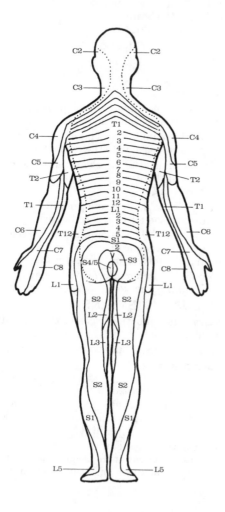

Figure 3B

THE SENSORY ORGANS

- **The ear**
- Vehicle for receiving auditory stimulation
- Consists of three principal parts: the outer ear, middle ear, and the inner ear (Figure 3C)
  - Outer ear
    - Has two parts: the pinna and the ear canal
    - Responsible for the following functions: protection of the ear drum, maintenance of a constant temperature, and the collection of sound waves from the environment
  - Middle Ear
    - Contains the ear drum and three bones: the malleus (hammer), incus (anvil) and the stapes stirrup)
    - Functions include: transmission and amplification of sound waves, protection of the inner ear from loud sounds, and maintenance of equal pressure within the inner ear
  - Inner ear
    - Has two major parts: the cochlea and the auditory nerve
    - Primary function is the translation of vibration from sound waves into nerve impulses and the subsequent transmission to the brain
- **The eye**
- Complex vehicle for receiving visual stimulation (Figure 3D)
- Contains seven major components
  - Sclera (white outer coating of the eye)
    - Gives the eye it's shape and protects the inner eye contents
  - Cornea (transparent covering for the iris)
    - Is bent to receive light rays
    - Is visible to the naked eye from the side
  - Choroid (lines the sclera's inner surface)
    - Absorbs light rays
  - Iris (located between the cornea and the pupil)
    - Colored portion of eye, brown or dark iris have more pigment while blue iris have no pigment
    - Regulates the amount of light entering the eye
    - Contracts with dim light allowing the pupil to receive more light

The Ear

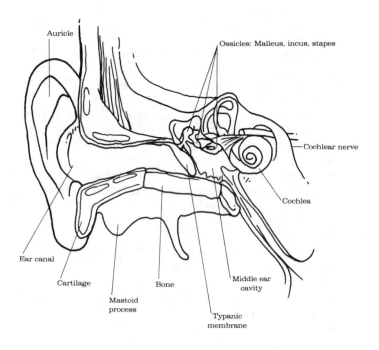

Figure 3C

- Pupil (black portion of the eye)
  - Light enters the eyeball via the pupil
- Lens (transparent disk behind the pupil)
  - Has the ability to change shape
- Retina (covers the choroid)
  - Primary function is image formation

The Eye

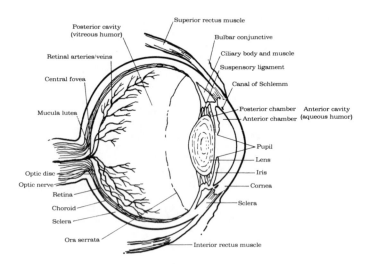

Figure 3D

Section II — ASSESSMENT

HEALTH HISTORY

Chief complaint

- Common chief complaints for this system include:
  - Mental confusion
  - Impaired memory or loss of mental abilities
  - Dizziness
  - Tinnitus (ringing sensation in ears)
  - Numbness or tingling in extremities
  - Unsteady gait, tremors and/or weakness
  - Hypotonia (loss of muscle tone)
  - Hypertonia (spasticity of muscles)
  - Double vision, impaired visual acuity
  - Pupil constriction or dilation
  - Difficulty in swallowing, impaired speech
  - Seizures

Family and personal history

- Good history is vital, many disorders have no abnormal physical or laboratory findings (seizures, headaches), history may be the foundation for the diagnosis
- Assess patients overall appearance, mood, and emotional state while taking the history, be alert for expressions of depression or suicidal thoughts
- Some neurological disorders involve changes in consciousness, perception, memory, language or loss of mental abilities, complete history may need to be obtained from both patient and significant others
- Obtain specific diagnoses and age at diagnosis when known
- Determine the order of appearance of symptoms and progression of patients complaint
- Many neurologic conditions are familial or inherited so family history is important to diagnosis
- Assess for presence and past treatment of the following:
  - Psychiatric illness
  - Multiple sclerosis
  - Alzheimers
  - Headache
  - Migraines (often confused with a severe headache)
  - Seizures

Head and/or spinal cord injury (cause and any disabilities)
Cancer (metastases can lead to neurological S&S)
- If above condition exists assess for required life style changes and current treatment of condition to include medications

Headache

- Common complaint with varitety of etiologies
- Headaches may be caused by organic disease such as brain tumor, brain abscess, meningitis, hemorrhage, vascular changes, alcoholism, poisonings, or hypertension
- While most patients who present with headache do not have a brain tumor it is the initial symptom in one third to one half of patients with brain tumors
- Severe headaches in a previously well patient, headaches that disturb sleep, exertional headaches, headaches with drowsiness, visual problems, limb problems, seizures or altered mentation may indicate subarachnoid hemorrhage, meningitis or brain tumor
- Chronic headaches may be due to migraine, tension or depression
- Tension headache symptoms include poor concentration, daily headaches that are generalized and most intense in neck or back of head, they are exacerbated by emotional stress, fatigue, noise or glare
- Cluster headaches usually affect middle-aged men, symptoms include unilateral periorbital pain, often nasal congestion, rhinorrhea, lacrimation, eye redness, occurs daily
- Migraines have similar periodic attacks over an extended length of time, may be unilateral or general and often originates in or about the eye and then spreads. Migraines are often accompanied by nausea, vomiting, photophobia and blurred vision
- Headaches may be caused by trauma from head injury, usually appearing within a day of injury, worsening over weeks ahead, usually a dull ache with throbbing often with nausea and vomiting
- Headaches may be psychogenic and caused from anxiety, hysteria or muscle tension headaches
- Important to obtain information on the location, severity, frequency and duration of headaches

Neurological system testing

- Assess for tests completed and patient's knowledge and understanding of any test procedures or results

NEUROLOGIC ASSESSMENT

Chief Complaint

Patient's statement_____ Onset_____

Frequency_____ Duration_____ Other areas affected_____

Have you had this before?_____ Date_____

What treatment was given?_____

What do you think caused this?_____

What lifestyle changes have you had to make?_____

Personal and Family History

	Patient	Family member	Patient
Psychiatric Illness	_____	_____	Seizures_____onset_____
			Type_____
Migraines	_____	_____	Frequency_____
Multiple Sclerosis	_____	_____	Head injury_____date_____
			Disability_____
Alzheimers	_____	_____	Spinal cord injury_____
			Date_____disability_____

Do you have numbness or tingling sensations (location)_____

Difficulty walking, talking, swallowing or chewing_____

Muscle weakness/spasm_____ Tremors_____ Visual problems_____

Headache (location, severity, frequency, duration)_____

Dizziness_____ Me mory or concentration loss _____ Insomnia_____

Describe your mood_____

Neurological system testing

EEG_____ Scan of brain (types)_____ Spinal tap_____

Cerebral angiogram_____ Electromyography_____ Myelogram_____

Hearing/vision testing_____ Skull x-ray_____ Blood tests_____

Current treatments/medications

Who is your physician?_____Phone_____

Name_____Dose_____Frequency_____Route_____

Name_____Dose_____Frequency_____Route_____

Name_____Dose_____Frequency_____Route_____

Is there anything else you want me to know?_____

PHYSICAL ASSESSMENT
* Neurological system is done in the following order:
    1. Inspection
    2. Palpation
* Assessment begins during the history intake
    * Observe the patient carefully for tremors and motor movements
    * Assess the ability to understand questions, recall medical history information and to reply appropriately

INSPECTION
General appearance/affect
* Assess posture, behavior, coordination and grooming as well as the ability to interact with the examiner
* Affect refers to the emotional state, is the patient elated, happy, quiet, confident, thoughtful, depressed, angry, or hostile?

Level of consciousness
* There are several levels of consciousness or responsiveness.
    * Fully conscious (Normal state)
      Alert and awake
      Responds quickly and appropriately to verbal questions
      Orientated to time, place, person and situation (X4)
    * Confused
      Provides an inappropriate response to questions
      Decreased memory and attention span
      May follow simple commands (raise your arm)
    * Lethargic
      Very drowsy affect with longer sleep periods noted
      Responds slowly and appropriately after a delay
      Difficult to awake, may return to sleep immediately
    * Delirious
      Anxious with marked confusion, perceptions are distorted, sleep wake patterns are altered
      Attention span is decreased
      Reactions to stimulus are inappropriate
    * Stuporous
      Early coma, unconscious
      Can arouse for short periods with intense, vigourous, direct external stimulation

Able to follow some simple commands, responses slow
Pupillary reflexes are sluggish
- Light coma
Moans in response to painful stimuli
Unarousable unresponsiveness even with strong stimuli
Flexion motor response or mass movement
- Deep coma
Decerebrate posturing to painful stimuli
- Deeper comatose state
Muscles are flaccid, no spontaneous respirations
No pupillary reaction to light
Some deep tendon reflexes may be present
- Brain death (Check agency guidelines)
Absence of brain waves on two EEG's (24 hours)
No cerebral function detected, failure of cerebral perfusion
Expert rules out hypothermia or drug toxicity

Speech quality

- Receptive speech is the ability to comprehend what is said follow commands)
- Expressive speech is the ability to communicate (speak, gesture, sign)

Orientation/memory/judgment

- Orientation is the awareness of what is going on, does the patient know his/her name, today's date, where they are and why (situation)? If so they are orientated X 4
- Memory questions can include immediate memory (repeating a sequence of numbers), recent memory (what was eaten for breakfast) or remote memory (mother's maiden name)
- Judgment questions are indicators of higher brain function, a sample question might be what do you if you are tired?

Motor function

- Assess posture (erect or bent over)
- Assess gait (normal, halting, ataxic, or shuffling)
- Romberg test is completed by having patient stand with feet together with eyes open and then closed. Stay near to protect patient if fall occurs. Only minimal body swaying should be present. Record how long the patient can stand on one foot in seconds.

Cranial nerve testing

- CN I, can patient with eyes closed identify coffee, alcohol or soap?
- CN III, test cardinal fields of vision by having the patient track a pen that makes an imaginary H in the air, assess for bilateral eye movement, note any nystagmus or paralysis
- PERL stands for pupils equal and reactive to light
- CN VII, have patient smile, frown, and puff out his/her cheeks
- CN VIII, tested during interview, can the patient hear you speak? Whisper while covering one ear (patients) at a time, record response
- CN IX, have patient taste and identify sugar and salt
- CN IX and X, observe the uvula while patient says "ah" is it symmetrical?
- CN XII, observe tongue in mouth for fasciculations (fine tremors) and usual resting point at midline (record deviations)

PALPATION

Cranial nerve testing

- CN V, patient clenches his teeth while you place your fingertips on his temples and then at the base of the jaw on the masseter muscle, feel for an asymmetry
- CN XI, patient raises shoulders while you push them down, is movement and strength equal? Test head movement by holding your hand to one side of the cheek while patient pushes with his head against it, assess movement and strength of sternomastoid on opposite side

Deep tendon reflexes

- Record response on figure provided (see next page)using numeric guide.

    4+   Hyperactive very brisk
    3+   Above average response but not abnormal
    2+   Average
    1+   Diminished to low normal
    0   No response

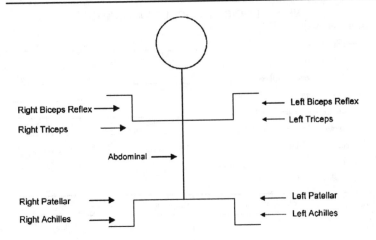

NEUROLOGIC PHYSICAL EXAMINATION

INSPECTION:

General appearance_____ Affect_____

Level of Consciousness_____ Speech quality_____

Orientation (name/date/place/situation)_____

Memory (address/president/state)_____ Judgment_____

Motor function: (posture/gait/romberg)_____

CN I:(olfactory) Identify: alcohol_____ soap_____

CN II: read print from 12 inches: rt eye_____ / lt eye_____

CN III: PERL_____

CN IV: Fields of gaze (below)

Rt.	Right eye	Lt	Rt.	Left eye	Lt.
Up					Up
(CN. III)		(CN III)	(CN III)		(CN III)
(CN VI)	(CN III)	(CN III)	(CN III)	(CN III)	(CN VI)
(CN III)		(CN IV)	(CN IV)		(CN. III)
Down					Down

CN VII: facial _____ CN VIII: hearing _____ CN IX: taste_____

CN IX, X: swallow_____ symmetry palate/uvula_____ Gag reflex_____

CN XII: tongue position_____ fasiculations_____

PALPATION

CN V:(trigeminal) temporal_____ masseter_____ equal sensation_____

CN XI:(spinal accessory) raise shoulders_____ head movement_____

Assessment Notes   Deep Tendon Reflexes

_____   Rt ____   ____ Lt

_____   ____   ____

_____   ____

_____   ____   ____

_____   ____   ____

Section III — LABORATORY & DIAGNOSTIC TESTS

In the following section traditional laboratory values and SI units are given, it is important to recognize that "normal" values vary from laboratory to laboratory. Check the normal values at the agency or institution where a test is performed. Most labs print their normal values on the laboratory reporting slip or page.

Table of Common Laboratory Tests

Test Name	Indications	Comments
Acetylcholine receptor Blood test **Normal:** Negative	Myasthenia gravis	**Regarding collection:** Collect 5-10ml in red top tube List all medications on lab slip **Results:** Positive in myasthenia gravis Negative result does not exclude myasthenia gravis
Cerebrospinal fluid analysis Fluid analysis **Normal:** Color: clear Blood: none Cells: No RBCs WBC 0-5 C&S: No organisms Protein: 15-45 mg/dl Chloride: 700-750 mg/dl Glucose: 50-75 mg/dl Lactic acid: 10-25 mg/dl	Brain tumor Cerebral hemorrhage Encephalitis Meningitis Myelitis NeurosyphilisRDegenerative brain diseases Autoimmune disorder Coma Cerebral abscess Multiple sclerosis Subarachnoid bleed Reye's syndrome Encephalopathy Spinal cord tumor	**Regarding collection:** Collected by primary care provider See lumbar puncture for details **Results:** See also lumbar puncture later in this chapter for complete listing of values and results

Table of Common Diagnostic Tests

Test Name	Indications	Comments
Audiometric testing Hearing testing **Normal:** Hearing adequate for speech	Suspected or confirmed hearing loss	**Pre-procedure:** Assess ability of patient to follow directions Earphones will be placed on head & deliver a series of tones at varying intensities; results are plotted on audiogram **Post-procedure:** No restrictions Hearing loss will be recorded in decibels (dB)
Brain Scan Nuclear Scan **Normal:** Normal brain, no areas of increased radionuclide uptake	Brain tumor Brain abscess Cerebral infarction Subdural hematoma Cerebral hemorrhage AV malformation Aneurysm HydrocephalusM	**Pre-procedure:** Explain procedure to patient Assess for allergy to iodine Procedure takes about 35-45 min & and repeated in 30-120 mins **Post-procedure:** Radioactive material is excreted within 6-24 hrs; no precautions are needed Encourage fluids
Cerebral angiogram AKA Cerebral arteriography X-ray with contrast dye **Normal:** Normal cerebral vascular structure & blood flow	Aneurysm Occlusion AV malformation Brain tumor Brain abscess Hematoma Cerebral fistula Cerebral thrombosis	**Pre-procedure:** Signed consent form is required Explain procedure to patient NPO for 8-12 hrs before testing Record baseline vital signs Assess for allergy to iodine Remove dentures, metallic jewelry Pre-medication will be ordered Mark peripheral pulse locations Perform baseline neurological exam Check orders for IV fluids **Post-procedure:** Assess site for bleeding or edema Assess pulses in extremities Assess vital signs frequently Bedrest for 12-24 hrs post-op Repeat neurlogical exam & compare Encourage fluids
Computed tomographic x-ray (CT or CAT scan) **Normal:** Normal brain structure	Brain tumor Cerebral infarction Congenital anomaly Cortical atrophy Cerebral aneurysm Intracranial hemorrhage Hematoma AV malformation Multiple sclerosis Hydrocephalus Trauma	**Pre-procedure:** Signed consent form may be required Assess orders for with or without dye, assess for iodine allergy Assess pt for ability to lie still during procedure Remove all metal jewelry or hairpins **Post-procedure:** Encourage fluids Assess for allergic reaction to dye if contrast CT was done No activity restrictions

Test Name	Indications	Comments
Digital subtraction angiography (DSA) X-ray with contrast dye **Normal:** Normal arterial blood flow & vasculature	Arterial stenosis Aneurysm Brain tumor Arterial occlusion Cerebrovascular accident (stroke) Emboli	**Pre-procedure:** Signed consent form is required Explain procedure to patient Assess pt's ability to hold their breath during procedure Assess for allergy to iodine NPO for 2 hrs Assess for anticoagulant use Procedure takes about 1 hr **Post-procedure:** Assess site for bleeding, redness Encourage fluids Assess for allergic reaction to dye Assess vital signs as ordered
Electroencephalography (EEG) **Normal:** Tracing showing normal frequency, amplitude & chracter of brain wave patterns	Seizure disorders Brain tumors Brain abscesses Head trauma Brain death Encephalitis Intracranial hemorrhage Cerebral infarction Alzheimer's disease	**Pre-procedure:** Assess orders for type of EEG: awake, drowsy, asleep, with stimuli or combination types Hair should be clean and free of oils, hairsprays or lotions For sleep EEG, assess policy for time patient may sleep night before No coffee, tea, cola, cocoa before No sedatives or hypnotics before Assess pt's ability to lie still during testing Procedure takes 45-120 mins **Post-procedure:** Remove collodion from hair; acetone or witch hazel may aid in removal Pt may shampoo hair as desired Keep siderails up as needed
Electromyography (EMG) **Normal:** No neuromuscular abnormalities found	Muscular dystrophy Myopathies Multiple sclerosis Sarcoidosis Polymyositis Traumatic injury Myasthenia gravis Guillain-Barre	**Pre-procedure:** Check policy for signed consent Coffee, tea, cocoa, colas and tobacco may be restricted before testing (2-3 hrs) Explain that a needle will be inserted into specific muscle and its response will be recorded Procedure takes about 20 mins **Post-procedure:** Assess for hematoma No activity restrictions
Electroneurography (ENG) **Normal:** No injury/disease to peripheral nerves	Nerve injury Nerve disease Muscular dystrophy Myasthenia gravis Tumor Guillain-Barre Carpal tunnel Diabetic neuropathy	**Pre-procedure:** Usually done with electromyography Check policy for signed consent Explain that electrodes will be placed on skin and that a mild shock is given and nerve response time will be recorded Procedure takes about 15 minutes **Post-procedure:** No activity restrictions

Test Name	Indications	Comments
Evoked potential studies: Brainstem auditory evoked response (BAER) Visual-evoked response (VER) Somatosensory-evoked responses (SERs) **Normal:** Normal neural conductions	Congenital brain anomaly Multiple sclerosis Parkinson's Tumors Auditory or visual disorders Spinal cord injury or dysfunction Cerebrovascular accident	**Pre-procedure:** Assess ability to lie still Patient should shampoo hair before Electrodes are placed on scalp Earphones are worn for BAER Procedure takes about 30 mins **Post-procedure:** No activity restrictions
Magnetic resonance imaging (MRI) Magnetic study **Normal:** Normal brain & spinal cord structure	Cerebral tumor Cerebral lesion Stroke (CVA) Vertebral disk degeneration Arteriovenous malformation Cerebral hemorrhage Subdural hematoma Multiple sclerosis Dementia Hydrocephaly	**Pre-procedure:** Explain procedure to patient Lie on a platform that will move head/spine into magnetic field so image can be made Assess for & remove all metallic items (prosthetics, hair pins, dental bridges, jewelry, credit cards, watches); if pt has plates or metal implants, MRI is contraindicated Assess pt's ability to lie still Procedure takes 30-90 mins and steady rhythmic pounding will be heard, earplugs may be worn **Post-procedure:** No activity restrictions
Myelogram X-ray with contrast dye **Normal:** Normal spinal canal	Spinal cord tumor Herniated disks Neurofibromas Meningiomas Lumbar stenosis Astrocytomas	**Pre-procedure:** Signed consent form is required Explain procedure to patient: a lumbar puncture will be done & dye injected into spine Assess for allergy to iodine Check agency policy for fluid/food restrictions Assess patient ability to lie still Procedure takes about 45 minutes **Post-procedure:** Bedrest with position as ordered by physician Monitor vital signs frequently Increase fluid intake

Test Name	Indications	Comments
Oculoplethys-mography (OPG) Manometric **Normal:** Equal blood flow in both carotid arteries	Carotid atherosclerotic stenosis	**Pre-procedure:** Explain procedure to patient: EKG electrodes are applied, eye drops are instilled & small suction cups (like contacts) are applied to eyes; tracings are then recorded Procedure takes about 20-30 mins **Post-procedure:** Anesthesia wears off in 30 minutes Patient should not rub eyes or insert contact lenses for 2 hours Sunglasses may be required
Positron-emission tomography (PET) Nuclear scan, X-ray **Normal:** Normal tissue meta-bolism	Stroke (CVA) Epilepsy Parkinson's Dementia Alzheimer's Schizophren i a Brain tumor Huntington's	**Pre-procedure:** Signed consent form may be required Start 1 or 2 IV lines as ordered No alcohol, caffeine or tobacco for 24 hrs before testing No sedatives or tranquilizers may be taken Procedure takes 60-90 mins **Post-procedure:** Monitor for postural hypotension Assist with position changes Encourage fluids
Skull X-ray X-ray **Normal:** Normal skull struc-ture	Trauma to head Tumor Sinusitis Hematoma Congenital cranial anomalies	**Pre-procedure:** Remove all objects above neck (dental bridges, jewelry, hairpins, glasses) Procedure takes 10-15 mins with another 10-15 mins to be sure films are readable Assess for pregnancy in females **Post-procedure:** No activity restrictions
Spinal X-ray X-ray **Normal:** Normal spine struc-ture	Trauma to back/neck Degenerative arthritis of spine Spondylosis Tumor	**Pre-procedure:** Remove all metal objects in area Procedure takes about 10-15 mins with addl. 10-15 mins to be sure films are readable Assess for pregnancy in females **Post-procedure:** No ativity restrictions

Test Name	Indications	Comments
Ventriculography X-ray **Normal:** No ventricular abnormalities	Brain tumors Cerebral anomalies No usually done if CT or MRI are available	**Pre-procedure:** Signed informed consent is required Explain procedure to patient Surgical procedure, burr holes will be made in skull and air/contrast material will be injected directly into ventricles of brain Contraindicated in increased ICP Procedure takes about 30 mins Performed by a neurosurgeon **Post-procedure:** Monitor vital signs frequently Head of bed 10-15 degrees for 1 day Assess dressing and reinforce PRN Encourage fluids once alert Administer analgesics as ordered Headache is a common reaction

LUMBAR PUNCTURE & CSF EXAMINATION

Definition:
- A lumbar puncture consists of a needle placed into the subarachnoid space by a primary care provider
- Also known as spinal puncture

Purpose:
- A lumbar puncture may be done for a variety of reasons:
    - To measure pressure in the subarachnoid space
    - Obtain fluid for cerebrospinal fluid analysis
    - Medication administration directly into spinal space
    - To inject diagnostic agents into the spinal space

Contraindications:
- Lumbar puncture should not be performed on:
    - Patients with increased intracranial pressure
    - Patients with severe degenerative vertebral joint disease
    - Patients with infection near the puncture site

Procedure:
Before
- Obtain signed informed consent per agency protocol
- Have patient void prior to procedure
- Explain that it will be necessary to lie or sit still during the puncture and any related procedures
- Assess patients ability to lie or sit still and obtain other personal to assist as needed

- Obtain lumbar puncture tray, additional spinal needles

During
- Procedure usually takes about 20 minutes
- Assess primary care providers preference for patients positon and assist patient into fetal position with back bowed or a sitting position with back arched like a "C"
- Explain what is happening to help patient relax and remain still, assist the patient in holding still
- Maintain sterile precautions during lumbar puncture
- Usually if CSF is examined, three sterile tubes of fluid will be collected, label them with name, hospital number, time, date, and number them for collection order
- Each tube contains about 3ml of CSF, transport to lab ASAP

After
- Apply bandaid to site and apply pressure with fingertips
- Position patient in prone with pillow under abdomen, head of bed flat to help prevent postpuncture spinal headache
- Encourage fluids, offer straw so patient can drink with head flat
- Assess the patient for numbness, tingling, ability to move all extremities, pain at site, drainage of blood or fluid from site and patients ability to void

Components of CSF examination
Results of CSF examination

Expected	Other findings	Comments
Crystal clear colorless CSF	Red or pink CSF	Traumatic lumbar puncture Subarachnoid hemorrhage Cerebral hemorrhage
	Xanthochromia CSF (yellow colored)	Old blood in CSF (hours to days old) previous subarachnoid hemorhage previous cerebral hemorrhage Discoloration may remain for 3 wks
	Cloudy CSF	Infection with increased WBCs meningitis neurosyphillis
CSF pressure (mmH$_2$O)	Pressure decrease	Dehydration Hypovolemia
Adult 75-175 Chile 50-100	Pressure increase above 200	Increased intracranial pressure meningitis or encephalitis subarachnoid hemorrhage brain tumor or abscess

Expected	Other findings	Comments
Cell count (WBCs) 3 (cu mm mm) Adult 0-5 Child 0-5 Newborn 0-15 Premature infant 0-20	Increased count	Viral infection poliomyelitis Aseptic meningitis Syphilis of the central nervous system Multiple Sclerosis Brain tumor Brain abscess Subarahnoid hemorrhage
Protein (mg/dl) Adult 15-45 Child 14-45 Infants: Premature <400 Newborn 30-200 1-6 mos 30-100	Increased protein	Meningitis Guillain-Barre syndrome Subarachnoid hemorrhage Brain tumor or abscess Syphilis of the central nervous system Trauma or traumatic lumbar puncture with blood in CSF
Chloride (MEq/L) Adult 118-132 700-750 mg/dl	Decreased level	Tuberculosis meningitis Bacterial meningitis IV saline or electrolyte infusions may cause an inaccurate result
Glucose (mg/dl) Adult 40-80 Child 35-75 Newborn 20-40	Decreased glucose	Purulent meningitis Fungi, protozoa, pyogenic bacteria Subarachnoid hemorrhage Lymphoma or leukemia
	Increased glucose	Trauma Diabetes hyperglycemia Always compared to blood glucose level Usually 2/3 of blood glucose level
Lactic acid content 10-25 mg/dl	Increased content	Hypoxic or ischemic cerebral injury Bacterial or fungal meningitis Brain tumor
CSF culture No organism found in CSF	Positive culture	Causative organism is identified Meningitis-bacterial pneumococcal meningococcal H. influenzae streptococca

Section IV — PROCEDURES

COMA IDENTIFICATION / MANAGEMENT

Definition
- A prolonged impairment of consciousness where the patient is unarousable and unresponsive in an abnormally deep sleep
- A symptom, not a disease in itself

Prevalence
- Up to 3% of hospital admissions to emergency department involve disorders of consciousness

Etiology
- May be due to illness or injury
- Traumatic head injury from accident or assult
- Circulatory disorders within the brain due to:
  - Cerebral hypertension
  - Cerebrovascular accidents (CVA)
  - Increased intracranial pressure
  - Insufficient blood flow to brain tissues
  - Intracerebral or subarachnoid hemorrhage
  - Thrombus formation
  - Uncontrolled seizures
- Infections
  - Acute botulism
  - Brain abscesses
  - Encephalitis or meningitis
- Drug overdoses (alcohol, barbiturates, insulin)
- Metabolic Causes
  - Acid-based imbalances
  - Diabetic coma (due to a lack of insulin)
  - Hepatic or kidney disease
  - Hypothermia

Symptoms
- Neurological Assessment's are generally repeated every 1-4 hrs. to assess for changes in neurological status
- Glascow coma scale used to assess the level of consciousness, the higher the score the higher the level of consciousness

- Eyes open
  - Spontaneously 4
  - To speech 3
  - To pain 2
  - No response 1
- Verbal response
  - Oriented to person, place and time 5
  - Disoriented/responds to questions 4
  - Random words, inappropriate response 3
  - Incomprehensible, groaning, moaning 2
  - No response 1
- Motor response
  - Obeys command correctly 6
  - Localizes pain 5
  - Withdrawal of limb from painful stimuli 4
  - Decorticate posture, flexion to pain 3
  - Decerebrate posturing, rigidity 2
  - No response 1
- Posturing (see figure)
  - **Decorticate**   Adduction of arm
                        Flexion of elbow
                        Flexion of wrist

  - **Decerebrate**   Adduction of arm
                        Internal rotation & extension of arm

Decorticate posturing

Decrebrate posturing

- Pupillary response
  - Normally contract briskly in strong light and dilate in dim light
  - Assess size, may range from 2-6mm
  - Assess pupil reaction time, brisk, slow or fixed
  - Pupils should react equally to light
  - Direct pupil reaction is the constriction of the pupil in the same eye that the light shines in
  - Consensual pupil reaction is the constriction of the pupil in the opposite eye that the light shines in

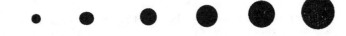

- Muscle strength should be equal bilateraly. Record as absent, weak, moderate or strong
  - Test upper extremities by having the patient grasp and squeeze one of your fingers
  - Test lower extremities by having the patient push with his/her leg while the foot rests against your hand

Care for the comatose patient

- Comatose patient is totally dependent upon others for care
- Needs should be prioritized from basic life needs to comfort measures
- Establish and maintain patent airway
  - Place oropharyngeal airway or assist with endotracheal intubation (ET) as needed
  - Position patient on side to prevent aspiration of secretions
  - Suction frequently to remove secretions which may block the airway
  - Restrain arms if needed to prevent accidental dislodgment of oropharyngeal or ET airway device
- Assess respirations
  - Establish baseline respiratory rate and rhythm
  - If no spontaneous breathing, provide oxygenation via ambu bag or rescue breathing to maintain oxygenation until ventilator can be obtained
  - Provide oxygen as needed and ordered

- If on mechanical ventilation, assess ordered and actual settings and compare with actual settings
- Assess level of ET tube and check that tubing is secured
- Check all alarms for function, be sure alarms are on
- Suction as needed to maintain patency of airway
- Monitor respiratory rate and rhythm on regular basis
- Assess pattern of respirations
  - Cheyne-Stokes   Rapid deep breathing alternating with slow shallow breathing
  - Hyperventilation   Rapid deep breathing
  - Atactic breathing   Irregular pattern with deep/shallow breaths
- Monitor pulse oxyimeter and arterial blood gas values to assess oxygenation status
- Assess and maintain circulation
  - Monitor pulse, blood pressure and temperature regularly
  - Connect patient to cardiac monitor and assess for heart arrhythmias
  - Monitor laboratory values and report any abnormal values
  - Administer medications as ordered to promote cardiac output/circulation
  - Maintain intravenous catheter to provide route for fluids and medications as ordered
  - Establish and maintain urinary catheter to assess renal blood flow and monitor output
  - Monitor all intake and output for any imbalances
- Provide for nourishment
  - Maintain nasogastric, gastrostomy tube, or total parental nutrition as ordered
  - Assess weight at least every other day and record
  - Consult with physician and dietian if weight loss is uncontrolled
- Provide for elimination needs
  - Assess frequency and character of stools
- Provide for activities of daily living
  - Reposition patient every two hours to prevent skin breakdown
  - Provide range of motion exercises regularly to increase blood circulation and prevent contractures of joints

- Provide meticulous skin care to prevent skin breakdown
- Provide meticulous oral care to prevent skin breakdown and reduce halitosis
- Provide for sensory stimulation
  - Talk to patient frequently, even if totally unresponsive to provide auditory stimulation
  - Touch the patient often during care to provide tactile stimulation
  - Play music or taped recording of family and friends to provide familiar auditory stimulation
  - Place brightly colored posters in room, hang mobiles from ceiling to provide visual stimulation

Section V — CONDITIONS

Increased Intracrainal Pressure (ICP)

Definition

- Not a disease in itself
- Intracrainal pressure (ICP) is the pressure the cerebrospinal fluid exerts within the ventricles of the brain
- Normal ICP in the ventricles is between 0-15 mm Hg
- When the ICP rises above 15 mm Hg it is increased
- Increased ICP is a life threatening condition

Etiology

- Results from a change within the contents of the skull
- The adult skull cannot expand, it is a rigid structure
- Normally brain tissue makes up about 80% of the skulls contents, cerebrospinal fluid makes up about 10%, the other 10% is blood volume
- If any of the three components within the skull increases the ICP increases
- Causes of increased ICP include:
  - Increased size of brain tissue
    - Brain tumor growth
    - Brain trauma, when injured the brain swells (cerebral edema)
    - Cerebrovascular accident (CVA), may lead to brain tissue hypoxia and cerebral edema secondary to insufficient blood flow to the brain tissue such as occurs with embolism or thrombosis of the cerebral arteries
  - Increase in cerebrospinal fluid
    - Obstruction in the flow of cerebral spinal fluid (CSF) causing hydrocephaly
    - Failure of the body to reabsorb CSF, allowing for a collection of this within the ventricles (hydrocephaly)
  - Increase in cerebral blood volume
    - Brain trauma, trauma to head may rupture or injure cerebral vessels leading to an accumulation of blood within the skull which increases ICP

- Cerebrovascular accident (CVA) from cerebral hemorrhage, cerebral arteriovenous malformation or aneurysm

Pathophysiology of Increased ICP

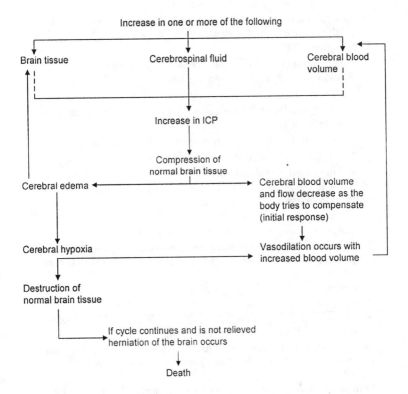

Symptoms of ICP

- The severity of symptoms depends on how high the ICP is and which area of the brain is being compressed, not all symptoms may be present in every patient
- Decreased level of consciousness (LOC), one of the earliest signs results from compression of brain tissue
  - Early restlessness or lethargy may be present
  - Disorientation often occurs, disorientation is first to time, then to place and finally to person
  - Untreated increased ICP will result in coma with decorticate or decerebrate posturing and then death
- Vital signs (VS):
  - Early in increased ICP the VS should be normal
  - Slowing respiratory rate occurs early
  - Later as the brainstem is compressed then
    - Bradycardia and a widening pulse pressure may occur (Cushing's response)
    - Eventually the blood pressure will decrease sharply
    - Cheyne-Stokes or ataxic breathing may occur
    - Increased rectal temperature
- Visual disturbances due to pressure on the cranial nerves that control eye movement to include:
  - Diplopia (double vision)
  - Blurred vision, or loss of visual acuity
  - Fixed pupillary dilatation or very sluggish pupils if the brain has begun to herniate due to compression of the third cranial nerve
- Headache
  - Onset may be vague
  - Later as ICP rises headache will be more severe especially when coughing, straining or bending
- Vomiting, if present assess frequency and if projectile, may occur without nausea due to compression of the vomiting regulatory center
- Muscle weakness due to pressure on the cortical tracts of the brain, remember any weakness you see on one side of the body will reflect brain compression on the opposite side

- Seizures may occur due to abnormal electrical activity within the brain secondary to compression of tissues

Components of initial examination for increased ICP

- Untreated increased ICP will continue to damage the brain's tissues so early recognition and treatment are vital

Complete medical history:

- Due to patient's condition it may not be possible to obtain a complete health history from patient
- If possible obtain previous medical records
- When possible and patient's condition permits obtain health history from significant other
- Any trauma, present or recent illness should be explored if etiology of increased ICP is unknown
- All current medications and any allergies known

Physical examination to include:

- General appearance for obvious signs of trauma
- Neurological assessment to include level of consciousness, speech quality, orientation, memory, motor function, pupillary reactions, cranial nerve testing and deep tendon reflexes as appropriate
- Airway for patency and adequacy
- Blood pressure, respiratory rate and rhythm, pulse rate. Should be taken initially and then monitored continuously until recovery, compare with patient's baseline if known
- Assessment of urinary output in ml/hour
- Core body temperature (rectal or ear probe, not axcillary)
- Pulse oximeter readings for oxygen saturation level

Laboratory and diagnostic testing:

- The single best diagnostic indicator of increased ICP is direct measurement of Intracrainal pressure via intraventricular catheter, subdural bolt or epidural sensor, normal pressure is 0-15mm Hg
- Complete blood count
- Arterial blood gases
- Computed tomography (CT) or Magnetic resonance imaging (MRI) to diagnose or rule out cerebral lesions, cerebral infarction, arteriovenous malformations, cerebral hemorrhage, brain tumors and cerebral edema
- Electroencephalography (EEG) to detect any abnormality in frequency, amplitude and patterns of brain waves

Treatment of increased ICP

- The primary goal is to maintain ICP within normal limits, to achieve this ICP must be monitored
- Establishment and maintanice of an adequate airway, may include need for mechanical ventilation and supplemental oxygenation
- Intracranial pressure can be measured continuously via one of three basic monitoring systems, all require surgical intervention:
  - The ventricular catheter — A cannula is implanted via burr holes into the anterior horn of the lateral ventricle, this allows for the meaurement of ICP and the ability to drain off large amounts of CSF if needed
  - The subarachnoid bolt — A metal screw with a sensory tip is inserted through a drill hole into the subdural or subarachnoid space, the cerebrum is not penetrated, allows for measurement or ICP and sampling of CSF
  - The epidural sensor — Placement of a fiberoptic sensor, radio transmitter or tiny balloon with radioisotopes in the epidural space through a burr hole, it allows for measurement of ICP it does not allow for sampling or draining of CSF
- Placement of intraventricular shunt to drain excess CSF
- Establishment and maintaince of intravenous lines
- Urinary catheter to determine renal perfusion

Medications for increased ICP

- Corticosteroid agents such as Dexamethasone (Decadron) to reduce cerebral edema
- Anticonvulsant agents to prevent or treat seizure activity related to increased ICP
- Laxative agents to prevent an increase in ICP assoicated with straining to have a bowel movement
- Antiemetic agents to eliminate or reduce vomiting
- Anti-infective agents to prevent infection from invasive intercrainal pressure monitoring devices

Seizure Disorders

Definition

- Seizure disorder, convulsive disorder and epilepsy are all terms used to describe chronic, recurrent, unpredictable, transient attacks of seizure activity

- A seizure is a change in neurological function caused by an abnormal surge of electrical activity within the brain
- A seizure is a symptom, not a disease, like any other symptom (fever) it may result from a variety of health problems, unlike fever a seizure does not have a constant factor that can be recognized by all persons at all times
- A seizure is convulsive if it is accompanied by motor movement
- A seizure may consist of sensory, cognitive or emotional function changes with or without convulsions
- May affect the entire body with loss of consciousness and tonic clonic movements, or it may only appear as lip smacking, ringing in the ears or the purposeless movement of one extremity
- A classification system was devised to group seizures into categories because of the variety of seizure manifestations, not all seizure activity fits into one category some patients have mixed seizure disorders with symptoms from more than one
- The type of seizure may even change from one episode to another, or begin with one type and go into another

Prevalence
- Estimated to affect 0.5-2% of the population
- Estimated that up to 10% of individuals will have at least one seizure in their lifetime
- Onset may occur at any age although childhood is most common

Etiology
- 50% of seizures have no identifiable cause (idopathic), other causes include:
- Structural brain damage from:
  - Congenital abnormalities of the brain
  - Brain tissue death from anoxia or compression of brain tissue
  - Head injury (Accidents, gunshot wounds or other cerebral trauma)
  - Primary brain tumors (Benign or malignant growths)
  - Metastatic tumors from lung, breast or other tissue
- Degenerative Brain Disorders
  - Generally associated with aging, however may also be found in younger patients
  - Dementia is a progressive decline in intellectual function may be caused by Alzheimer's disease, Huntington's chorea, multiple sclerosis, or acquired immunodeficiency syndrome

- Central nervous system infections
  - Bacterial infections (meningitis) to include *Neisseria meningitidis, Hemophilus influenzae and Streptococcus pneumoniae*
  - Viral infections (encephalitis or aseptic meningitis) to include *poliovirus, coxsackie virus,* or *herpes zoster*
  - Fungal infections (subacute meningitis) to include *Cryptococcus, Candida,* or *Aspergillus*
  - Acquired immunodeficiency syndrome (AIDS) with opportunistic infections such as toxoplasma encephalitis, cryptococcal and tuberculous meningitides and multifocal leukoencephalopathy
- Metabolic Imbalances
  - May cause a single seizure which is usually corrected when the underlying problem is corrected or lead to onset of seizure disorder if damage to brain tissues occurs
  - Oxygen deprivation with cerebral hypoxia
  - Hypovolemia - Dehydration
  - Increased temperature, febrile seizure in child < age 6
  - Electrolyte, mineral, or acid-base imbalance's

Classification and symptoms of epileptic seizures

- The following classification is summarized from the International League Against Epilepsy (ILAE)
- *Partial or Focal seizures*
  - Begin in one area of the brain with symptoms unique to the specific lesion site
  - Causes include:
    - Birth injury or postnatal trauma
    - Brain tumor, abscess or infarction
    - Vascular malformation or structural abnormality
  - Classified as simple or complex
  - *Simple partial seizures* (No alteration in consciousness)
    - May have motor, sensory, autonomic or psychic symptoms without loss of consciousness
    - Symptoms may be confined to one area or progress to other areas

- May have sensory symptoms such as distorted vision, flashing lights, ringing in ears or unusual sensations in one or more body parts
- May have autonomic symptoms such as sweating or dilation of pupils
- *Complex partial seizures* (Consciousness is altered)
  - Episodic behavior changes of which the patient is unaware
  - Aura occurs
  - Cessation of conscious activity with other motor activity occurring (smacking lips, walking aimlessly)
  - May have cognitive symptomatology such as mental confusion, may resist help
  - May have affective symptomatology such as auditory or visual hallucinations or illusions
  - Psychosensory symptomtology such as intense emotions (anger, fear) or forced thinking may occur
  - Post-seizure amnesia from minutes to hours
- *Secondary generalization of partial seizures*
  - Simple or complex partial seizures can progress to generalized seizures with loss of consciousness and convulsions
  - Partial paralysis or another specific neurologic focal deficit may occur following the seizure
- *Primary generalized seizures*
  - *Tonic-clonic (grand mal)*
    - Begin with no aura or warning if primary
    - Epileptic cry may be present
    - Sudden loss of consciousness and postural control
    - Brief rigid muscular contraction (tonic phase) followed by recurrent muscular contractions of all four limbs (clonic phase) for 1-2 minutes
    - Tongue or lips may be bitten
    - Urinary or fecal incontinence may occur
    - Postical sleep or headache usually follows
  - *Tonic*
    - Sudden onset of rigid muscular contraction

- Deviation of head or eyes to one side
- Not followed by clonic phase
- Shorter in duration than tonic-clonic seizure
- *Clonic*
  - Rhythmic jerking of extremities
  - No tonic phase
- *Absence seizure (petit mal)*
  - Momentary sudden loss of consciousness without convusions and usually without loss of posture
  - Last seconds or minutes
  - No aura is present
  - Sudden return to full consciousness without confusion
  - Onset usually in childhood
- *Atypical absence*
  - Patient also has other forms of generalized seizures and some other form of neurologic dysfunction
- *Myoclonic seizures*
  - Sudden, brief onset of a single or repetitive muscle contraction of one body part or the entire body
  - If entire body is involved patient will fall
  - No loss of consciousness
- *Atonic seizures*
  - Sudden, brief loss of muscle tone and consciousness
  - No tonic muscular contractions are noted
  - No aura, patient just drops to the floor
- *Infantile spasms*
  - Brief contractions of neck, torso and both arms
  - Onset between birth-1 year in infants who usually have underlying neurologic disorder, may occur in apparently healthy infant
  - 90% will develop mental retardation
  - Disappears between 3-5 years of life and other forms of seizures often replace the spasms
- *Status Epilepticus*
  - Prolonged or repetitive attack of any seizure type without a recovery period

- Life-threatening if tonic-clonic seizures occur
- May go unrecognized in absence seizures for some time
- *Recurrence patterns*
  - Recurrent seizures occur sporadically or randomly
  - May have no triggering event or can occur cyclically as with the menstrual cycle (catamenial epilepsy) or in response to a specific stimuli such as light changes, music, reading, hypoventilation or tactile stimulation
  - Emotional stress, drowsiness, sleep deprivation, alcohol or drug withdrawal may be the precipitating factor
  - Seizures may occur only at night or only during the day
  - Seizure types include absences, myoclonic jerking, partial seizures, and occasional generalized convulsions

Components of initial examination for seizure disorder

- *Complete medical history to include:*
- Personal history of seizure activity from patient or significant other (patient may have no memory of activity or be unable to respond following seizure)
  - Onset of seizures to include age, any illness or trauma that preceded onset
  - Frequency of seizures to include frequency at onset, current frequency of seizures and date of last seizure
  - Type(s) of seizure(s) if known
  - Description of last seizure to include duration, loss or retention of consciousness, any motor movements or loss of postural tone, pupillary reaction, urinary or fecal incontinence, emotional or behavior changes
  - Ask if last seizure was typical of most of the seizures patient has, if not obtain description of typical seizure
  - Presence of auras or reoccurance factor that is known to precede seizure activity, some seizures are triggered by the following stimuli:

Loss of sleep	Menstrual period	Missed medication
Illness	High fever	Loud noise
Emotional stress	Flashing lights	Missed meal

  - Postictally (following the seizure), assess time before full consciousness is returned, muscular aches, weakness, paralysis or headaches following seizures
- Previous and current treatment of seizures to include medication history and lifestyle changes

- Patient's understanding of diagnosis and treatment
- Patient's willingness to make lifestyle changes
- Attention span and ability to recall information, this may be affected by recent seizure or by medication used to control seizures
- Family history of seizure disorder or neurological diseases
- Birth history for any congenital birth defects, anoxia during labor or delivery
- If onset of seizures in neonatal period assess for history of developmental delays or other neurological impairments
- Medical history is vital to the diagnosis as seizures are not in themselves a conditon, they are only a symptom, a complete medical history is vital to determining underlying cause and should include any known medical problems or history of trauma
- History of alcoholism, seizures may present secondary to old cerebral contusion (from fall), chronic subdural hematoma, undernutrition, liver disease or alcohol withdrawal
- *Physical examination to include:*.
- Adequacy of airway and ventilation if ongoing seizure
- Presence of ongoing seizure activity to include description of seizure, duration and post-seizure responsiveness
- Current level of consciousness and awareness
- General appearance and posture, assess for any paralysis or weakness of extremities following seizure
- PERLA, pupils equal and reactive to light and accomadation
- Complete physical examination to rule out systemic disease responsible for the seizure activity
- Motor responses for asymmetry, clumsiness, posturing and deep tendon reflex assessment
- *Laboratory and diagnostic testing:*
- Electroencephalography is the most useful diagnostic test for seizure disorders, although 20% of patients with epilepsy will have normal random EEG's
- Lumbar puncture with cerebrospinal fluid analysis if cerebral infection or subarachnoid hemorrhage is suspected
- Complete blood count, liver function tests, blood urea nitrogen, and urinalysis to rule out systemic diseases and to establish a baseline before antiepileptic drugs are begun
- Therapuetic drug levels if antiepileptic drugs are taken

- Computed tomography (CT) or magnetic resonance imaging (MRI) to detect or rule out brain lesion, structural anomaly, tumor or cerebral changes from trauma
- Cerebral angiography if vascular malformation is suspected
- Psychometric testing to include IQ, memory, language, attention, motor performance and personality tests may be helpful if abilities are changing or impaired

Treatment of seizure disorder

- Goals of treatment during a seizure are to:
  - Stablilize the patient and ensure adequate airway and ventilation
    - Stay calm
    - Move any objects away that may cause injury
    - Do not attempt to restrain the patient
    - Do not insert an airway if teeth are clenched
    - If teeth are not clenched place oral airway or soft washcloth between teeth
    - Turn head to side to prevent aspiration of saliva
    - Place soft pad under patients head
    - Loosen any tight clothing
    - Remain with the patient until seizure activity stops and consciousness if regained
    - Assess vital signs and perform neurological checks
  - Stop the current seizure activity and determine it's cause
  - Observe characteristics of seizure
    - Motor activity, pupillary changes, incontinence, behavior changes and respiratory changes
  - Goals of treatment for the patient with chronic epilepsy are:
  - Protect the patient from subsequent seizures while minimizing interference with cognitive function and intellectual development
  - Provide for patient safety (institute seizure precautions)
    - Padded side rails, up at all times to prevent accidental fall and injury if seizure occurs
    - Oral airway kept at bedside
    - Frequent checks on patients condition
  - Monitor for harmful systemic side effects from medications

- Primary treatment modality is medication, 60% of all patient's with epilepsy can be controlled with medications
- Surgical intervention if epilepsy remains uncontrolled

Medications for seizure disorder

- Anticonvulsants to control or reduce seizure activity
- Whenever possible the lowest dose of a single medication is used to limit harmful systemic side effects
- Monitor medication serum drug levels and report abnormal results
- Monitor related laboratory studies, report abnormal values
- Monitor for and report side effects from seizure medications
- Instruct patient in importance of compliance with medication regime, noncompliance is the primary cause of status epilepticus

Section VI — DIETS

• No diets specific for this system

Section VII — DRUGS

The table's supply only general information, a drug handbook or the physicians desk reference (PDR) should be consulted for details. Each classification includes detailed information about the example drug, this drug is representative of the other drugs in the classification and can be used as a model.

Every effort has been made to include the major classes of drugs used in the treatment of central nervous system diorders.

ANALGESICS — NARCOTIC AGONISTS

Action: Cause analgesia, thought to inhibit pain in the substantia gelatinosa of the spinal cord, brain stem, reticular formation, thalamus, and the limbic system. Narcotic action provides pain relief, sedation, euphoria, mental clouding, respiratory depression, miosis, decreased peristalsis and orthostaic hypotension. Generally schedule II drugs.

Indications: Moderate to severe pain of an acute nature.

Example: Morphine Sulfate (*Astramoroph PF, Duramorph, Roxanol*)

Route: PO, IM, SQ, IV, Epidural

Pharmacokinetics: Peak 60 min PO, 50-90 min SQ, 30-60 min IM, 20 min IV

Contraindications: Seizure disorder, respiratory depression, asthma, COPD, increased intracrainal pressure, acute colitis, Addison's disease, acute alcoholism, acute abdominal conditions, pancreatitis, hypothyrodism, head injury, increased intraocular pressure or loss of consciousness

Common adverse effects: Pruritus, constipation, nausea

Life threatening adverse effects: Respiratory depression

Other adverse effects: Rash, urticaria, edema, euphoria, insomnia, visual disturbances, dysphoria, convulsions, decreased cough reflex, drowsiness, dizziness, miosis, bradycardia, palpitations, syncope, facial flushing, orthostatic hypotension, anorexia, dry mouth, vomiting, urinary retention, dysuria, oliguria, sweating

Interventions:

Before administration assess respiratory rate, depth and rhythm,

RR <12/min indicates toxicity, withhold drug and report, monitor RR on regular basis

Assess respirations for 24 hours after intrathecal or epidural medication

Monitor patient for degree of pain, elevated pulse, respiratory rate, or increased restlessness may indicate poor pain relief

In post-operative patients encourage turn cough and deep breathing as drug depresses cough and sigh reflexes which may induce atelectasis

Encourage patient to void every 4 hours, drug may dull feelings of bladder distention and promote urinary retention

Nausea and orthostatic hypotension may occur, change positon slowly and assist with ambulation, bedside rails should be up at all times

Avoid alcohol and over the counter drugs during drug use

Potential for psychologic or physical dependence, Rx required and cannot be renewed, high abuse potential (Schedule II drug)

Examples of other drugs in this classification:

Alfentanil hydrochloride (*Alfenta*), IV general anesthetic for surgery Codeine, PO/IM/SQ, Used also to supress nonproductive or hyperactive cough, analgesic potency is about 1/6th that of morphine

Fentanyl citrate (*Duragesic, sublimaze*), Short acting analgesic during surgery and perioperative periods, IM/IV, Duration 30-60 min IV

Hydrocodone bitartrate (*Dihydrocodeinone bitartrate, hyacetamino-phen*), Schedule III drug, PO, Used primarily for cough control

Hydromorphone hydrochloride (*Dilaudid, Dilaudid-HP*), PO/SQ/IM/IV, 8-10 times more potent than morphine with more rapid onset and shorter duration, Used for analgesia and cough control

Levorphanol tartrate (*Levo-Dromoran*), PO/SQ, Used for analgesia and pre-operatively for apprehension relief

Meperidine hydrochloride (*Demerol*), PO/SQ/IM/IV, SQ route is painful and may cause local irritation

Methadone hydrochloride (*Dolophine*), PO/SQ/IM, Also used in detoxification programs for patients with narcotic addiction

Opium alkaloids hydrochlorides (*Pantopon*), IM/SQ, For relief of severe pain, largely been replaced by other narcotics today

Opium tincture, PO, Used to treat acute diarrhea and for neonates born to women addicted to opiates

Oxycodone hydrochloride, Oxycodone terephthalate (*Percodan, Roxicet*), PO, Has little or no effect on cough reflex, administer after meals, Percodan contains aspirin, percocet contains acetaminophen

Oxymorphone hydrochloride (*Numorphan*), SC/IM/IV, 1 mg is equal to 10mg of morphine

Paregoric (*Camphorated opium tincture*), PO, Used for acute diarrhea and abdominal cramps, Schedule III drug

Propoxyphene hydrochloride (*Darvon, Novopropoxyn*), PO, Capsules contents may be mixed with food or water

Sufentanil citrate (*Sufenta*), IV, Used in general anesthesia

ANALGESICS, NARCOTIC (OPIATE)
AGONIST — ANTAGONISTS

Action: Cause analgesia by acting on the central nervous system, possibly at the limbic system. Antagonizes the action of narcotics and are less likely to cause physical dependence than narcotic agonists. Generally schedule IV drugs

Indications: Moderate to severe pain

Example: Pentazocine hydrochloride (*Talwin*)

Route: PO, IM, IV, SQ, Laboring women IM

Pharmacokinetics: Onset 15-30 mins PO/IM/SQ or 2-3 mins IV
                  Peak 1-3 h PO/IM, 15 mins IV
                  Duration 3 h PO/IM, 1 h IV

Contraindications: Head injury, increased intracranial pressure, history of drug abuse, emotionally unstable patients

Common adverse effects: Drowsiness, dizziness, lightheadedness, euphoria, nausea, vomiting

Life-threatening adverse effects: Respiratory depression

Other adverse effects: Sweating, flushing, dry mouth, taste alterations, urinary retention, visual disturbances, allergic reactions, rash, pruritus

Interventions:

Rotate injection sites and assess for irritation or inflammation (IM)

May be given direct IV or diluted with 1ml sterile water for q 5 mg, give 5mg over 1 minute

May cause withdrawal symptoms in patients who have been recieving opioids

Examples of other drugs in this classification:

Buprenorphrine hydrochloride (*Buprenex*), IM/IV/Epidural
    Butorphanol tartrate (*Stadol*), IM/IV/Intranasal, Do not administer if RR <12 bpm, report marked changes in BP or bradycardia, causes sedation and dizziness assist in position changes and ambulation as needed

Nalbuphine hydrochloride (*Nubain*), SC/IM/IV 10mg over 3-5 minutes, Assess for sulfite sensitivity may cause allergic reaction if present

ANALGESICS, NARCOTIC ANTAGONIST
Action: Pure narcotic opiate antagonist free of analgesic activity. Reverses respiratory depression, analgesia and drowsiness.
Indications: Narcotic overdose, to reverse respiratory depression
Example: Naloxone hydrochloride (*Narcan*)
Route: IV
Pharmacokinetics: Onset 2 minutes, duration 45 minutes
Contraindications: Respiratory depression due to nonopioid drugs
Common adverse effects: Excessive or too rapid reversal may result in reversal of analgesia, increased BP, tremors, hyperventilation, drowsiness, nausea, vomiting, sweating and tachycardia
Interventions:
Give 0.1-0.2 mg q 2-3 minutes until reversal is achieved
Surgical and obstetric patients should be closely monitored for bleeding after administration (may cause abnormal coagulation test results)
Examples of other drugs in this classification:
Naltrexone hydrochloride (*Trexan*), PO, Used in detoxified addicts, has many more side effects than Narcan and can cause hepatotoxicity

ANALGESICS, NONNARCOTIC ANALGESIC
Action: Produces analgesia without narcotics, perhaps by action on the peripheral nervous system. Also used for fever reduction.
Example: Acetaminophen (*Acephen, Anuphen, Dolanex, Halenol, Liquiprim, Panadol, Tempra, Tylenol, Valadol*)
Route: PO
Pharmacokinetics: Peaks 0.5-2.0 hours, Duration 3-4 hours
Contraindications: Hypersensitivity to acetaminophen or phenacetin, repeat use in anemia or hepatic disease
Common adverse effects: Generally negligible, rash, anorexia, nausea, vomiting, dizziness, lethargy, diaphoresis, chills, epigastric or abdominal pain, diarrhea, hepatotoxicity in alcoholics, liver damage with over dosage
Interventions:
May be crushed and taken with fluids
High abuse potential with psychologic dependence
Example: Aspirin (*Alka-Seltzer, ASA, Aspergum, Bayer, Cosprin, Easprin, Ecotrin, Empirin, Halfprin, Measurin, ZORprin*)

Route: PO
Pharmacokinetics: Peak 15 minutes — 2 hours
Contraindications: Sensitivity to aspirin, oil of wintergreen,
NSAIDS, history of GI ulceration, bleeding, vitamin K deficiency,
hemophilia or other bleeding disorders, not for use in pregnancy or
nursing mothers, not for use in children under 2 or in children with
flulike symptoms or chickenpox
Common adverse effects: Heartburn, nausea, stomach pains
Life-threatening adverse effects: Agranulocytosis, anaphylactic shock
Other adverse effects: Dizziness, confusion, drowsiness, tinnitus,
hearing loss, vomiting, diarrhea, anorexia, ulceration, occult
bleeding, GI bleed, thrombocytopenia, leukopenia, neutropenia,
hemolytic anemia, urticaria, bronchospasm, laryngeal edema,
petechiae, easy bruising, rash, sweating, thirst, hypoglycemia,
impaired renal function, iron-deficiency anemia, prolonged bleeding
time, prolonged pregnancy and labor with increased bleeding,
hepatoxicity
Interventions:
Administer with full glass of fluid to minimize gastric irritation or
with food, do not crush enteric coated tablets or administer them
with milk
Monitor therapuetic ranges if administered for specific activity
Rheumatic disease range is 250-300 ug/ml, antiplatelet range is 100
ug/ml, antiinflammatory range is 150-300 ug/ml
Toxic range is greater than 300 ug/ml
Usually discontinued one week before any surgical procedures
including oral surgery
Tablets that have a vinegarlike odor should be discarded
Examples of other drugs in this classification:
Magnesium salicylate (*Doan's pills, Magan, Mobidin*), PO, Used for
   relief of pain and inflammation in rheumatoid arthritis
Methyl salicylate (*Oil of wintergreen, betula oil, gaultheria oil, sweet
   birch oil*), Topical, for relief of minor discomforts from low back
   pain, osteroarthritis and rheumatoid arthritis

ANALGESICS, NONSTERIODAL ANTIINFLAMMATORY DRUG (NSAID)

Action: Group of drugs that have analgesic, anti-inflammatory and
antipyretic effects, the exact mode of action is unknown, believed to
work through inhibition of the synthesis of prostaglandins
Indications: Rheumatic diseases, degenerative joint diseases, acute
joint diseases, musculoskeletal problems, osteoarthritis,
dysmenorrhea, relief of mild to moderate pain

Example: Ibuprofen (*Advil, Haltran, Ibuprin, Medipren, Motrin, Nuprin, Pamprin-IB, Pediaprofen, Rufen, Trendar*)
Route: PO
Pharmacokinetics: Onset 1 hour, Peak 1-2 hours, Duration 6-8 hours
Contraindications: Sensitivity to aspirin or NSAIDs, active peptic ulcer, bleeding abnormalities
Common adverse effects: Heartburn, nausea, occult blood loss
Life-threatening adverse effects: Aplastic anemia, toxic hepatitis, anaphylaxis
Other adverse effects: Headache, dizziness, lightheadedness, anxiety, emotional lability, paresthesias, hallucinations, fatigue, malaise, drowsiness, anxiety, confusion, depression, aseptic meningitis, amblyopia, hypertension, palpitations, peripheral edema, nystagmus, visual problems, tinnitus, impaired hearing, dry mouth, gingival ulcerations, dyspepsia, vomiting, anorexia, diarrhea, constipation, bloating, flatulence, GI ulceration, epigastric or abdominal pain, thrombocytopenia, neutropenia, leukopenia, decreased Hgb, Hct, acute renal failure, polyuria, azotemia, cystitis, hematuria, nephrotoxicity, pruritus, rectal itching, acne
Interventions:
Administer on an empty stomach, 1 hour before meals or 2 hours after meals
If stomach upset occurs may take with meals or milk
Tablet may be crushed and mixed with food or liquids
Assess for occult blood loss- dark tarry stools, coffee ground emesis or frank bleeding, report blood loss immediately
Notify surgeon or dentist that NSAIDS are being taken
Examples of other drugs in this classification:
Diclofenac sodium (*Voltaren*), PO, Dose adjustment common for first 2 weeks of therapy, prothrombin time is used for dose adjustment

Fenoprofen calcium (*Nalfon*), PO, Baseline Hgb, renal and liver studies are recommended

Flurbiprofen sodium (*Ansaid, Ocufen*), PO

Indomethacin (*Indameth, Indocin*), PO, Also IV for premature infants to close patent ductus arteriosus, Administer with meals to prevent GI upset, Monitor weight in patients with cardiovascular disease for possible water retention, frontal headache should be reported

Meclofenamate sodium (*Meclofen, Meclomen*), PO, Diarrhea is a common side effect and is dose related, weight should be bi-weekly to assess for edema, a weight gain of 3 pounds in any one week should be reported

Mefenamic acid (*Ponstan, ponstel*), PO, Administer with meals or milk, use of drug for more than 1 week is not recommended by manufacturer

Naproxen (*Naprosyn*), PO, Also available as naproxen sodium

Oxaprozin (*Daypro*), PO, Usually one daily dose although divided dose may be given, Monitor for edema, assess Hgb, renal and hepatic functioning

Piroxicam (*Feldene*), PO, Administer at same time daily, incidence of GI bleeding is relatively high, assess for signs of occult bleeding

Sulindac (*Clinoril*), PO, Tablet may be crushed

Tolmetin sodium (*Tolectin*), PO, Usually morning dose and bedtime dose, Capsule may be emptied and contents swallowed with water or mixed in food

ANESTHETICS — LOCAL ANESTHETIC
Action: Anesthesia affects a local area only, the anesthetic asts upon nerve or nerve tracts in the local area to prevent nerve conduction

Indications: To facilitate placement of a needle into the skin or spine, surgical removal of skin tags, warts, or non-melanotic moles with use as peripheral nerve block, some can also be used for spinal anesthesia and epideral nerve blocks by injection.

Example: Procaine hydrochloride (*Novocain*)

Route: SC, Epideral

Pharmacokinetics: Onset 2-5 minutes, Duration 1 hour

Contraindications: Known sensitivity to Procaine or other similiar drugs sepsis at injection site, generalized septicemia, meningitis, syphilis as a cerebrospinal disease, heart block, hypotension, hypertension, bowel pathology

Life-threatening adverse effects: Respiratory arrest, anaphylactoid reaction

Other adverse effects: Anxiety, nervousness, dizziness, tinnitus, blurred vision, tremors, drowsiness, sedation, convulsions, myocardial depression, arrhythmias, hypotension, nausea, vomiting, urticaria, pruritus, sweating, syncope

Other adverse effects with epidural anesthesia: urinary retention, fecal or urinary incontinence, loss of perineal sensation, slowing of labor, increased use of forceps delivery, headache, backache, high spinal block

Other adverse effects with spinal anesthesia: Postspinal headache, palsies, arachnoiditis, nerve paralysis, meningism

Interventions:
Do not use solutions that are cloudy or discolored
Inject slowly with frequent aspirations to prevent accidental IV use
Inform patient that there will be loss of sensation in area injected
Use with caution in areas with limited blood supply (toes, ears, nose)
as reduced perfusion may occur (pale, cold skin)
Monitor for hypotension after spinal anesthesia

Examples of other drugs in this classification:

Benzocaine (*Americaine, Anbesol, Benzocol, Biocozene, Biocozene, Dermoplast, Hurricaine, Oracin, Orajel, Solarcaine, T-caine, Unguentine*), Topical, for minor burns, wounds or insect stings, perianal discomforts

Bupivacaine hydrochloride (*Marcaine, Sensorcaine*), IM/Epidural/ Spinal, Sensation to lower extremities during spinal administration may not return for 2.3-3.5 hours

Chloroprocaine hydrochloride (*Nesacaine*), Nerve Block/Caudal/ Epidural, Not used for spinal, topical or IV anesthesia, Monitor VS carefully

Dibucaine (*Nupercainal*), Topical, Used for relief of pain and itching of hemorrhoids and other anorectal disorders or for insect bites, cuts, burns

Etidocaine hydrochloride (*Duranest*), IM, used for central neural blocks such as lumbar or caudal epidural blocks, if restlessness, anxiety, tinnitus, dizziness, blurred vision, tremors, or drowsiness occur then administer oxygen (CNS toxicity)

Lidocaine hydrochloride (*Anestacon, Dilocaine, L-Caine, Lida-Mantle, Nervocaine, Octocaine, Xylocaine*), IV/IM/SQ/Nerve Block/ Epidural/Caudal/Spinal/Saddle Block/Topical, Also used to control ventricular arrhythmias

EMLA — Eutectic Mixture of Lidocaine and Prilocaine (*EMLA cream*), topical, Cream is applied and covered with occlusive dressing 1-2 hours before analgesia is desired

ANTICONVULSANTS — BARBITURATES

Action: Control seizure activity through depression of abnormal neuronal discharges. Barbiturates act by interfering with impulse transmission of the cerebral cortex thereby increasing the threshold for motor cortex stimuli and decreasing the spread of seizure activity.

Indications: Management of tonic-clonic and partial seizures, as well as status epilepticus, febrile convulsions and eclampsia. Some medications are used as sedatives.

Example: Phenobarbital (*Barbita, Gardenal, Luminal, Solfoton*)

Route: PO, IM, IV

Pharmacokinetics: Peak 8-12 hours PO or 30 minutes IV, Duration 4-6 h IV

Contraindications: sensitivity to barbiturates, porphyria, severe renal or respiratory disease, history of addiction to hypnotics, uncontrolled pain

Common adverse effects: Somnolence

Life-threatening adverse effects: Laryngospasm with IV, agranulocytosis, respiratory depression or death with overdose

Other adverse effects: Nightmares, insomnia, headache, anxiety, thinking problems, dizziness, nystagumus, irritability, confusion, depression or excitment, ataxia, bradycardia, syncope, hypotension, nausea, vomiting, constipation, diarrhea, epigastric pain, rash, fever, urticaria, hypoventilation, apnea, bronchospasm, liver damage, megaloblastic anemia, hypocalcemia, osteomalacia, rickets, thrombocytopenia, folic acid deficiency, vitamin D deficiency

Interventions:

PO drug may be crushed and mixed with fluid or food

IM should be injected deep into muscle, IV administration mix with at least 10 ml of dilutent, administer 60 mg/minute or less, extravasation of IV solution may require skin graft so patency of IV site is cruical

Monitor laboratory values for therapeutic response 15-40 µg/ml, monitor patient for any sign of seizure activity and take appropriate precautions

Assess for signs of drug toxicity to include ataxia, slurred speech, poor judgments, irritability, nystagmus, confusion and insomnia, drug levels >50 ug/ml may produce coma, drug levels >80 ug/ml are potentially deadly

Assess for drowsiness, inform patient that this side effect should diminsh over the first few weeks of therapy, patient should avoid activities such as driving or operating potentially hazordous machinery if drug response is not known or drowsiness occurs

Patient may need Vitamin D, B12 or B9 dietary supplements as indicated

Drug should not be stopped or decreased without medical advice/ supervison as withdrawal symptoms may occur and can be fatal

Report any fever, sore throat, malaise, bleeding, petechiae or rash

Examples of other drugs in this classification:

Mephobarbital (*Mebaral, Methylphenobarbital*), PO, Used for tonic clonic & absence seizures

Paraldehyde (*Paracetaldehyde, Paral*), PO/Rectal, Used more for
  alcohol withdrawal or convulsions from tetanus, eclampsia,
  status epilepticus and drug poisonings, Do not use plastic to
  measure or administer this drug as it can decompose drug to
  toxic compound, do not use if drug is colored or smells like
  vinegar, rubber catheter used for rectal administration, IM
  injection is sometimes done by physicians

ANTICONVULSANTS — BENZODIAZEPHINES
Action: Stop seizure activity by suppressing the spike and wave
discharge in seizures and by decreasing the frequency, amplitude,
duration and spread of the discharges in minor motor seizures
Indications: Seizure activity, also for anxiety
Example: Diazepam (*E-Pam, Meval, Valium, Valrelease*)
Route: IV, IM, PO
Pharmacokinetics: Onset 30-60 min PO, 15-30 min IM, 1-5 min IV
Peak 1-2 hours PO, Duration 3 hours PO, 15-60 min IV
Contradindications: IV/IM-shock, coma, acute alcohol intoxication,
vital sign depression, obstetric patients, PO-acute angle glaucoma or
with MAO inhibitor therapy
Common adverse effects: Drowsiness
Life-threatening adverse effects: Cardiovascular collapse,
laryngospasm
Other adverse effects: Fatigue, ataxia, confusion, dizziness, vertigo,
amnesia, vivid dreams, headache, slurred speech, tremors,
hypotension, tardive dyskinesia, tachycardia, edema, blurred vision,
diplopia, nausea, nystagmus, xerostomia, constipation, incontinence,
urinary retention, menstrual irregularities, hiccups, coughing,
throat and chest pain, jaundice, venous thrombosis
Interventions:
Tablets may be crushed and mixed with food or fluids
Administer IM injection deep into large muscle, inject slowly
Administer IV slow with each 5 mg over at least 1 minute, direct
injection into vein is preferred to infusion tubing injection
Assess patient receiving IV/IM drug for hypotension, tachycardia
and respiratory depression
Monitor patients response to drug and supervise during ambulation
Examples of other drugs in this classification:
Clonazepam (*Klonopin, Rivotril*), PO, Used for absence, myoclonic,
  akinetic seizures, infantile spasms and restless legs. Monitor
  I&O, often given in combination with other anticonvulsants
  assess for drug interactions, liver function studies, platelet

counts, blood counts are recommended, loss of seizure control may occur after 3 months and require dose adjustment

ANTICONVULSANTS — HYDANTOINS

Action: Primary site of action is the motor cortex. The spread of seizure activity is inhibited by either increasing or decreasing the sodium ions across the motor cortex during nerve impulse generation.

Indications: Clonic tonic and psychomotor seizure activity

Example: Phenytoin (*Dilantin*)

Route: PO, IV

Pharmacokinetics: Peak 1.5-3.0 hours, 4-12 hours for extended release

Contraindications: sensitivity to hydantoin products, rash, seizures due to hypoglycemia, sinus bradycardia, heart block, Adams-Stokes syndrome

Common adverse effects: Drowsiness, gingival hyperplasia

Life-threatening adverse effects: Cardiovascular collapse, agranulocytosis, aplastic anemia, toxic epidermal necrolysis

Other adverse effects: (generally dose related) Nystagmus, ataxia, tremors, dizziness, mental confusion, insomnia, headache, seizures, bradycardia, hypotension, ventricular fibrillation, phlebitis, photophobia, diplopia, conjunctivitis, blurred vision, nausea, vomiting, constipation, epigastric pain, dysphagia, loss of taste, weight loss, hepatitis, liver necrosis, thrombocytopenia, leukopenia, leukocytosis, pancytopenia, eosinophilla, megaloblastic anemia, hemolytic anemia, fever, hyperglycemia, glycosuria, weight gain, edema, alopecia, hirsutism, rash, keratosis, renal failure, ostermalacia, rickets, pneumonitis, pulmonary fibrosis, periarteritis nodosum, acute systemic lupus erythematosus, craniofacial abnormalities, Peyronie's disease, lymphadenopathy

Interventions:

Tablet may be crushed and mixed with food or fluid, drug is alkaline and needs to be taken after a small amount of fluid and followed with a full glass of fluid

For IV administration, administer slowly 25-50 mg/minute, venous patency should be assured as drug may cause serious irritation if infiltration occurs, follow injection with saline flush to minimize irritation

Monitor respiratory rate and vital signs during and after IV dosage

Monitor for therapeutic laboratory values 10-20 µg/ml, toxic level 30-50 µg/ml and lethal level is 100 µg/ml

Patients on prolonged therapy may require Vitamin D and folic acid supplementation

Urine may be pink, red or red-brown during use of this drug

Assess for jaundice and monitor liver function studies

Assess for measles-like rash and report immediately if appears

Examples of other drugs in this classification:

Carbamazepine (*Epitol, Tegretol*), PO, Used for tonic-clonic, psychomotor, temporal lobe epilepsy or mixed seizures, also used for trigeminal neuralgia, administer with meals, recommed CBC, electrolytes, iron, liver function studies, BUN and UA at start of treatment

Felbamate (*Felbatol*), PO, Used for partial seizures, Monitor WBC, sodium, potassium levels, monitor weight

ANTICONVULSANTS — SUCCINIMIDES

Action: Elevate seizure threshold in the cortex and basal ganglia and reduces synaptic response to low frequency repetitive stimulation. Will also suppress the wave pattern of EEG.

Indications: Absence or myoclonic seizures

Example: Ethosuximide (*Zarontin*)

Route: PO

Pharmacokinetics: Peak 4 hours

Contraindications: hypersensitivity to succinimides, severe liver or renal disease

Common adverse effects: Anorexia, epigastric distress, weight loss

Life-threatening adverse effects: Agranulocytosis, pancytopenia, aplastic anemia, exfoliative dermatitis

Other adverse effects: Drowsiness, hiccups, ataxia, dizziness, headache, euphoria, restlessness, irritability, anxiety, hyperactivity, aggression, depression, difficulty concentrating, fatigue, muscle weakness, lethargy, confusion, sleeping disorders, night terrors, hypochondriacal behavior, blurred vision, myopia, photophobia, periorbital edema, nausea, vomiting, abdominal pain, diarrhea, constipation, swelling of the tongue, increased libido, vaginal bleeding, eosinophilia, leukopenia, thrombo- cytopenia, hirsutism, alopecia, erythema multiforme, Stevens-Johnson syndrome, pruritic erythematous skin eruptions, urticaria, hyperemia, gingival hyperplasia

Interventions:

Monitor patient closely for any behavioral changes, provide supervision

Monitor patient until drug response is known; may impair mental or physical abilities (driving skills may be affected)

Monitor weight for changes and report

Examples of other drugs in this classification:

Methsuximide (*Celontin*), PO, Used for absence seizures, Drug should be slowly withdrawn if depression or aggression occurs

ANXIOLYTICS — SEDATIVE HYPNOTICS, BARBITURATES

Action: Central nervous system depressant acting primarily on brainstem reticular formation, reducing nerve impulses to the cerebral cortex. Also depresses respiratory, muscle and nerve function. They also raise the seizure threshold

Indications: Short-term treatment of anxiety, agitation and insomnia

Example: Secobarbital (*Seconal*)

Route: PO, IM, IV, Rectal form may be used for a child

Pharmacokinetics: PO onset 15-30 min, IM onset 7-10 min, IV onset 1-3 min

Duration: PO 1-4 hours, IV 15 minutes duration

Contraindications: sensitivity to barbiturates, uncontrolled pain, pregnancy, parturition

Life-threatening adverse effects: Respiratory depression, laryngospasm

Common adverse effects: Drowsiness, lethargy, hangover, paradoxical excitement in the elderly

Interventions:

Pills may be crushed and mixed with fluid or food

Administer IM injection deep into large muscle mass, aspirate carefully

IV administration, use only clear solution, administer 50 mg/60 seconds, with rapid IV administration BP may fall, monitor BP, pulse, respiratory rate every 3-5 minutes

When given to pregnant women, carefully assess fetal heart tones (slowing or irregularities)

Long-term use may result in nutritional deficiencies or in dependence and abuse

Monitor and assist patient with ambulation and other activities that require alertness, maintain side-rails in up positon

Examples of other drugs in this classification:

Chloral hydrate (*Aquachloral, Supprettes, Noctec, Novochlorhydrate*), PO, Rectal

Glutethimide (*Doriglute*), PO, Withdrawal should be gradual, report onset of rash

Pentobarbital (*Nembutal*), PO/IM/IV, IV is for preoperative sedation
and should be given slowly, extravasation may result in tissue
necrosis

ANXIOLYTICS — SEDATIVE HYPNOTICS, BENZODIAZEPINES

Action: Central nervous system depression, thought to act on the
hypothalamus and limbic system of the brain, decreasing the pressor
response and increasing the arousal threshold

Indications: Used for the treatment of insomnia restoration of
normal sleep patterns. Used for patients with acute or chronic
medical problems.

Example: Lorazepam (*Ativan*)

Route: PO, IV, IM

Pharmacokinetics: IV onset 1-5 minutes, IM onset 15-30 minutes
IM peak 60-90 minutes, PO peak 2 hours
Duration 12-24 hours

Contraindications: sensitivity to benzodiazepines, acute glaucoma,
shock, depression, psychosis, coma, acute alcohol intoxication,
pregnancy, breast feeding

Common adverse effects: Drowsiness, sedation

Other adverse effects: Usually disappear with continued medication,
anterograde amnesia, dizziness, weakness, unsteadiness,
disorientation, depression, sleep disturbances, restlessness,
confusion, hallucinations, hypertension, hypotension, blurred vision,
diplopia, depressed hearing, nausea, vomiting, abdominal
discomfort, anorexia

Interventions:

Administer IM injection deep into a large muscle mass

Administer IV slowly no more than 2 mg/minute with repeated
aspiration to prevent extravasation, monitor patient on IV drug
carefully and have airway at bedside

Supervise ambulation and other activities to prevent injury and
provide for patients safety, keep siderails up at all times

Monitor CBC and liver function tests, report any abnormal findings

Monitor patient and assess for evidence of depression, provide for
patient safety as indicated, monitor patient for dependence with
long-term use

As with all sedatives, patient should avoid alcohol use and
self-medication

Examples of other drugs in this classification:

Buspirone hydrochloride (*BuSpar*), PO, Used for management of
anxiety, give with food, if given with digoxin may increase

potential for toxic serum levels of digoxin, report any involuntary movements, assess for edema and decreased urinary output and report

Clorazepate dipotassium (*Tranxene*), PO, Used for management of anxiety, partial seizures and alcohol withdrawal, do not administer with antacids

Oxazepam (*Serax*), Used for management of anxiety and for acute alcohol withdrawal symptoms, PO

ANXIOLYTICS — SEDATIVE HYPNOTICS, CARBAMATES

Action: Non-barbiturate central nervous system depressants, works on multiple sites in the CNS and appears to block corticothalamic impulses.

Indications: Relief of anxiety and tension (psychoneurotic states), sleep promotion in patients who are tense

Example: Meprobamate (*Equanil, Meprospan, Miltown*)

Route: PO

Pharmacokinetics: Onset 1 hour, Peak 1-3 hours

Contraindications: hypersensitivity to carbamates, prophyria, pregnancy, breast feeding

Common adverse effects: Drowsiness, ataxia

Life-threatening adverse effects: Exfoliative dermatitis, anaphylaxis, agranulocytosis, aplastic anemia, thrombocytopenia, respiratory depression and circulatory collapse

Other adverse effects: Rash, petechiae, purpura, ecchymoses, eosinophilia, peripheral edema, angioneurotic edema, adenopathy, fever, chills, oliguria, bronchospasm, anuria, Stevens-Johnson syndrome, dizziness, vertigo, slurred speech, headache, weakness, paresthesias, paradoxic euphoria and rage, impaired visual accommodation, seizures in epileptics, syncope, panic reaction, hypotensive crisis, palpitation, tachycardia, arrhythmias, anorexia, nausea, vomiting, diarrhea, leukopenia

Interventions:

Assess patients response to medication, assist with postion changes and supervise ambulation as needed, side rails up at all times for safety

Physical or psychic dependence may occur with long term use, drug should be withdrawn slowly to prevent withdrawal reactions

Monitor therapeutic blood levels of medication 0.5-2 mg/dl, blood levels of 3-10 mg/dl usually correspond to mild to moderate overdose, levels of 10-20 mg/dl have severe overdose symptoms with levels >20 mg/dl being lethal

Report onset on skin rash, sore throat, fever, bruising, or bleeding

PSYCHOTHERAPEUTIC AGENTS — ANTIDEPRESSANTS, TRICYCLIC

Action: Thought to inhibit the uptake of norepinephrine and/or serotonin by the presynaptic neuronal membrane in the central nervous system, increasing the concentration of these biogenic amines at the synapse

Indications: Relief of depression (oldest class of antidepressants)

Example: Imipramine hydrochloride or Imipramine pamoate (*Janimine, Tofranil, Tofranil-PM*)

Route: PO, IM

Pharmacokinetics: PO peak 1-2 hours, IM peak 30 minutes

Contraindications: hypersensitivity to tricyclic drugs, recovery from MI, bundle branch conduction defects, severe renal disease, severe hepatic impairment, pregnancy, children under age 12 except for enuresis treatment

Common adverse effects: Sedation, drowsiness, orthostatic hypotension, arrhythmias, heart block, blurred vision, slight mydriasis, dry mouth, urinary retention

Life-threatening adverse effects: Agranulocytosis, myocardial infarction

Other adverse effects: Dizziness, headache, fatigue, numbness, tingling of extremities, incoordination, ataxia, tremors, peripheral neuropathy, EEG pattern alteration, extrapyramidal symptoms, lowered seizure threshold, delirium, disturbed concentration, confusion, hallucinations, anxiety, nervousness, insomnia, vivid dreams, restlessness, agitation, mania, mild sinus tachycardia, psychoses exacerbation, hyperpyrexia, hypertension or hypotension, palpitation, ECG changes, stroke, flushing, cold cyanotic hands and/or feet, testicular swelling, gynecomastia, galactorrhea and breast enlargement, increased or decreased libido, ejaculatory/ erectile disturbances, delayed or absent orgasm, increased or decreased blood glucose levels, nasal congestion, tinnitus, disturbances of accommodation, nystagmus, aggravation of glaucoma, constipation, heartburn, excessive appetitie, weight gain, nausea, vomiting, diarrhea, flatulence, abdominal cramps, slowed gastric emptying, esophageal reflux, anorexia, stomatitis, increased salivation, black tongue, peculiar tastes, paralytic ileus, delayed urination, nocturia, paradoxic urinary frequency, bone marrow depression, eosinophilia, thrombocytopenia, skin rash, erythema, urticaria petechiae, pruritus, photosensitivity, edema of the face, tongue, edema that is generalized, drug fever, excessive perspira- tion, cholestatic jaundice, porphyria, dyspnea, changes in heat and cold tolerance, hair loss, SIADH

Interventions:
Administer with food, single daily dose should be given at bedtime to minimize drowsiness unless insomnia occurs with drug use

Monitor pulse for tachycardia, hold drug if sudden increase in pulse rate

Monitor BP for fall >20mmHg, hold drug and notify physician if occurs

Monitor laboratory values to assess hepatic, renal and hematologic status report any abnormal results

Weigh patient at least twice weekly, report a gain of 1.5-2 pounds within a 2-3 day period, edema should be reported, weight gain may be related to an increase in appetitie

Monitor intake and output to detect urinary retention or frequency

Monitor bowel elimination for constipation or paralytic ileus

Report jaundice, dark urine, light colored stools, yellow sclearae or skin

Assess for history of glaucoma and report in positive patients headache, halos around lights, dilated pupils, eye pain, or nausea from acute attack

Report tremors, twitching, ataxia, incoordination, hyperreflexia, drooling, these may be reported to extrapyramidal symptoms

Assess for aspirin sensitivity, some patients with ASA allergys have allergy to imipramine compounds

Assist with position changes and ambulation until response to drug is known, avoid hazardous tasks and activities (driving)

Limit exposure to strong sunlight

Smoking and over-the-counter drug use is not recommended with this drug

Dry mouth is a frequent problem and may require saliva substitue

Examples of other drugs in this classification:

Amitriptyline hydrochloride (*Amitril, Elavil, Emitrip, Endep, Enovil, Meravil*), PO/IM, Tablet may be crushed, May be ordered for migraine prophylaxis

Amoxapine (*Asendin*), PO, Tablet may be crushed, report neuroleptic malignant syndrome fever, sweating, rigidity, unstable BP, rapid irregular pulse, change in level of consciousness or coma. Encourage fluids to 2000 ml per day

Clomipramine hydrochloride (*Anafranil*), PO, used for obsessive-compulsive disorder, taken in divided doses with meals, monitor for and report signs of neuroleptic malignant syndrome (see above), drug may cause impotence

Desipramine hydrochloride (*Norpramin, Pertofrane*), PO, Take with food

Doxepin hydrochloride (*Adapin, Sinequan*), PO, Used for psychoneurotic anxiety as well as depression, oral concentrate form must be diluted with 120 ml of fluid, capsule may be mixed with food or fluid

Nortiriptyline hydrochloride (*Aventyl, Pamelor*), PO, Oral solution does not require dilution, administer with food

Protriptyline hydrochloride (*Vivactil*), PO, Tablets may be crushed or can be mixed with food, last dose of day should be taken no later than mid-afternoon to prevent insomnia

Trimipramine maleate (*Surmontil*), PO

PSYCHOTHERAPEUTIC AGENTS — ANTIDEPRESSANTS, SEROTONIN-REUPTAKE INHIBITOR

Action: Inhibition of presynaptic neuronal uptake of serotonin in the central nervous system, chemically unrelated to other antidepressants.

Indications: Depression

Example: Fluoxetine hydrochloride (*Prozac*)

Route: PO

Pharmacokinetics: Onset 1-3 weeks, Peak 4-8 hours

Contraindications: sensitivity to prozac

Common adverse effects: Headache, nervousness, anxiety, insomnia, nausea, diarrhea

Other adverse effects: Drowsiness, fatigue, tremor, dizziness, hypomania, mania, palpitations, hot flushes, chest pain, anorexia, dyspepsia, dry mouth, increased appetite, rash, pruritus, sweating, blurred vision, flu-like symptoms, myalgias, arthralgias, hyponatremia, sexual dysfunction, menstrual irregularities

Interventions:

Generally administered in single am dose, may be given in two doses, one am and one at noon to prevent insomnia

Approximately 2-3 weeks before the therapeutic effect is noted

Weigh weekly to assess for weight loss, report any significant loss

Assess for rash, fever, leukocytosis, arthralgias, carpal tunnel syndrome, edema, respiratory distress, proteinuria and report

Assess for patient's response to the drug and implement safety measures as indicated such as assisted ambulation, side rails up on bed

Assess for seizures in any patients with history of seizure activity

Monitor sodium levels for hyponatremia

Patient should avoid over-the-counter medications during prozac use

Examples of other drugs in this classification:
Paroxetine (*Paxil*), PO, Monitor patients with a history of mania for a return of symptoms, alcohol use may increase risk of adverse effects

Sertraline hydrochloride (*Zoloft*), PO, used for major depression, May be given in the morning or evening, not for concurrent use with MAO inhibitor, Assess for use of warfarin therapy, if taken assess laboratory reports and report prolonged PT or any signs of bleeding

PSYCHOTHERAPEUTIC AGENTS — ANTIDEPRESSANTS, MONOAMINE OXIDASE INHIBITORS

Action: Monoamine oxidase (MAO) is an enzyme found in the mitochondria of cells located in nerve endings and other body tissues. MAO acts as a catalyst and inactivates dopamine, norepinephrine, epinephrine and serotonin. MAO inhibitors block MAO and lead to an increase in dopamine, norepinephrine, epinephrine and serotonin at the neuronal synapses, thus having an antidepressant effect.

Indications: Severe depression that has not responded to other medications or psychotherapy.

Example: Phenelzine sulfate (*Nardil*)

Route: PO

Pharmacokinetics: Onset 2 weeks

Contraindications: sensitivity to MAO inhibitors, pheochromocytoma, CHF, hyperthyroidism, cardiovascular disease, cerebrovascular disease, impaired renal function, hypernatremia, atonic colitis, glaucoma, severe headache history, liver disease, abnormal liver function studies, elderly, paranoid schizophrenia, debilitated patients

Common adverse effects: Constipation, dry mouth, orthostatic hypotension, insomnia, nausea, anorexia

Life-threatening adverse effects: Hypertensive crisis, coma, circulatory collapse, respiratory depression

Other adverse effects: Dizziness, vertigo, headache, drowsiness, weakness, fatigue, vomiting, weight gain, edema, tremors, twitching, hyperreflexia, mania, hypomania, confusion, memory impairment, blurred vision, skin rash, hyperhidrosis, glaucoma, nystagmus, incontinence, dysuria, galactorrhea, urinary frequency or retention, transient impotence, gynecomastia, black tongue, hypernatremia, transient respiratory and cardiovascular depression, jaundice, delirium, hallucinations, euphoria, acute anxiety reaction, akathisia, ataxia, precipitation of schizophrenia, convulsions, peripheral neuropathy, photosensitivity, normocytic and normochromic anemia, leukopenia

Interventions:

Foods that must be avoided during drug use include red wine, some beers, cheese, smoked or pickled fish, beef or chicken liver, summer sausage, fava or broad bean pods, yeast vitamin supplements these foods may lead to hypertensive crisis. Other foods that are questionable include overripe avocados and bananas, sour cream, yogurt and soy sauce. Be sure dietary order restricts tyramine-containing foods, caffeine beverages and alcohol.

MAO inhibitors should be stopped at least 10 days before surgery whenever possible, rapid withdrawal should be avoided to prevent rebound effects.

Prior to onset of therapy assess BP in standing and lying for baseline BP and pulse should be monitored between doses, hypotension may occur

Baseline blood counts and liver function studies should be performed, report any abnormal results

Monitor I&O and assess for edema and urinary dysfunction, report if found

Hypomania may occur as depression is resolved, report immediately

Monitor diabetic patient for hypoglycemia, reduced insulin may be required

Patient should avoid over the counter medications unless cleared by health care provider

Assess for hypertensive crisis to include intense occipital headache, marked hypertension, palpitations, stiff neck, nausea, vomiting, sweating, fever, photophobia, dilated pupils, bradycardia or tachycardia, chest pain and intracrainal bleeding, report immediately can be lethal

Assist patient with position changes as needed and assess for orthostatic hypotension, dangle patient before standing, avoid hot showers or baths

MAO inhibitors may mask angina, patient should avoid over exertion

Examples of other drugs in this classification:

Isocarboxazid (*Marplan*), PO, therapeutic effect may be seen in 1-4 weeks

PSYCHOTHERAPEUTIC AGENTS — ANTIMANIC AGENTS

Action: Mechanism of action is unknown, neurotransmitter hyperactivity is corrected. May act by it's ability to alter sodium transport at the nerve endings, inhibit cyclic AMP formation in nerve cells and enhances the uptake of serotonin and norepinephrine by nerve cells

Indications: Used for patients with manic-depressive psychosis in an acute manic phase, also for prevention of manic episodes

Example: Lithium (*Eskalith, Lithane, Lithobid, Lithonate, Lithotabs*)

Route: PO

Pharmacokinetics: Peak 0.5-3.0 hours carbonate, 15-60 mins citrate

Contraindications: severe cardiovascular disease, severe renal disease, brain damage, severe debilitation, dehydration, sodium depletion, patients on low salt diets, patients on diuretics, breastfeeding, children <12 years

Common adverse effects: Headache, lethargy, fatigue, recent memory loss, nephrogenic diabetes insipidus, nausea, vomiting, anorexia, abdominal pain, diarrhea, dry mouth, fine hand tremors, muscle weakness, reversible leukocytosis

Life-threatening adverse effects: Peripheral circulatory collapse

Other adverse effects: Dizziness, drowsiness, slurred speech, psychomotor retardation, giddiness, incontinence, restlessness, seizures, confusion, blackout spells, disorientation, stupor, coma, EEG changes, arrhythmias, hypotension, vasculitis, ECG changes, impaired vision, transient scotomas, tinnitus, thyroid enlargement, hypothyroidism, transient hyperglycemia, glycosuria, hyponatremia, metallic taste, coarse tremors, choreoathetotic movements, fasciculations, clonic movements, incoordination including ataxia, hyperreflexia, encephalopathic syndrome, pruritus, maculopapular rash, hyperkeratosis, chronic folliculitis, transient acneiform papules, anesthesia of skin, cutaneous ulcers, drying and thinning of hair, edema, allergic vasculitis, albuminuria, oliguria, urinary incontinence, polyuria, polydipsia, increased uric acid excretion, weight gain or loss, flu-like symptoms, exacerbation of psoriasis

Interventions:

Administer drug with meals, dosage is determined by drug serum levels

Therapeutic drug levels are 0.6-1.6 mEq/L during maintenance treatment and 1.0-1.5 mEq/L for treatment of acute mania, levels between 1.5-2.0 mEq/L may lead to signs of lithium intoxication which include vomiting, lack of coordination, diarrhea, drowsiness, muscular weakness & slurred speech

Report symptoms and withhold the next dose until consultation

Drug levels above 2.0 mEq/L may lead to ataxia, blurred vision, giddiness, tinnitus, muscle twitching, coarse tremors, and diluted urine

Hospitalization is usually required until dose adjustment is complete
Weigh patient daily and assess for edema, monitor I&O ratio
Periodic monitoring of urine specific gravity is recommended,
polyuria and polydipsia are common adverse effects esp. in the
elderly
Encourage fluids, it is recommended that individuals drink 1.0-1.5
liters/day during therapy, normal salt intake is required to keep
lithium blood levels in the therapeutic range (Na intake of 6-10
grams/day)
Monitor patients response to drug, may impair physical and mental
ability

PSYCHOTHERAPEUTIC AGENTS — ANTIPSYCHOTICS (TRANQUILIZERS), BUTYROPHENONE

Action: Act to block dopamine at receptor sites in the brain, thereby
enhancing the turnover of this neurotransmitter. Acts as a mild-
moderate blocker of alpha-adrenergic receptors located in the
sympathetic nervous system.
Indications: Relief of symptoms of psychoses to include schizo-
phrenia and manic-depressive diorders. Also used for the control of
tics and verbal utterances associated with Gilles de la Tourette's.
Example: Haloperidol (*Haldol*)
Route: PO, IM
Pharmacokinetics: IM onset 30-45 minutes, peak 10-20 minutes
PO peak is 2-6 hours
Haloperidol decanoate IM peak is 6-7 days
Contraindications: Parkinson's disease, parkinsonism, seizure
disorders, coma, alcoholism, severe mental depression, CNS
depression, thyrotoxicosis
Common adverse effects: Extrapyramidal reactions (long-term use)
Life-threatening adverse effects: Tardive dyskinesia (long-term use),
neuroleptic malignant syndrome, agranulocytosis, laryngospasm,
respiratory depression
Other adverse effects: Insomnia, restlessness, anxiety, euphoria,
mental depression, agitation, drowsiness, lethargy, fatigue, weakness, tremor, ataxia, headache, confusion, vertigo, hyperthermia,
tonic-clonic seizures, exacerbation of psychotic symptoms, tachycardia, ECG changes, hypotension, hypertension, menstrual
irregularities, galactorrhea, lactation, impotence, gynecomastia,
increased libido, hyponatremia, hyperglycemia, hypoglycemia,
blurred vision, dry mouth, anorexia, nausea, vomiting, constipation,
diarrhea, hypersalivation, urinary retention, priapism, mild leukopenia, anemia, bronchospasm, broncho- pneumonia, diaphoresis,

rash, decreased serum cholesterol, liver function study variations, cholestatic jaundice

Interventions:

Obtain baseline BP measurements before treatment is started, a high diastolic reading may be predictive of potential for neuroleptic syndrome

Administer with fluid or food, do not mix with coffee or tea

IM administer injection deep into the gluteus muscle

Monitor patient's on IM drug for orthostatic hypotension, assist with position changes as needed, recommended to have patient with side rails up for 1 hour after injection in recumbant position for safety

Monitor patient's mental status, hallucinations, insomnia, hostility, delusions and agitation should decrease

Monitor patient for onset of neuroleptic malignant syndrome with muscle rigidity, BP changes, increased temperature, pulse and respirations, diaphoresis and mental changes, NMS if untreated can lead to coma, acute respiratory failure, renal failure and cardio-vascular collapse

Assess patient for history of seizures, haloperidol may lower the seizure threshold

Monitor complete blood counts and liver function studies for patients on long-term therapy

Monitor patient until drug response is known may impair mental or physical abilities (driving skills may be affected)

Assess patient for dry mouth, encourage fluids and good oral care

Patient should avoid overexposure to sunlight or sunlamps

Examples of other drugs in this classification:

Droperidol (*Inapsine*), IM/IV, Used for tranquilizing effect during surgery and diagnostic procedures, may be ordered as a premedi-cation, monitor VS closely during use, hypotension and tachycardia are common adverse effects

PSYCHOTHERAPEUTIC AGENTS — ANTIPSYCHOTIC (TRANQUILIZER), PHENOTHIAZINE

Action: Block dopamine at the postsynaptic receptor sites in the brain, enhances the turnover of this neurotransmitter. Also decreases the uptake of other neurotransmitters, norepinephrine and serotonin by the neurons. Decrease the sensory stimulation of the reticular activating system in the brain stem, thereby producing a sedative effect.

Indications: Relief of symptoms of acute and chronic psychoses including those from schizophrenia, schizoaffective disorders and involutional psychosis. Also used for the relief of nausea and vomiting and for the reduction of agitation.

Example: Chlorpromazine hydrochloride (*Ormazine, Promapar, Promaz, Sonazine, Thorazine, Thor-Prom*)

Route: PO, IM, IV, Rectal

Pharmacokinetics: Onset 30-60 minutes, Peak 2-4 hours PO, 15-20 min IM

Duration 4-6 hours

Contraindications: sensitivity to phenothiazines, withdrawal from alcohol comatose states, brain damage, bone marrow depression, Reye's syndrome

Common adverse effects: Sedation, drowsiness, extrapyramidal symptoms, EEG changes

Life-threatening adverse effects: Neuroleptic malignant syndrome, hypothermia, adynamic ileus, agranulocytosis, pancytopenia, sudden unexplained death

Other adverse effects: Dizziness, restlessness, tardive dyskinesias, tumor, syncope, headache, weakness, insomnia, reduced REM sleep, dizarre dreams, cerebral edema, convulsive seizures, inability to sweat, depressed cough, reflex, orthostatic hypotension, hypertension, palpitation, tachycardia, bradycardia, ECG changes, blurred vision, dry mouth, mydriasis, photophobia, constipation, cholestatic jaundice, peptic ulcer aggravation, dyspepsia, increased appetite, anovulation, infertility, pseudopregnancy, menstrual irregularity, gynecomastia, galactorrhea, priapism, ejaculation inhibition, reduced libido, urinary retention and frequency, thrombocytopenic purpura, nasal congestion, laryngospasm, bronchospasm, respiratory depression, depressed cough reflex, urticaria, reduced perspiration, contact dermatitis, exfoliative dermatitis, photo-sensitivity, eczema, anaphylactoid reactions, hypersensitivity vasculitis,hirsutism, weight gain, hypoglycemia, hyperglycemia, glycosuria, enlarged parotid glands, idiopathic edema, muscle necrosis (after IM injection), SLE-like syndrome

Interventions:

Concentrate should be mixed with 120 cc of fluid or food just prior to administration

IM injection administration should be made slowly deep into large muscle, massage site well, avoid SQ administration as it causes tissue irritation

Rotate injection sites, patient should lie down, side rails up for 0.5 hr following IM injection, assess for hypotensive reaction

IV administration, dilute each 25 mg with 24 ml of normal saline, yielding 1mg drug per 1 ml, administer 1mg over 2 minutes, monitor

BP during IV infusion, may be diluted in up to 1000 ml of normal saline for continuous infusion

Prior to administration obtain baseline BP, pulse and respiratory rate

Assess patient for neuroleptic malignant syndrome symptoms include fever, altered mental status, muscle rigidity, irregular or increased pulse, BP changes and sweating

Monitor I&O, urinary retention may occur, elevate legs when sitting and use support hose for hypotension, urine may be pink to red-brown in color

Monitor CBC, liver function studies, EEG and results from any ocular exams

Report any abnormalities

Provide oral care and assess patient for dry mouth, oral candidiasis may occur

Monitor patient's response to drug, mental and physcial abilities may be impaired, caution should be exercised during driving and other activities

Examples of other drugs in this classification:
Loxapine hydrochloride (*Loxitane*), PO/IM

Section VIII — GLOSSARY OF TERMS

Acuity loss Inability to see clearly, objects are (vision) blurred

Akathisia Strong desire to move or an inability to sit May be an extra-pyridial symptom of antipsychotic medications

Alexia Inability to read

Alzheimer's disease Progressive degeneration of brain tissue usually in persons over 50 years of age

Amblyopia "lazy eye" Dim vision in one eye with no apparent anatomical cause

Anticonvulsant Medication used to prevent seizure activity

Aphasia Inability to understand spoken messages (receptive language) or communicate by speaking (expressive language) may be due to stroke (CVA) or brain injury

Ataxia Incoordination of muscle movements

Auditory Pertaining to hearing

Audiologist A person trained to assess and provide interventions for persons with hearing loss

Autonomic nervous system Part of the nervous system that cannot be controlled voluntarily, the autonomic nervous system is divided into the sympathetic and parasympathetic systems

Aura Subjective warning seconds to hours prior to a seizure, may be accompanied by hallucinations

Brain abscess Pus collected within the brain's tissue

Cerebrovascular accident (CVA) Condition generally caused by a blockage in or rupture of a vessel in the brain, often results in residual disability, "Stroke"

CNS Central Nervous System

Conductive hearing loss Sound waves are blocked from reaching the inner ear

Cortical hearing loss	Brain is unable to interpret nerve impulses and/or translate them into a meaningful message
Cortical vision loss	Brain is unable to interpret nerve impulses from the eye into a meaningful message
Crainiectomy	Surgical removal of part of the skull
Delusion	A belief that is false, and is not supported by external stimuli
Diplopia	Double vision
EEG	Electroencephalography, the process of assessing and recording the brain's electrical activity
Encephalitis	Inflammation of the brain
Encephalomyelitis	Inflammation of the brain and spinal cord
Epileptic cry	Sound which may occur with the onset of a tonic-clonic seizure, due to air being forced out of the vocal cords with the first contraction of the body's muscles
Epilepsy	Another term for seizure disorder, a condition where recurrent seizure activity occurs
Euphoria	A feeling of well being
Febrile seizure	A seizure occurring in a child less than six years old associated with fever
Field visual loss	Unable to see in one or all of the six visual fields
Gingival	Swollen enlarged tender gums. May be hyperplasia associated with medications such as dilantin
Hallucination	A visual, auditory or olfactory experience that has no basis in reality. A false sensation without any external stimulation
Hyperopia	Far sighted, unable to see objects close up as well as objects far away

Insomnia	Condition where one or more of the following occur; inability to fall asleep, maintain state of sleep, or early morning wakefulness
Intraventricular hemorrhage	Bleeding within a ventricle inside the brain
Meninges	The term given to the three membranes that cover the brain and spinal cord, the dura mater, the arachnoid and the pia mater
Meningitis	Inflammation of the meninges
Myopia	Near sighted, able to see objects close up better than objects far away
Olfactory	Pertaining to the sense of smell
Pseudo-parkinsonism	A combination of side effects that are similar to Parkinson's disease, these include; a mask like face, arm tremors, and pill rolling movements
Sensorineural hearing loss	Sound waves are not translated into nerve impulses in the cochlea
Status epilepticus	A life threatening condition where seizure activity continues for more than 30 minutes, or patient has one seizure after another
Tardive dyskinesia	A side effect of some psychotic medications characterized by involuntary movements of the mouth, tongue, face, jaw, and possibly movements of the extremities
Tinnitus	Ringing in the ears

Hematologic System
Immune System

HEMATOLOGIC SYSTEM
IMMUNE SYSTEM

Table of Contents

Section I — THE OVERVIEW

The hematologic and the immune system are two different body systems that are included under one chapter in this manuscript because they share some of the same components and functions.

Primary functions

- The manufacture and development of blood cells
  - Red blood cells (RBCs or erythrocytes)
  - White blood cells (WBCs or leukocytes)
  - Platelets (thrombocytes)
- The filtering of blood to remove non-functioning blood cells, bacteria, viruses, and toxins
- Transport of nutrients, minerals, enzymes, hormones, vitamins and antibodies to the cells of the body where needed
- Transport of waste products from cells to the kidneys, sweat glands and lungs for removal from the body
- Dysfunction of the immune system leads to a variety of disorders

Components

Composed of bone marrow, blood cells, platelets, plasma, lymph, lymph vessels, lymph nodes, the thymus, the spleen and the liver

Bone marrow

- Consists of red and yellow bone marrow (yellow not needed for hematopoiesis)
- Red bone marrow is where hematopoiesis (formation of blood cells) occurs, this includes production of RBCs, WBCs, and platelets

Red blood cells (RBCs)

- Contain millions of hemoglobin molecules
  - Transport oxygen from the lungs to the body tissues. Each hemoglobin has four atoms of iron (heme) which can each hold one oxygen molecule, oxygen is picked up in the lungs and transported to the individual cells of the body
  - Transport carbon dioxide from the body to the lungs. The globin part of the hemoglobin molecule picks up carbon dioxide from the body's cells and transports it to the lungs for removal via exhalation
- Have antigens on their surface that determine blood type: A, B, AB, and O (absence of antigens)

- O is the universal donor, AB is the universal recipient

White blood cells (WBCs)

Composed of several different types, they have a nucleus (RBCs and platelets do not)

- Combat toxins and infection from bacteria and viruses
- Induce inflammation to destroy foreign invaders
- Lymphocytes constitute about 20-44% of all WBC's
- Main components of the immune system are the T-lymphocyte and B-lymphocyte, both originate in the same stem cells that all blood cells arise from

Platelets

- Prevent excessive and life threatening blood loss from occurring when a blood vessel is damaged (needed for blood clot formation)

Plasma

- Liquid part of blood, blood cells float in this medium
- Blood plasma consists of water, electrolytes, glucose, proteins (albumin and globulin), nonprotein nitrogenous compounds, fats, bilirubin and gases
- Transports minerals, hormones, vitamins, and antibodies
- The albumin in plasma prevents leakage of fluids from capillaries
- Bicarbonates, carbon dioxide, chlorides, phosphates and ammonia are components of plasma that are important in maintaining the acid-base balance of blood

Lymph

- Clear, transparent, colorless or slightly yellow fluid
- Formed in tissue spaces throughout the body and transported by lymph vessels
- Composed of water, protein, fats and the end products of cell metabolism, lymph formed/derived from different parts of the body may have a slightly different composition

Lymph vessels

- Carry lymph in a one-way direction into the venous blood system
- Consists of small lymphatic capillaries and larger lymphatic vessels which have valves
- The walls of lymphatic vessels are thinner than those in blood vessels

Lymph nodes
- Encapsulated areas of lymphatic tissue found along the lymph vessels where bacteria and foreign cells are filtered out of the lymph fluid
- New lymphocytes are formed in lymph nodes

Thymus
- Located between the sternum and the great vessels of the heart
- Essential for the maturation of T-cells needed for the immune response

Spleen
- Dark red organ in the upper left abdomen just below the stomach
- Forms all of the blood cells in the fetus
- Forms lymphocytes from bone marrow precursors in the adult
- Reservoir for blood storage
- Filters blood; removes bacteria and old blood cells

Liver
- Largest and one of the most versatile organs in the body
- Manufactures clotting factors needed for hemostasis
  - Including factor V, VII, IX, X, and prothrombin

Concepts

Erythropoiesis (production of RBCs)
- Figure 4-1 shows the life cycle of a RBC, erythropoiesis is important in assessing and understanding laboratory values
- Reticulocyte counts may be ordered to assess the number of maturing RBCs
  - Normally only about 1% of all RBCs should be reticulocytes
  - A high reticulocyte count indicates an increase in RBC production which may occur when RBCs are being:
    - Destroyed (hemolytic anemia)
    - Lost (hemorrhage)
    - Replaced, once anemia has been corrected
  - A low reticulocyte count indicates bone marrow dysfunction

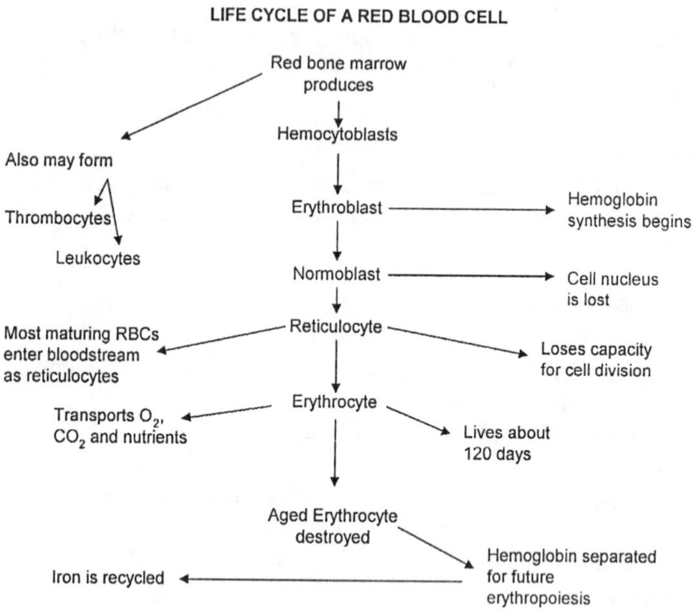

LIFE CYCLE OF A RED BLOOD CELL

Figure 4-1

Immune response

- Normal adaptive response to protect the body from destruction by foreign invaders (materials, bacteria, viruses, mutant cells)
- An immune response results from an antigen and antibody having contact with one another
- Immunity is passive or active
  - Passive immunity is temporary and borrowed from another source
    - Passed from mother to infant in utero
    - Passed from mother to infant in breast milk
    - Transferred from injection of antiserum or gamma globulin that contains antibodies from blood plasma

- Active immunity is acquired
  - Antibodies are made from having the disease
  - Antibodies are formed from immunization against the disease
  - There are three main types of cells involved in the immune response: macrophages, T lymphocytes and B lymphocytes

Antigen

- Protein marker for identification found on the surface of cells
- Identifies the cell as own body cells (autoantigens) or foreign antigens (not from own body)
  - A damaged autoantigen may appear foreign to the body and start an immune response
  - Matching certain tissue antigens is essential for successful organ transplant to prevent tissue rejection
- Identifies the type of cell (skin etc.)
- Identification of a foreign antigen leads to immune response
  - Stimulates the production of antibodies (B-lymphocytes)
  - Stimulates cytotoxic responses by granulocytes, monocytes and lymphocytes

Macrophages

- A type of WBC that circulates in the blood stream as a monocyte (2 days) and then moves into tissues such as the spleen, lymph nodes, liver and tonsils where they mature into macrophages
- One of the first lines of defense when the body is attacked by foreign invaders
- One of the major phagocytic cells of the immune system
- They have receptors on their surface that enable them to identify foreign antigens and ingest them
- They process foreign antigens and secrete a chemical marker that activates the immune response via the T-lymphocytes

Lymphocytes

- A type of white blood cell that is found primarily in lymphatic tissue
- Also present in blood (less than 1% of total)
- Main components of the immune system are the T-lymphocyte and B-lymphocyte, both originate in the same stem cells that all blood cells arise from

T-lymphocyte

- Develop in the bone marrow and then they migrate to the thymus, so they are thymus-derived
  - Immature T-cells are called thymocytes
  - Once mature, T-cells circulate between the blood and lymph systems
- Mature T-cells are antigen specific (differentiated or sensitized) so that each one responds to only one antigen
- Involved with cell-mediated immunity which results from activation of antigen specific T cells to destroy or neutralize specific foreign antigens that have invaded the body
  - Cell-mediated immunity is important in
    - Delayed hypersensitivity reactions
    - Transplant reactions
    - Protection against viruses and cancer cells
    - Not easily transferred from one individual to another
  - There are different types of T-cells that have different immune functions
- T-cells are unable to recognize foreign antigens on their own
- A macrophage must engulf and process the foreign antigen first displaying part of the antigen and then secreting a chemical marker (interleukin-1) which then activates the helper T/4 cell
- Once identified as a foreign antigen by the macrophage the T-cells direct the immune response

Helper T4 cells (CD4 cells)

- Major regulatory cells, control activity of other T cells
- Secrete interleukin-2 (IL-2) which stimulates the activity of cytotoxic T cells, killer T cells and B cells
- Secrete gamma interferon to inhibit the growth of viruses and to simulate macrophages cytotoxicity and processing of antigens
- Activate suppressor T8 cells
- T4 cells are the primary target of the HIV virus

Suppressor T8 cells

- After several days into an immune reaction these cells inhibit or suppress the responses of T4 cells and B cells
- Protective feedback mechanism to prevent excessive lymphocyte activity

- Create memory cells
  Cytotoxic T cells and killer T cells
- Directly kill other cells

B-lymphocytes

- Formed in the bone marrow and then they migrate to the spleen, lymph nodes and other lymph tissue
- Mature B cells can recognize antigens independently or they can be stimulated by T4 release of IL-2
- The primary function of B cells is to produce antibodies to a large variety of antigens, all antibodies are immunoglobulins
- Differentiate into anti-body producing plasma or memory cells
- Humoral immunity results from these antibodies in plasma or lymph
  - Two responses: primary and secondary humoral immunity
  - Primary humoral immunity occurs when antigen is introduced into the body
    - First there is a latent period when antigen is recognized and antibodies are produced (48-72 hours)
    - Memory cell records the information for future antibody production
    - Antibody titer will rise for 10-14 days then recovery from illness will occur
  - Secondary humoral immunity occurs when antigen is reintroduced
    - Memory cell recognizes the antigen and prompts plasma cells to produce specific antibody needed
    - Titers rise faster and reach higher level than in primary humoral immunity
  - Immunoglobulins have been divided into five major classes
    - IgG, 75% of total, present in of B-cells
      - Contains antiviral, antitoxin and antibacterial antibodies
      - Crosses the placenta to provide protection for the newborn
      - May be given as gamma globulin to provide temporary resistance to diseases (hepatitis)
      - Activates complement
      - Binds to macrophages
    - IgA, 15% of total, present in saliva, nasal secretions, respiratory secretions, tears and breast milk

- One of the primary defenses against local infections
- Found in colostrum (first breast milk) and helps protect the newborn from infections
- IgM, 10% of total
  - Contains the A, B, O blood group antibody responses
  - Does not cross the placenta to the fetus
  - Prominent in early immune response
  - Most efficient antibody for complement activation
- IgD, 0.2% of total,
  - Previously called Rho(D) immune globulin, prepared from the plasma of persons with a high concentration of Rh antibodies
  - Given to Rh negative mothers who have Rh positive infants within 72 hours of birth to prevent isoimmunization
  - Trade names include RhoGAM
- IgE, 0.004% of total, present in respiratory and intestinal tracts
  - Involved in allergic and hypersensitivity reactions
        50% of patients with allergic diseases have elevated IgE levels
  - Binds to mast cells and basophils

Section II — ASSESSMENT

Looks at the body in general for signs of immune system activation or failure as well as for blood component abnormalities

HEALTH HISTORY

Chief complaint

- Common chief complaints for this system include:
    Excessive tiredness, lack of energy or weakness
    Inability to do some activities
    Bleeding easily from nose, rectum or gums
    Fainting or dizziness
    Night sweats
    Fevers
    Swollen glands
    Frequent infections

Family and personal history

- Family history is a significant factor in many anemias and bleeding disorders
    - Hemophilia, most common hereditary bleeding disorder due to clotting factor deficiencies
    - Anemia, some anemia's are genetic or inherited
        - Cooley's anemia (thalassemia major)
        - congenital hemolytic anemia
        - erythroblastic anemia
        - sickle cell anemia
- Personal history is vital to diagnose some hematologic and immune disorders
    - HIV status if known and date of last testing, check agency policy regarding HIV status disclosure
    - History of transfusions, some immune disorders are transmitted via the blood (HIV), assess date and reason for transfusion
    - Assess for history of multiple sexual partners, increased risk of HIV infection
    - History of intravenous drug abuse, increased risk of HIV
    - Toxins, exposure to occupational radiation or radiation therapy is a possible risk factor in the development of certain hematologic or immune disorders (leukemia, lymphoma, aplastic anemia, or multiple myeloma)

- Acute or chronic hemorrhage that may lead to anemia
- History of frequent or unusual infections which may indicate immune system dysfunction
- History of chronic disease which may precipitate anemia such as cancer or diseases that lead to nutritional deficiencies
- Obtain specific diagnoses and age at diagnosis when known
- Assess for presence and past treatment of the following:
  - Anemias: Achlorhydric, acquired hemolytic, pernicious, aplastic, iron-deficiency, deficiency and macrocytic

Hematologic and immune system testing

- Assess for tests completed or ordered and patient's knowledge and understanding of any test procedures or results

ASSESSMENT FORM

Chief Complaint

Patient's statement_____   Onset_____

Frequency_____ Duration_____ Other areas affected_____

Have you had this before?_____   Date_____

What treatment was given?_____

What do you think caused this?_____

What lifestyle changes have you had to make?_____

Personal and Family History

	Patient date	Family member		Patient Only date
Hemophilia (type)	_____	_____	HIV positive/AIDS	_____
Anemia (type)	_____	_____	Fatigue	_____
Immune system problem:	_____	_____	Night sweats	_____
Cancer, Lupus, etc.			Frequent fevers	_____

Weight loss_____   Lumps under arm pits, neck or groin_____

Frequent infection_____   Types_____

Bleeding from gums, rectum, nose, between periods_____

Easy bruising_____   Fainting_____   Dizziness _____

Blood transfusions_____   Exposure to radiation/toxic agent_____

Number of sexual partners_____   IV drug use_____

Hematologic and immune system testing

Blood tests_____   Urine tests_____

Lymphangiogram_____   Biopsy_____

Bone marrow exam_____   Bone scan_____

Current Treatments/Medications

Medication_____ Dose_____ Frequency_____ Route_____

Medication_____ Dose_____ Frequency_____ Route_____

Medication_____ Dose_____ Frequency_____ Route_____

PHYSICAL ASSESSMENT

Inspection:

General appearance_____

Shortness of breath or activity intolerance_____

Syncope_____ Skin color_____ Skin temperature_____

Ecchymosis_____ Petechiae_____

Skin lesions: Location_____ Size_____ Color_____

Temperature of surrounding skin_____ Drainage_____

Mucous membrane color_____ Gum condition_____

Mouth ulcerations/infections_____

Bleeding: Nose, gums, sores, rectum, hematuria_____

Ophthalmoscopic exam_____

Sclera color_____ Conjunctiva color_____

Palpation:

Temperature_____ Route_____ Pulse_____ Resp_____ B/P____/_____

Nodes: head, neck, axillary, epitrochlear, inguinal, popliteal

Location/size/tenderness_____

Palpable spleen_____ Liver_____

Tender or painful areas_____

Assessment Notes_____

_____

_____

_____

_____

PHYSICAL ASSESSMENT

- Assessment of the hematologic and immune systems should be done in the following order:
  1. Inspection
  2. Palpation
  3. Auscultation
- Patient should be undressed, gowned and covered with a sheet
  - Expose each area as it's examined and then re-drape
- As with any examination gloves should be worn when exploring areas of broken skin or areas with frank infection present
- When palpating lymph nodes use a gentle rotating motion

INSPECTION

General appearance

- Assess for appearance of weakness
  - If anemia is present there may not be enough RBCs to transport oxygen and fatigue or syncope may result
  - Does it require excessive effort for simple position changes?
- Visually assess body appearance for cachexia
  - May occur in immune disorders or cancer related to:
    - Poor appetite
    - Chronic diarrhea
    - Fatigue
    - Increased nutritional needs of body fighting off infection or neoplasm
- Assess patient's chosen positioning
  - Patient who is short of breath from anemia may best tolerate a sitting position
- Assess current comfort and pain level
  - Malaise is a common complaint for these systems
  - Severe abdominal pain may occur with some infections
  - Bone pain may be present in patients with some anemias, multiple myeloma

Skin

- Color—Pallor, cyanosis, or jaundice may be present in patients with hematologic or immune system disorders
- Ecchymosis (bruising) may be present with low platelets

- Petechiae (small circular purple discolorations) may be present related to thrombocytopenia of any cause
- Purpura (larger cutaneous areas of hemorrhage) may also be found in thrombocytopenia
- Hematoma (bleeding into tissues) occurs with coagulation disorders
- Skin lesions or rashes, note location, color and drainage if present
    - Multiple red, purple plaques or nodes on the skin may be related to Kaposi's sarcoma (AIDs)
    - Immune system dysfunction may lead to severe outbreaks of herpes zoster (shingles)
    - Candidiasis infection can infect skin, nails, vagina, vulva, or penis
        - Skin lesions are red and macerated
- Temperature — Hot, reddened, dry, edematous skin may indicate infection, intermittent elevated temperatures may occur
- Mucous membranes may have lesions, spots or color changes
    - Candidiasis (thrush) may occur in the patient with immune dysfunction
        - Painless white plaques that adhere to the tongue and oral mucosa
    - Multiple herpes simplex lesions may be found on oral mucosa
    - Cyanosis in mucous membranes indicates lack of oxygen
    - Bleeding gums may indicate low platelets
- Increased mucous secretions with nasal stuffiness, sneezing, frequent itching of the nose, eyes and throat are common in allergic reactions
- Assess the tongue, atrophy of the tongue may occur in some anemias related to deficiencies of cobalamin, folate, or iron
- Assess for bleeding from any orifice due to low platelets, clotting factor abnormality or other hematologic dysfunction

Neck

- Assess for visible evidence of masses or swelling indicating swollen lymph nodes
    - Lymph nodes may be swollen in acute infections or in chronic disorders such as lymphomas

Eyes

- Ophthalmoscopic examination may reveal bleeding fundi in coagulation disorders
- Sclera should be white without jaundice or hemorrhage
  - Jaundice may indicate hemolytic anemia
  - Retinal hemorrhages may be present in some anemias (aplastic)
- Pale conjunctiva may indicate anemia, normally rose colored

PALPATION

- Warm hands to avoid startling patient
- Assess pulse, rapid pulse may indicate the body is compensating for anemia by increasing the cardiac output or that infection is present
- Elevated temperature may indicate infection
- Palpate lymph nodes, lymph node enlargement is a common finding on physical examination, if enlarged assess for the following:
  - Location, the location of enlarged lymph nodes may aid in the diagnoses of disorders or infections and should be listed
    - Cervical node enlargement is often related to acute infections of sinuses, ears, pharynx, head, neck and mononucleosis
    - Supraclavicular lymph node enlargement is associated with malignancies, lymphoma, and thoracic infections
    - Axillary node enlargement is associated with infections or trauma to hands or arms, cat-scratch fever, lymphomas, breast cancer and melanoma
    - Inguinal node enlargement is associated with infections of the leg or foot, lymphoma, pelvic malignancies and venereal diseases
    - Generalized lymph node swelling is associated with infections (Epstein Barr, toxoplasmosis, tuberculosis, hepatitis, syphilis, HIV, histoplasmosis), malignancies (lymphomas, leukemia) and drug reactions
  - Size, enlarged lymph nodes may measure 1 cm to size of tennis ball
  - Mobility, fixed immobile nodes may indicate malignancy

- Pain, generally lymph node enlargement due to an infectious process will occur rapidly causing pain as nodes stretch
- Firm, fixed, nontender lymph nodes are frequently associated with metastatic tumors
- Large, firm, mobile, nontender, rubbery lymph nodes are associated with lymphomas
- Palpate abdomen gently to prevent trauma
  - Palpate spleen, in the adult the spleen is not palpable unless enlarged, if the spleen is palpated note location and any tenderness
  - Enlarged spleen may occur in hemolytic anemia
  - Palpate the liver note location and tenderness

AUSCULTATION

- Auscultate for presence of heart murmurs or palpitations these may indicate the body is compensating for anemia by increasing the cardiac output
  - Heart palpitations may be a complaint if patient has hemolysis with a rapidly falling hemoglobin

Section III — LABORATORY AND DIAGNOSTIC TESTS

In the following section traditional laboratory values and SI units are given, it is important to recognize that "normal" values vary from laboratory to laboratory. Check the "normal" values at the agency or institution where the test is performed. Most labs print their normal values on the laboratory reporting slips or page.

Table of Common Laboratory Tests

Test Name	Indications	Comments
AIDS serology Immune system Blood test **Normal:** No HIV antigens or antibodies	R/O HIV infection	**Regarding collection:** Signed informed consent may be required, check agency policy Use red-top tube collect 7-10 ml Follow agency policy regarding the labeling of specimen (number may be assigned for confidentiality) **Results:** ELISA test is repeated if first is positive. If both are positive the Western Blot test is completed to validate the results Check agency policy regarding the reporting of any positive results
AIDS T-lympho-cyte cell markers (CID4 marker, CD4%, CDF:CD8 ratio) Immune system Blood test **Normal:** CD4 >1000/mm3	HIV infection AIDS	**Regarding collection:** Use green-top tube collect 10 ml Use purple-top tube collect 5 ml Record collection time on lab slip Do not refrigerate sample **Results:** CD4 cell counts are used to assess the infection progress in HIV pts
Antideoxyribo-nuclease-B titer (Anti-DNase-B) Immune system Blood test **Normal:** < or = 85 units	Rheumatic fever Poststreptococcal glomerulonephritis	**Regarding collection:** Use red-top tube for collection **Results:** Increased titer of two or more increments between acute and convulsants indicates that streptococcal infection occurred

Test Name	Indications	Comments
Anti-DNA antibody Immune system Blood test **Normal:** No or low antibody levels	Systemic lupus erythematosus (SLE)	**Regarding collection:** Use red-top tube for collection **Results:** 40-80% of patients with SLE have high titers Titers may also be high in some rheumatic & liver disorders
Antimitochondrial antibody (AMA) & anti-smooth muscle antibody (ASMA) Immune system Blood test **Normal:** No AMA's at titers >1.5 No ASMA's at titers >1:20	Biliary cirrhosis Obstructive jaundice Chronic hepatitis	**Regarding collection:** Use red-top tube collect 7-10 ml **Results:** Increased levels in Cirrhosis, hepatic obstruction, autoimmune diseases, pernicious anemia, Thyroiditis, Addison's disease
Antinuclear antibody (ANA) Immune system Blood test **Normal:** No ANA titer in a titer dilution >1:32	Systemic lupus erythematosus (SLE) Suspected autoimmune disorders Rheumatoid arthritis	**Regarding collection:** Use red-top tube collect 7-10 ml List any of the following drugs on lab slip: acetazolamide, anino-salicylic acid, chlorprothixene, chlorothiazides, griseofulvin, hydralazine, penicillin, phenyl-butazone, phenytoin sodium, pro-cainamide, streptomycin, sulfonamides, steroids and tetracyclines **Results:** Increased in autoimmune disorders, chronic hepatitis, mononucleosis, leukemia or cirrhosis
Anti-thrombin III (AT-III, Heparin cofactor) Hematologic system Blood test **Normal:** Plasma: >50% of control value Serum: 15-34% lower than plasma Immunologic: 17-30 mg/dL Functional: 80-120%	Disseminated intravascular coagulation (DIC) Hypercoagulation Heparin therapy Deep vein thrombosis	**Regarding collection:** Check agency policy — Use blue or red-top tube **Results:** Increased in kidney transplant Decreased in coagulation disorders, familial deficiency of AT-III

Test Name	Indications	Comments
Bleeding time Hematologic system Blood test **Normal:** 1-9 minutes (Ivy)	History of bleeding Easy bruising Familial bleeding	**Regarding collection:** Usually performed by lab personal Cleanse inner forearm with alcohol Place BP cuff on upper arm, inflate to 40 mm Hg Puncture cleansed site 1mm deep Record time of puncture Blot blood drops every 30 seconds until bleeding stops (not site) Record time bleeding stops Determine bleeding time in mins Remove BP cuff & apply dressing If bleeding >10 mins, stop test Record on lab slip any aspirin, anticoagulants, dextran, cold indomethacin or streptokinase use **Results:** Prolonged bleeding in bone marrow failure, DIC, thrombocytopenia, clotting factor deficiencies, liver disease
Blood typing **ABO group** Hematologic system Blood test **Normal:** Compatibility	Blood transfusion Pregnancy Pre-operative surgical patients Newborns	**Regarding collection:** Use red-top tube collect 7-14 ml **Results:** Type A has A antigens on RBCs Type B has B antigens on RBCs Type AB has A & B antigens on RBCs Type O has neither A nor B antigens Whether Rh antigens are present (Rh positive) or absent (Rh negative)
Coagulating **factor** concentration Hematologic sys- tem Blood test **Normal:** 50-200% of normal levels found	Suspected coagulation factor deficiency Hemophilia	**Regarding collection:** Use blue-top tube collect 7-10 ml **Results:** Test measures the following factors I – fibrinogen II – prothrombin V – proaccelerin VII – proconvertin stable factor VIII – antihemophilic factor IX – Christmas factor X – Stuart factor XI – plasma thromboplastin factor XII – Hageman factor
Complement **assay** **Immune system** Blood test **Normal:** 75-160 u/ml or 75-160 u/L (SI)	Autoimmune diseases Serum sickness	**Regarding collection:** Use red-top tube collect 7-10 ml **Results:** Increased levels in MI, cancer, colitis and rheumatic fever Decreased levels in autoimmune disorders, serum sickness, kidney transplant rejections, rheumatoid arthritis, hepatitis & cirrhosis

Test Name	Indications	Comments
Complete blood count (CBC) Hematologic system Blood test with 6 major components **Normal:** Hemoglobin: Male 14-18 g/dL or 8.7-11.2 mmol/L Female 12-16 g/dL or 7.4-9.9 mmol/L Hematocrit: Male 42-52% or Female 37-47% RBC count: Male 4.7-6.1 million/mm3 Female 4.2-5.4 million/mm3 WBC count: 5,000-10,000/mm3 See also WBC differential	Routine test done for a variety of reasons to include: R/O anemia R/O blood loss R/O infection R/O blood cell changes Hospital admission Pending surgery	**Regarding collection:** Use lavender-top tube collect 3 ml Keep tourniquet on <90 seconds to prevent hemolysis **Results:** A variety of disorders and diseases may alter any one or all of the components of the CBC See section on complete blood count at the end of this chapter for more detailed information
Coomb's test, direct Immune system Blood test **Normal:** Negative	Suspected reaction to transfusion Suspected Rh incompatability in newborn	**Regarding collection:** Use lavender-top tube collect 5-7ml Cord blood is used in newborn List any medications patient is taking on lab slip **Results:** Positive results reported as trace to +4 depending on severity of the reaction (4 being most severe)
Coomb's test, indirect Immune system Blood test **Normal:** Negative	Preparation for blood transfusion to determine compatibility	**Regarding collection:** Use red-top tube collect 7 ml List any medications taken on the laboratory slip **Results:** "Screen" part of type and screen If positive then antibody screening to prevent incompatible transfusion will be done
D-dimer test Hematologic system Blood test **Normal:** Negative	Suspected DIC	**Regarding collection:** Use blue-top tube for collection **Results:** Increased in DIC above 250 ng/ml May also be increased in deep-vein thrombosis, pulmonary embolism, malignancy, sickle cell anemia

Test Name	Indications	Comments
Euglobulin lysis time Hematologic system Blood test **Normal:** 1.5-6 hrs	MI patients who are on streptokinase or urokinase therapy Suspected DIC	**Regarding collection:** Patient should not exercise before Use blue-top tube collect 5 ml Avoid agitation of blood sample Place on ice and send to lab ASAP **Results:** Shortened lysis time means increase in fibrinolysis and may indicate: Incompatible blood transfusion, leukemia, shock, streptokinase or urokinase therapy, thrombocytopenia trauma, cirrhosis
Ferritin Hematologic system Blood test **Normal:** Male 12-300 ng/mL or 12-300 ug/L Female 10-150 ng/l or 10-300 ug/L	Iron deficiency Anemia Protein deficiency	**Regarding collection:** Use red-top tube collect 5-7 ml **Results:** Decreased levels in iron deficiency anemia or protein deficiency Increased levels in megaloblastic or hemolytic anemia, hemosiderosis, hemochromatosis, hepatocellular disease, Hodgkin's disease
Fibrinogen Hematologic system Blood test **Normal:** 200-400 mg/dL or 2.0-4.0 g/L	Suspected bleeding disorders	**Regarding collection:** Use blue-top tube for collection **Results:** Decreased in disseminated intra-vascular coagulation, fibrinolysis, coagulation deficiencies, liver disease, trauma, and eclampsia
Folic acid Hematologic system Blood test **Normal:** 5-20 ug/mL or 14-34 mmol/L	Suspected hemolytic disorder Suspected folic acid deficiency	**Regarding collection:** Use red-top tube collect 7-10 ml Avoid hemolysis during collection List medications taken on lab slip **Results:** Decreased in malnutrition, liver disease, pregnancy, alcoholism, hemolytic and folic acid deficiency anemias Increased in pernicious anemia or vegetarianism
Hemoglobin electrophoresis Hematologic system Blood test **Normal:** Hgb A1 = 95-98% Hgb A2 = 2-3% Hgb C = 0% Hgb D = 0% Hgb F = 0.8-2% Hgb S = 0%	Sickle cell anemia or other abnormal forms of hemoglobin	**Regarding collection:** Use lavender-top tube collect 10 ml **Results:** Hgb C 90-100% with Hgb C disease Hgb F 1-3% with Thalassemia minor Hgb F 65-100% Thalassemia major Hgb H 5-30% with Hgb H disease Hgb S 20-40% with Sickle cell trait Hgb S 80-100% with Sickle cell disease Abnormalities of Hgb are known as hemoglobinopathies

Test Name	Indications	Comments
Human T-cell lymphotrophic I/II antibody (HTLV) Immune system Blood test **Normal:** Negative	T-cell leukemia Hairy cell leukemia	**Regarding collection:** Use red-top tube collect 7 ml **Results:** Positive result indicates infection which is associated with T-cell & hairy cell leukemia in adults, however, infection can occur with no malignancy
Immunoglobulin electrophoresis Immune system Blood test **Normal:** IGA 85-385 mg/dL IgD minimal IgE minimal IGG 565-1765 mg/dL IgM 55-375 mg/dL	Immune deficiencies Autoimmune diseases Chronic infections Multiple myeloma Hypersensitivity Intrauterine fetal infections	**Regarding collection:** Use red-top tube collect 7-10 ml List any immunizations/vaccinations within 6 months on lab slip List gamma globulin, hydralazine, isoniazid, phenytoin, procainamide, tetanus toxoid or antitoxin on lab slip if taken by patient **Results:** Increased IgA levels with cirrhosis rheumatic fever, alcoholism, GI or hepatic cancer & chronic infections Decreased IgA with malignancies, agammaglobulinemia, chemotherapy, & inflammatory bowel disease Increased IgE with allergies, IgE decrease with agmmaglobulinemia Increased IgG with liver disease, chronic infection, malnutrition, sarcoidosis, rheumatic fever, multiple myeloma, hyperimmunization Decreased IgG with amyloidosis, leukemia, preeclampsia, lymphoid hyperplasia & agammaglobulinemia Increased IgM levels with viral infections, macroglobulinemia, rheumatoid arthritis, brucellosis, malaria or fungal infections Decreased IgM with leukemia, agammaglobulinemia, lymphoid hyper-plasia and amyloidosis
Iron level & total iron-binding capacity (TIBC) Hematologic system Blood test **Normal:** Iron 60-190 ug/dL or 13-31 umol/L TIBC 25-420 ug/dL or 45-73 umol/L Transferrin 200-400 ug/dL	Iron deficiency or Iron excess	**Regarding collection:** Assess for recent blood transfusion NPO except water for 12 hrs before testing Use red-top tube collect 5-7 ml Avoid hemolysis of sample List medications taken on lab slip **Results:** Increased levels with lead toxicity iron poisoning, hemolytic anemia, hemosiderosis, hemochromatosis and hepatitis Decreased in malnutrition, chronic blood loss, iron deficiency anemia

Test Name	Indications	Comments
Lupus (LE cell) **erythematosus test** Immune system Blood test **Normal:** No LE cells found	System lupus erythematosus (SLE)	**Regarding collection:** Use red-top tube collect 7-10 ml List medications taken on lab slip **Results:** 70-80% of patients with SLE have positive test (LE cells found) Usually ordered daily for 3 days as may be negative then positive Also positive in rheumatic diseases
Lyme disease test Immune disease Blood test **Normal:** Negative	Suspected lyme disease	**Regarding collection:** Use red-top tube collect 7-10 ml **Results:** Positive — lyme disease
Mononucleosis spot test Immune system Blood test **Normal:** Negative	Suspected infectious mononucleosis	**Regarding collection:** Use red-top tube collect 7-10 ml **Results:** Positive result with infectious mononucleosis, chronic Epstein-Barr virus infection, chronic fatigue syndrome, Burkitt's lymphoma
Partial thrombo-plastin time (PTT) Hematologic system Blood test **Normal:** 60-70 seconds acti-vated time is 30-40 seconds-APTT	Suspected clotting deficiencies Heparin therapy	**Regarding collection:** If on heparin, draw 30-60 mins before next dose is due Use blue-top tube, collect 10 ml **Results:** Therapeutic range during heparin therapy is 1.5-2.5 times normal <50 seconds APTT on heparin is below therapeutic >100 seconds APTT risk of serious bleeding, report either to primary care provider Decreased levels with extensive CA or early DIC Increased levels with clotting factor deficiency, DIC, leukemia, hemophilia, cirrhosis of liver, heparin therapy

Test Name	Indications	Comments
Protein electro-phoresis Immune system Blood test **Normal:** Total protein 6.4-8.3 g/dL or 64-83.0 g/L (SI) Albumin 3.5-5.0 g/dL or 35-50 g/L Alpha1 globulin 0.1--0.3 g/dL or 103 g/L (SI) Alpha2 globulin 0.6-1.0 g/dL or 6-10 g/L (SI) Beta globulin 0.7-1.1 g/dL or 7-11 g/L (SI)	Inflammation Nephrotic syndrome Hypoprotein problem	**Regarding collection:** Use red-top tube collect 7-10 ml List any medications on lab slip **Results:** Decreased albumin with malnutrition and nephrotic syndrome Increased Alpha 1 with inflammatory diseases or malignancy, decreased Alpha1 with Childhood emphysema Increased Alpha2 with nephrotic syndrome or acute inflammation, decreased Alpha2 with hemolysis Increased Beta1 with lipoprotein disorders, decreased Beta1 with malnutrition and hypoprotein Increased gamma globulin with acute infection, multiple myeloma, chronic inflammatory diseases, malignancy, dysproteinemias
Platelet count Hematologic system Blood test **Normal:** 150,000-400,000 mm3	Part of CBC Bleeding Easy bruising Leukemia, anemia Chemotherapy	**Regarding collection:** Use lavender-top tube collect 5ml List meds taken on lab slip **Results:** Increased indicates thrombocytosis Decreased indicates thrombocyto-penia
Prothrombin time (PT) Hematologic system Blood test **Normal:** 11.0-12.5 seconds 85-100%	Coumarin therapy Liver disease	**Regarding collection:** Use blue-top tube collect 5-7 ml If warfarin is being taken, draw before daily dose List any medications on lab slip **Results:** Increased levels with hepatitis, cirrhosis, Vit K deficiency, bile obstruction, coumarin, DIC
Rabies neutraliz-ing antibody test Immune system Blood test	Suspected rabies infection	**Regarding collection:** Use red-top tube collect 7-10 ml **Results:** Positive results indicate exposure to rabies virus or vaccine
Reticulocyte count Hematologic system Blood test **Normal:** 0.5-2%	Assess bone marrow function Anemia	**Regarding collection:** Use lavender-top tube collect 7 ml **Results:** Increased in hemolytic anemia, leukemia, hemorrhage Decreased in pernicious anemia, folic acid deficiency, cirrhosis of liver, aplastic anemia, bone marrow failure, chronic infection

Test Name	Indications	Comments
Rheumatoid factor Immune system Blood test **Normal:** Negative, <60U/mL	Rheumatoid arthritis Systemic lupus erthematosus	**Regarding collection:** Use red-top tube collect 7 ml **Results:** Increased in rheumatoid arthritis, autoimmune disease, viral infection subacute bacterial endocarditis, mononucleosis, leukemia, cirrhosis
Sickle cell test Hematologic system Blood test **Normal:** No sickle cells	Suspected sickle cell trait or anemia	**Regarding collection:** Use lavender-top tube collect 7ml **Results:** Only a screening test for sickle cell anemia or trait

Table of Common Diagnostic Tests

Test Name	Indications	Comments
Bone marrow aspiration **Normal:** Active blood cell production	Suspected or confirmed cancer Aplastic anemia Other hematologic problems	**Pre-procedure:** Signed consent form is required Review lab work for coagulation abnormality and report if found Pre-medication may be ordered Explain procedure to patient Place patient in prone or on side Local anesthetic will be given Large bore needle will be inserted into bone and bone marrow aspirated Mod-severe pain with aspiration **Post-procedure:** Apply pressure to site and bandage Bedrest for 30-60 minutes Assess for bleeding, shock & pain
Lymphangio-graphy X-ray with contrast dye **Normal** sized lymph nodes with normal function	Suspected cancer involving lymph nodes	**Pre-procedure:** Signed consent form may be required Assess for allergy to iodine or dye Inform patient contrast dye may be blue in color and result in blue nodes with normal tinge to urine Procedure requires patient to lie still for a long period of time, pre-medication may be ordered Dye will be infused using infusion pump over 90 minutes then x-rays will be taken, repeated in 24 hours **Post-procedure:** Assess vital signs and incision Skin may be bluish for 24 hours

THE COMPLETE BLOOD COUNT (CBC)

Definition:
- A laboratory test that includes six components:
  - RBCs   RBC indices (MCV, MCH, MCHC)
  - WBCs   WBC differential
  - Hemoglobin (Hgb)
  - Hematocrit (Hct)
- Platelets are often ordered or included automatically

Function/Uses of the CBC:
- Ordered routinely at admission or prior to surgical procedures
  - To detect anemias
- To determine blood loss during trauma, surgery or childbirth
- To detect blood cell changes or infections

CBC Values:

	Female	Male	Child	Newborn
RBC $X10^{12}$/L	4.2-5.4	4.6-6.2	3.8-5.5	3.8-7.2
WBCs $X10^{9}$/L	4.5-11.0	4.5-11.0	6.0-17.00	9.0-30.00
Hgb g/dl	12-16	13.5-18	11-16	14-24
mmol/L	1.86-2.48	2.09-2.79		
Hct	38-47%	40-54%	36-38%	42-54%
volume fraction	0.38-0.47	0.40-0.54		
MCV cu mcg	78-95	78-95	82-91	96-108
MCH pg	27-33	27-33	27-31	32-34
MCHC	32-36%	32-36%	32-36%	32-33%
concentration fraction	0.32-0.36	0.32-0.36	0.32-0.36	0.32-0.33
Platelets cu mm	150000-400000		150000-300000	
$X10^{12}$/L	0.15-0.4	0.15-0.4	0.15-0.3	0.15-0.3

Red Blood Cells (Erythrocytes):
- Make up 99% of blood cells
- Formed in red bone marrow, body produces over 2 million RBCs per second with approximately 35 trillion in the circulation
- The life span of a healthy RBC is approximately 120 days
- Contain hemoglobin which attracts oxygen and carbon dioxide
- RBC count is elevated in persons living at higher altitudes to compensate for a lower atmospheric oxygen concentration

Terms used to describe red blood cells:
Achromatic — colorless, hemoglobin has been dissolved
Erythroblast — immature precursor of erythrocyte
Erythrocytopenia — deficiency of RBCs
Erythrocytosis — increase in circulating RBCs
Polychromatic — uneven staining on laboratory examination
Macrocyte — abnormally large RBCs
Poikilocytosis — abnormal RBC shape

Decreased RBCs	Increased RBCs
Hemorrhage	Polycythemia vera
Aplastic anemia	Dehydration
Cooley's anemia	Increased altitudes
Iron deficiency anemia	Cor pulmonale
Leukemias	
Multiple myeloma	
Kidney disorders	
Pregnancy	
Excessive hydration	

White Blood Cells (Leukocytes):
- Make up less than 1% of all blood cells
- Primary function is to fight infection
- Two major types of WBCs with several subtypes
- Granulocytes which are formed in the bone marrow
  - basophils
  - eosinophils
  - neutrophils
- Agranulocytes which are formed in the lymph tissue and bone marrow
  - lymphocytes (includes B-lymphocytes and T-lymphocytes)
  - monocytes

Terms used to describe white blood cells
Leukopenia — decrease in WBCs
Leukocytosis — an increase in WBCs

Leukoblast — immature precursor of leukocyte
Leukocytopenia — deficiency of WBCs
Leukocytosis — increase in circulating leukocytes (infection)

Decreased WBCs	Increased WBCs
Aplastic anemia	Tuberculosis
Pernicious anemia	Pneumonia
Malaria	Meningitis
Alcoholism	Tonsillitis
Antibiotic use	Appendicitis
Some chemotherapeutic agents	Pe ritonit is
	Pancreatitis
	Gastritis
	Rheumatic fever
	Myocardial infarction
	Burns
	Peptic ulcer
	Leukemias
	Rheumatoid arthritis
	Trauma
	Sickle cell anemia
	Fever
	Convulsions

Hemoglobin (Hgb):

* Composed of heme (iron containing pigment) and globin (a protein)
* Function is to combine with oxygen to form oxyhemoglobin for transport to cells or to combine with CO_2 to form carboxyhemoglobin for transport from the cells to the lungs
* Gives blood its red color
* Elevated in persons living in higher altitudes to compensate for a lower atmospheric oxygen concentration

Terms used to describe hemoglobin

Achromatic — colorless RBCs due to hemoglobin dissolving.
Hemoglobins — found in sickle-cell disorders
Hemoglobinemia — excessive hemoglobin in plasma
Hemoglobinopathies — diseases of hemoglobin

Decreased Hgb	Increased Hgb
Anemias	Chronic obstructive pulmonary disease (COPD)
Hemorrhage	Congestive heart failure (CHF)
Kidney disease	Dehydration
Leukemias	Polycythemia
Lymphomas	Severe burns
Pregnancy	
Slow chronic blood loss	
Thalassemia	

Hematocrit (Hct):

- Measures the % of blood volume occupied by blood cells
- When drawn by capillary tube Hct may be falsely low
- Requires blood sample be centrifuged for 2-3 minutes to separate the plasma from the blood cells

Decreased Hct	Increased Hct
Anemias Hemorrhage Kidney disease Leukemias Lymphomas Multiple myeloma Peptic ulcer Systemic lupus erythematosus Vitamin deficiencies	COPD, Late Dehydration Polycythemia vera Transient cerebral ischemia (TIAs)

RBC Indices:

- MCV is the mean cell volume
  - Measures the size of RBCs in cubic microns
  - Calculated as follows: MCV = HCT X 1000/RBC Count
- MCH is the mean cellular hemoglobin
  - Measures the weight of hemoglobin in RBC
  - Calculated as follows MCH = Hb X 10/RBC Count
- MCHC is the mean cellular hemoglobin concentration
  - Measures the concentration of hemoglobin in the RBCs
  - Calculated by either formula below
  - MCHC = Hgb/Hematocrit   or   MCHC = (MCH/MCV) X 100

Terms used to describe the red blood cell indices

Microcytic — abnormally small RBCs less than 5 microns
Macrocytic — abnormally large RBCs greater than 10 microns
Megalocyte — abnormally large RBC

	Decreased	Increased
MCV	Anemia, iron def. Anemia, sickle cell Carcinoma Lead poisoning Radiation Thalassemia Rheumatoid arthritis	Anemia, aplastic Anemia, pernicious Hypothyroidism
MCH	Anemia, chlorotic Anemia, iron def. Anemia, microcytic	Anemia, blind loop Anemia, macrocytic Anemia, pernicious

	Decreased	Increased
MCH	Anemia, chlorotic Anemia, iron def. Anemia, microcytic	Anemia, blind loop Anemia, macrocytic Anemia, pernicious
MCHC	Anemia, hypochromic Anemia, iron def. Excessive hydration Thalassemia	Dehydration, severe

WBC Differential (Diff):

- Provides individual counts of various types of leukocytes to assist in diagnosis
- Values are expressed in percentages

The Granulocytes:

- Neutrophils — Most common leukocyte (50-70%)
  - First line of defense against infections through the inflammatory process by ingesting and killing bacteria and small particles via phagocytosis
- Eosinophil 1-3% of leukocytes
  - Release chemicals that aid in killing of infectious agents
- Basophils make up only 0.4-1% of leukocytes
  - Release histamine and heparin and other chemicals at sites of injury or infection

The Agranulocytes:

- Lymphocytes make up 25-35% of leukocytes and are divided into two major types:
  - B cells that produce antibodies
  - T cells that aide in cellular immunity
- Monocytes make up 4-6% of leukocytes
  - Largest of all leukocytes, they ingest large particles via phagocytosis
  - Respond late in illness but live longer than other WBC's

Terms used to describe white blood cell differential

Eosinophilia — abnormal increase in eosinophils in blood
Lymphocytopenia — decreased lymphocytes in blood
Lymphocytosis — increased lymphocytes in blood
Monocytopenia — decreased monocytes in blood
Monocytosis — increased monocytes in blood
Neutropenia — decreased neutrophils in blood
Leukolysis — destruction of leukocytes

	Decreased	**Increased**
Neutrophils	Anemia, aplastic Anemia, iron def. B_{12} and folate def. Dialysis Hypopituitarism Infectious mononucleosis Leukemia Malaria Septicemia, severe Systemic lupus erythematosus Viral illness	Appendicitis Bacterial infections Burns Carcinomas COPD Diabetic ketosis Hodgkin's disease Kidney failure Myocardial infarction Pancreatitis Peritonitis Pneumonia Pregnancy, late-labor Rheumatic fever Rheumatoid arthritis
Eosinophils	Burns Cushing's syndrome Post-steroid use Trauma	Addison's disease Allergic reactions Asthma Carcinomas COPD Gastritis Hodgkin's lymphoma Kidney disease Helminth infection Phlebitis Thrombophlebitis
Basophils	Hyperthyroidism Post-steroid use Pregnancy Rheumatic fever Stress	Chronic myeloid leukemia Hodgkin's lymphoma Polycythemia vera
Lymphocytes	Anemia, aplastic Carcinomas, selected Guillain Barre Kidney disease Multiple sclerosis Myasthenia gravis Systemic lupus erythematosus Trauma	Chicken pox Chronic infections Hepatitis Infectious mononucleosis Lymphocytic leukemias Measles Multiple myeloma Mumps Pertussis Viral illnesses
Monocytes	Anemia, aplastic Hodgkin's lymphoma Lymphocytic leukemia	Infectious mononucleosis Leukemia Multiple myeloma Parasitic infection Recovery period from acute bacterial infection Rheumatoid arthritis Sickle cell anemia Systemic lupus erythematosus Tuberculosis Typhoid Ulcerative colitis

Platelets:
- Primary function is to aide in blood coagulation: after tissue injury platelets stick or adhere to the endothelium and each other to form a plug
- Severe decrease leads to hemorrhage

Terms used to describe platelets
Thrombocyte — blood platelet
Thrombocytopenia — decrease in platelets

Decreased Platelets	Increased Platelets
Anemia, aplastic	Acute hemorrhage
Burns	Bone fracture
Chemotherapeutic agents	Carcinomas, selected
Eclampsia/Preeclampsia	Polycythemia vera
Infectious mononucleosis	Postpartum mothers
Leukemias	Trauma
Massive transfusions	
Thrombocytopenic purpura	

Section IV — PROCEDURES
BLOOD TRANSFUSIONS
Blood Products and Indications for Use:

Product	Indication	Comments
Whole blood, no elements removed	Hemorrhage Open heart surgery Exchange transfusion	450 cc/unit approximate
PRBC packed red blood cells	Most often used Chronic/acute loss GI bleeding Surgery, trauma	250-300 cc/unit approximate May dilute with saline Should infuse within 4 hrs
Platelets	Low platelet count <20,000-50,0000	50 cc/unit, IV push Ordered in multiple units
Washed RBCs WBCs almost completely gone	Renal failure Hx of transfusion reaction	300 cc/unit approximate Very expensive Less chance of reaction
Cryoprecipitate	Hemophilia A on Willebrand's fibrinogen deficiency	10 cc/unit approximate Contains factor VII & XIII
Fresh frozen plasma	Undx bleeding Liver disease >10 transfusions Immune globulin deficiency	150-250 cc/unit plasma Thaw about 1 hour Factors II, VII, IX, X,XI, XII, XIII, heat labile to V, and VII
Rho gam	Rh- mom with Rh+ baby to provide antibody to Rh factor	Given <72hrs of birth Rho D immune globulin
Albumin 5% no need for compatibility	Acute blood loss	Plasma expander made from plasma precipitate Available in most pharmacies
Albumin 25%	Burns Hypoalbuminemia	Plasma volume expander Draws ECF into circulation

General Guidelines for Transfusing Blood Products:
- Check orders for type, amount, and time of transfusion
- Obtain type and crossmatch laboratory work, patient band should be checked prior to drawing and sending sample
- Prepare the blood tubing according to manufactures instruction
  - Tubing has two connectors: one for blood product and one for normal saline (NS)
- Start the infusion of NS at a KVO (keep vein open) rate

- When blood arrives double check it with a second nurse, check for correct:
  - Type of blood product and time to be infused (orders)
  - Donor number (against tag and bag)
  - ABO group and compatibility
  - Expiration date of blood, and bag for punctures, product color and consistency
  - At bedside check the patient's identification band for correct name, hospital number and blood identification numbers (always check orders, band, blood tag, and bag)
  - Return the product if any discrepancies exist
- Obtain baseline vital signs and record
- Attach labeled bag to blood tubing, close off the NS and open clamp for blood
- Record date and time transfusion was begun
- Monitor patient closely:
  - Assess vital signs after first five minutes then every 15 minutes X2, and every 30 minutes thereafter
- Assess for any transfusion reaction to include:
  - Temperature increase greater than 1.8 degrees
  - Drop in blood pressure
  - Onset of back or chest pain
  - Skin rash
  - Sudden unexplained feelings of doom
  - Wheezing
  - Cyanosis
- If any adverse reaction occurs:
  - STOP THE TRANSFUSION, close the clamp to the blood
  - Open the clamp to the saline
  - Stay with the patient and assess the vital signs
  - Have someone call the primary care provider blood bank
  - Recheck the blood component with all the steps above
- Blood should be transfused within four hours, check orders for administration time
- If adverse reaction has occurred blood component and tubing are sent to the blood bank, blood and urine samples are obtained
- For allergic transfusion reactions (hives or skin rashes), an antihistamine may be ordered and the transfusion continued

Rules for Transfusion of Packed Red Blood Cells (PRBCs)

- Never add medications to blood components - hemolysis may occur
- Use only normal saline (NS) when transfusing blood
  - D5W may lyse the red blood cells being transfused
  - Lactated Ringers may cause clotting
- Never store blood in the unit refrigerator
  - If transfusion is delayed return blood to the blood bank
- Always use a peripheral line started with a large gauge needle
  - A central line is only used if ordered may lead to dysrhythmias
- For multiple transfusions, change filter every four hours to reduce the risk of bacterial growth
- Do not use a pressure bag for blood transfusions without an order as this increases hemolysis

HIV transmission risk:

- All prospective donors are screened to determine any risk factors
- If donor history shows any risk factor, the blood is discarded
- All donated blood is screened for HIV infection antibody
  - Any blood that is positive is discarded

Hepatitis transfusion risk:

- Post transfusion viral hepatitis is believed to occur in about 7-10% of all persons receiving blood transfusions

Charting Tips

- Chart all of the following during the blood transfusion
  - Reason for transfusion and total amount to be transfused
  - Blood unit number, donor number, ABO type, Rh type and expiration date of unit
  - Second person who checked blood component and title
  - Date and time transfusion begun
  - Vital signs at onset, after 5 min, 20 min, 35 min and then every 30 minutes, end of transfusion
  - Any reaction noted and actions taken
  - Time and Date of transfusion finish

Interventions for Hematolymphathic Problems

- When the immune and hematologic systems fail due to disease (AIDS or cancer) or from chemotherapeutic agents used to treat those disorders any of the conditions listed below may occur:
  - Anemia — reduction in RBCs

- Leukopenia — reduction in WBCs
- Thrombocytopenia — reduction in platelets
- Pancytopenia — reduction in all blood cells
- Interventions for each of these problems are listed below:

Anemia

- Monitor RBC level
- Monitor Hematocrit and Hemoglobin levels
- Assess for fatigue, dizziness, chills or shortness of breath, all of which are symptoms of a low red blood cell count
- Encourage periodic rest periods during the day
- Encourage the addition of foods high in iron to the diet such as green leafy vegetables, liver, and red meats
- Encourage getting out of bed slowly to prevent or reduce dizziness
- Assess the need for oxygen therapy and initiate if indicated
- Administer blood transfusions as ordered

Leukopenia

- Monitor white blood count and differential
- Inform physician of any abnormal values
- Assess for elevated temperature above 100 degrees F
- Assess for chills, sweating, diarrhea, burning on urination, sore throat or coughs
- Assess mouth for redness, open sores or ulcers, known as stomatitis or oral mucositis
- Instruct patient to report any of the above symptoms
- Instruct compromised patient how to avoid infection to include:
  - Washing hands frequently, especially before eating and after using the restroom
  - Avoiding crowds and anyone known to have respiratory or other contagious illnesses
  - Thorough cleansing of any cuts, scrapes, or wounds at once with soap and water
  - Use of an electric shaver to avoid abrasions from a razor
  - No cutting or tearing cuticles; a commercial preparation for cuticle removal should be used instead
  - Avoiding squeezing or scratching pimples or skin blemishes
  - Cleaning the anal area thoroughly after each bowel movement
  - Postponing elective dental work and surgical procedures

- If stomatitis is present instruct the patient to rinse mouth before and after eating with a normal saline solution: 1 tsp salt in 1 quart water

Thrombocytopenia:

- Monitor platelet count
- Assess for bruises and petechiae
- Assess for bleeding in stool, urine, saliva, phlegm, or sputum
- Apply pressure on any venipuncture sites for 5-10 minutes when low platelet count is present
- Avoid unnecessary venipunctures or intramuscular injections
- Monitor number of peri-pads during menstruation to assess for unusual amount of bleeding
- Instruct patient in how to avoid bleeding to include:
  - Use of an electric shaver, not a razor
  - Avoidance of any over the counter drug containing aspirin
  - Wearing shoes at all times, to prevent trauma to soles of feet
  - Instruct patient to avoid using dental floss
  - A soft foam toothbrush may be recommended to prevent trauma to gums, which may lead to bleeding
  - Avoid very hot or spicy foods, abrasive foods, such as tortilla chips, acidic foods or liquids
  - Encourage eating soft foods when ulcers are present

Pancytopenia

- All of the above interventions are appropriate for someone with pancytopenia
- The table below contains common problems and interventions that may be helpful when caring for a patient with problems in the hematologic or immune system

Problem	Intervention
Bad Breath (Halitosis)	Offer mints and gum Have normal saline available to use as a mouth rinse
Loss of Appetite	Provide small, frequent meals Provide attractive meals High calorie, high protein diet Encourage rest prior to meal
Nausea/Vomiting	Offer antiemetics as needed Remove bedpans or other offensive items immediately after use Serve foods at room temperature, better tolerated than hot or cold

Problem	Intervention
Nausea/Vomiting — cont'd	Don't serve liquids with meals or within 1 hour of eating Avoid foods that are fried, fatty or sweet as these increase nausea Avoid foods with strong odors Instruct patient to eat slowly and chew the food well to promote digestion Provide dry foods like toast, dry cereal, or crackers when nauseous Provide cool unsweetened drinks between meals (flat soda, ginger ale, or apple juice) Discuss relaxation techniques, music therapy or other non-traditional approaches
Dry Mouth	Provide ice chips Increase fluid intake Offer sugarless gum or hard candy Moisten dry foods with gravy or sauce prior to serving Offer lip balm for dry lips
Stomatitis	Assess condition of sores or ulcers daily Avoid serving highly spiced or acid foods Provide diet of soft unseasoned foods Discourage smoking which tends to irritate the problem Avoid commercial mouth washes, use saline instead to prevent irritation of tissues Brush teeth 3-4 times daily
Diarrhea	Increase fluids/force fluids include water, weak tea, broth or apple juice For severe diarrhea provide a clear liquid diet Provide a low residue diet Monitor input and output Avoid serving oily or greasy foods Avoid serving caffeine containing liquids Avoid milk and milk products, if they aggravate the diarrhea Encourage meticulous anal care after each bowel movement Provide anti-diarrheal agents as ordered
Constipation	Provide high fiber diet Increase fluid intake Increase physical activity Provide stool softener or laxative as ordered
Hair Loss (Alopecia)	Hair loss is usually temporary Encourage use of scarves, wigs, hats prior to severe hair loss
Sexual Dysfunction	Assess for loss of sexual function Encourage open discussion of fears with partner and physician Explain that fatigue, which often accompanies cancer treatment, can affect sexual desire Encourage rest periods if fatigue is a problem Cessation of menstruation or irregular menstrual cycles can occur with chemotherapy treatment Assess for dryness, itching of vaginal tissue, provide topical medication as ordered Encourage the use of birth control medications during chemotherapy to prevent pregnancy

Section V — Conditions

Human Immunodeficiency Virus (HIV) and Acquired Immune Deficiency Syndrome (AIDS)

Definition

- Infection with HIV-1 may result in an asymptomatic infected state to advanced AIDS, it is a broad spectrum disease
- AIDS stands for Acquired Immune Deficiency Syndrome
  - **Acquired**, meaning you did not inherit the disease
  - **Immune**, referring to the immune system
  - **Deficiency**, meaning the Immune system is impaired
  - **Syndrome**, a group of signs & symptoms that appear together
- The criteria for AIDS has undergone several revisions since the syndrome was first named, the current criteria is found below

CDC surveillance definition for AIDS (1993)

A. Indicator diseases diagnosed definitively in the absence of other causes of immunodeficiency and without laboratory evidence of HIV infection
- Candidiasis of the esophagus, trachea, bronchi or lungs
- Cryptococcoses, extra pulmonary
- Cryptosporidiosis with diarrhea persisting > 1 month
- Cytomegalovirus disease of any organ excluding liver, spleen, and lymph nodes in a patient >1 month of age
- Herpes simplex virus infection causing a mucocutaneous ulcer persisting >1 month; or bronchitis, pneumonia, or esophagitis in a patient > 1 month of age
- Kaposi's sarcoma in a patient < 60 years old
- Lymphoma of brain (primary) in a patient < 60 years old
- Lymphoid interstitial pneumonia and/or pulmonary lymphoid hyperplasia in a child < 13 years of age
- *Mycobacterium avium* complex or *M. kansaii* disease
- *Pneumocystis carinii* pneumonia (PCP)
- Toxoplasmosis of the brain in a patient > 1 month of age

B. Indicator diseases diagnosed definitively regardless of the presence of other causes of immunodeficiency and in the presence of laboratory evidence of HIV infection
- Any disease listed in section A

- Bacterial infections (multiple or recurrent) in children < 13 years of age caused by *Haemophilus*, *Streptococcus*, or other pyogenic bacteria
- Coccidioidomycosis, disseminated
- HIV encephalopathy
- Histoplasmosis, disseminated
- Isosporiasis with diarrhea persisting > 1 month
- Kaposi's sarcoma at any age
- Non-Hodgkin's lymphoma of B cell or unknown phenotype and having the histologic type of small noncleaved lymphoma or immunoblastic sarcoma
- Any mycobacterial disease, disseminated, excluding *M. tuberculosis*
- *M. tuberculosis*, extra pulmonary
- *Salmonella* (nontyphoid) septicemia, recurrent
- HIV wasting syndrome

C. Indicator diseases diagnosed presumptively in the presence of laboratory evidence of HIV infection
- Candidiasis of the esophagus
- Cytomegalovirus retinitis with loss of vision
- Kaposi's sarcoma
- Lymphoid interstitial pneumonia and/or pulmonary lymphoid hyperplasia in a child < 13 years of age
- Mycobacterial disease, disseminated
- *Pneumocystis carinii* pneumonia
- Toxoplasmosis of the brain in a patient > 1 month of age

D. Indicator diseases diagnosed definitively in the absence of other causes of immunodeficiency and in the presence of negative results for HIV infection
- *Pneumocystis carinii* pneumonia
- Other indicator diseases listed in section A and CD4+ T lymphocyte count < 400 cells/microliter

E. The 1993 expanded definition includes:
- All HIV-infected persons who have <200 CD4+ T lymphocyte counts/microliter, or a CD4+ T lymphocyte percentage of total lymphocytes of < 14
- Pulmonary tuberculosis
- Recurrent pneumonia
- Invasive cervical cancer

Prevalence

- HIV/AIDS is pandemic, the World Health Organization estimates 8-10 million persons are infected worldwide
- The CDC states that 1 in every 250 persons in the U.S. are infected with HIV-1
- Epidemic in the U.S.A., confirmed AIDS cases are on the rise:
  - In 1981, the first known cases were reported
  - By 1989 over 100,000 cases had been reported
  - By end of 1991 cases had reached 200,000
  - At the end of 1994 cases had reached 441,528
- At the end of 1994 the cumulative total deaths from HIV/AIDS in the U.S. was 270,870, with 3,391 deaths in children under 13
- HIV/AIDS is the 3rd leading cause of death in the 25-44 year old age group for males
- HIV/AIDS is one of the top five causes of death of women of childbearing age in the U.S.
- HIV/AIDS is the 6th leading cause of death among youths age 15-24 years of age in the U.S.
- HIV/AIDS is the leading cause of death for young males in San Francisco, Los Angeles and New York City

Etiology

- HIV-1 is the retro virus responsible for AIDS it contains a single strand of RNA and belongs to the subfamily lentiviruses
- In the usual cell DNA goes to RNA. Retro viruses contain the enzyme reverse transcriptase that can transcribe the viral RNA in the cytoplasm into DNA, the DNA with the virus can then splice itself to all the DNA cells of the body.
- HIV-1 does not directly cause the infections associated with AIDS it is lymphotropic (attacks the immune system), making the body too weak to fend off invaders
  - The bacteria and other infectious agents that the body could normally fight, now become life-threatening.
  - The symptoms are caused by opportunistic infectious agents and cancers that take advantage of the weakened body
- HIV is very specific when it attacks the immune system, preferring the T-cells (See also Immune response this chapter)
  - Prefers T4 lymphocytes (T4 helper cells), once inside a T-cell HIV-1 releases it's RNA strand which is converted to DNA

- The DNA then overtakes the T-cell nucleus where it manufactures more HIV
- The infected cell eventually dies and newly manufactured HIV are released to attack other T-cells
- The process continues until the body does not have enough T-cells to fight infection.
- HIV-1 is not transmitted by casual contact or even close nonsexual contact (social kissing, touching). Transmission requires an exchange of body substances containing cells infected with HIV
  - Blood or blood plasma
  - Semen or vaginal secretions
- The virus has been found in tears and saliva also but transmission from one person to another has not been reported.
- The three major routes of transmission are:
  - Sexual contact with an infected partner (may be vaginal, anal, or oral, heterosexual or homosexual)
    - Groups at particular risk include anyone who has had male to male sexual contact since 1977, any one having sexual contact with a prostitute or anyone who has had more than one sexual partner since 1977
  - Contamination with HIV infected blood
    - Contaminated hypodermic needles (intravenous drug abusers, accidental needle sticks in health care workers)
    - Transfusion of infected blood or blood products
    - Infected lymphocytes in blood can also be transferred through minute breaks in the skin or mucous membranes when blood contacts the skin, eyes, or mouth.
  - Transplacentally leading to congenital infection
    - The risk of an infected woman passing HIV onto her child is 15-40%
    - Approximately 80% of pregnant women with HIV infection are asymptomatic
    - Studies have also shown that HIV is present in breast milk and rare cases of transmission via breast milk have been reported

Symptoms of HIV infection

- HIV infection produces a broad spectrum of signs and symptoms based on the response of the individual, the presence of opportunistic infections and the CD4+ T cell count this produces stages of HIV infection.
- There are several different classification systems based on these stages
  - The Centers for Disease Control (CDC) Classification system:
    Group I Acute HIV syndrome
    Group II Asymptomatic infection
    Group III Persistent generalized lymphadenopathy
    Group IV Other diseases
    > Subgroup A Constitutional disease
    > Subgroup B Neurologic disease
    > Subgroup C Secondary infectious diseases
    > Subgroup D Secondary neoplasms
    > Subgroup E Other conditions
  - Another classification system depends on CD4+ T cell count
    - Early: CD4+ T cell count >500/ microliter
    - Intermediate: CD4+ T cell count 200-500/ microliter
    - Advanced CD4+ T cell count less than 200/ microliter
- Group I — Acute HIV syndrome
  - Occurs 3-6 weeks after primary infection in approximately 50-70% of those infected
  - Symptoms usually last 1-2 weeks and then subside
  - Fever, pharyngitis, headache, arthralgia, lethargy, malaise, anorexia, weight loss, rash, nausea, vomiting and diarrhea have been reported
  - Lymphadenopathy is reported in about 70% of patients
  - May develop meningitis, encephalitis, peripheral neuropathy or myelopathy during this period
- Group II — Asymptomatic infection
  - Amount of time spent in this stage varies with mode of infection, intravenous drug users generally have a shorter asymptomatic period than those infected sexually
  - Median time in one study for homosexual men was 10 years
  - While patient may be asymptomatic virus replication continues and the CD4+ T-cell count lowers

- Some patients have intermittent symptoms that are not persistent enough to be categorized as constitutional disease, these include malaise, lethargy, weakness and anorexia
- Group III — Persistent generalized lymphadenopathy
  - Lymph nodes >1 cm in two or more extringuinal sites for more than 3 months without an obvious cause
  - Nodes are discrete and freely moveable
  - Often the earliest symptom of HIV-1 infection
- Group IV — Other diseases
  Early Symptomatic disease — Constitutional disease
  - Usually when CD4+ T-cell count is < 500 the patient begins to develop signs and symptoms of clinical illness
  - In the past this was called AIDS-related complex (ARC)
  - Oral lesions are common to include thrush, hairy leukoplakia, and aphthous ulcers
  - Herpes zoster or shingles is seen in 10-20% of patients with HIV-1 infection
  - Other clinical conditions seen include molluscum contagiosum, basal cell skin carcinoma, headache, condyloma acuminata, oral or genital herpes
  Subgroup A — Constitutional disease
  - HIV wasting syndrome
    - Weight loss greater than 10%
    - Intermittent or constant fever
    - Chronic diarrhea or fatigue for more than 1 month in the absence of a defined cause
    - Major muscle wasting
    - Primary AIDS defining illness in Africa
    - 6th leading AIDS diagnosis in New York City
  Subgroup B — Neurologic Disease
  - May be related directly to HIV infection or to opportunistic infections or cancers
  - Neurologic disease related to opportunistic infections occurs in about 1/3 of all AIDS patients
    - Includes central nervous system infections from toxoplasmosis, cryptococcoses, multi focal leukoencephalopathy, CMV, HTLV-1, mycobacterium

tuberculosis, syphilis, and central nervous system lymphoma

- Aseptic meningitis may be seen throughout all stages of HIV infection
- Neurologic disease related directly to HIV infection may be demyelinating, inflammatory or degenerative.
- Most AIDS patients will have some type of neurologic problem
- Seizures may be a consequence of HIV infection
- AIDS dementia complex generally occurs late in HIV infection and presents with decline in cognitive ability, inability to concentrate, forgetfulness and motor problems such as gait disturbances, poor balance, and incontinence.
  - In about 10% of patients dementia is the initial problem

Subgroup C — Secondary infectious diseases

- Seen in advanced disease (CD4+ T cell count < 200)
- Leading cause of morbidity and mortality for AIDS patients
- 80% of AIDS patients die from secondary infectious diseases
- Caused by organisms that do not ordinarily cause disease unless the immune system is compromised
- Includes the following infections
  - *Pneumocystis carinii*
    Persistent nonproductive cough
    Shortness of breath, dyspnea, tachypnea
  - *Toxoplasma gondii*
    Disease caused by a protozoa
    Pneumonitis
    Hepatitis
    Encephalitis, brain abscess
  - *Isospora belli*
    A parasitic protozoan inhabiting small intestine
    Diarrhea lasting more than one month
  - *Crypto sporidia Micro sporidia*
    Disease caused by a protozoa
    Explosive diarrhea
    Diarrhea lasting more than one month
    Abdominal cramps
    Highly infectious

- *M. avium intracellulare*
  Disseminated disease may involve lung, bone
  marrow or liver
- *Mycobacterium tuberculosis*
  Mycobacterium avium (TB of birds) disseminated
  Chronic progressive pulmonary disease
  Extrapulomonary (found outside lungs as well)
- *Candida albicans*
  Thrush
  Vaginitis
  Esophagitis, may also be in trachea, bronchi, or lungs
- *Crytoptococcus neoformans*
  A systemic fungus infection
  May involve any organ of the body
  Pneumonia
  Brain or meninges often involved, brain abscess
- *Histoplasma encapsulatum*
  Histoplasmosis
  A systemic fungal respiratory disease
  Pneumonia
- *Cytomegalovirus*
  Herpes virus family infection
  Infection of an organ other than the liver, spleen, or
  lymph nodes in patient over 1 month of age
  Cytomegalovirus retinitis (loss of vision
  Esophagitis, colitis
  Pneumonia
- *Herpes simplex*
  Chronic mucocutaneous or disseminated herpes
  Perioral, perirectal or genital ulcers
  Mucocutaneous ulcer lasting longer than 1 month
  Bronchitis, pneumonitis or esophagitis over 1 month
- *Herpes zoster*
  May be local or disseminated
  Retinal necrosis
- *Treponema pallidum*
  Early syphilis
  Late or neurosyphilis

Subgroup D — Secondary neoplasms
- Kaposi's sarcoma (KS), a cancer
  - Most frequently diagnosed disorder in this subgroup
  - Diagnosed in patient under 60 years of age
  - Multiple red, purple plaques or nodes on skin
  - Elevated temperature
- Non-Hodgkin's lymphoma
  - B cell lymphoma or unknown phenotype
  - Burkitt on non-Burkitt lymphoma (noncleaved lymphoma)
- Primary lymphoma of the brain
  - Diagnosed in patient under 60 years of age

Components of initial examination for HIV

- *Complete medical history to include:*
- Assessment of risk factors for HIV/AIDS infection
  - History of sexual practices, this is important in both the etiology of HIV-1 infection and also for counseling to prevent the future spread of infection
  - History of any previous sexually transmitted diseases
  - History of intravenous drug use and needle sharing, important for etiology of infection and also to prevent spread of infection by counseling and education efforts
  - Blood transfusion history
- History of positive AIDS serology blood screening test with duration of time with known HIV-1 infection, previous treatments and illness related to HIV-1 infection
- History of previous TB skin tests and results or exposure to tuberculosis
- Due to the variety of opportunistic infections and the effects of primary HIV-1 infection a complete review of systems is needed
- History of weight loss, fatigue, frequent infections, night sweats, loss of appetite, intermittent elevations in temperature, skin rashes, diarrhea, swollen lymph nodes, chronic cough, shortness of breath, headache and seizures may all be reported
- Patient's understanding of diagnoses and treatment
- Patient's willingness to make required lifestyle changes
- *Physical examination to include:*
- General appearance, patient with active disease may have:
  - Muscle wasting and cachexia from HIV wasting syndrome

- Dyspnea on exertion and shortness of breath from PCP
- Seborrheic dermatitis may be present between eyebrows, forehead, and upper cheeks (common with PCP)
- Height and weight for baseline
- Vital signs
  - Temperature may be elevated from a variety of infections
  - Respiratory rate may be increased with PCP
- Thick white coating from thrush may be present on gums, tongue, or mouth due to thrush
- Difficulty swallowing may be related to esophagitis from candidiasis (esp. if thrush was found in mouth)
- Presence of skin rashes or ulcerations, unusual skin eruptions may occur due to more than one infection at the same time Possible infections include:
  - Scabies
  - Tinea infections
  - Common plantar warts
  - Condylomata
  - Herpesvirus infections
  - Herpes Zoster
  - Kaposi's sarcoma
  - Seborrheic dermatitis
  - Urticaria
- Assessment of lymph nodes for swelling, nodes are swollen in Group I to Group III disease but may not be swollen in Group IV when severe immune deficiency is present and nodes are hypoplastic
- Neurologic examination
- Mini-mental status examination to establish baseline mental functioning levels
- Presence of a non-productive cough (may occur for months)
- Auscultation of the lungs may be clear in PCP or rales may be noted
- Abdominal pain related to diarrhea or ascites may be present on abdominal palpitation
- Examination of the genitalia for ulcerations, skin lesion or discharges

- Examination of the rectum for ulcerations, condylomata, hemorrhoids, fistulas, abscesses or other skin lesions
- *Laboratory and diagnostic testing:*
- AIDS serology (ELISA) blood screening test is performed first and if positive twice the more sensitive Western Blot test is performed to determine infection with HIV-1
  - A negative test result does not mean that the person has not been exposed to HIV-1: It can take from 1-18 months for antibodies to appear in the blood
  - The test does not show whether the person has AIDS, it only shows whether they have antibodies to HIV
  - A positive HIV even without symptoms does mean the person can spread HIV
- CD4+ T cell count is the most accepted indicator of the progression of HIV-1, Normal level > 1000 per microliter
  - Patients with HIV-1 infection should have CD4+ T cell counts at least every 6 months and more often if condition indicates
  - CD4+ T cell counts under 500 per microliter indicates a need for antiviral therapy
  - CD4+ T cell counts under 200 per microliter with HIV infection is diagnostic for AIDS and also indicates a high risk of infection from Pneumocystits carinii
  - CD4+ T cell counts under 100 per microliter with HIV infection is diagnostic for AIDS and also indicates a high risk of infection from CMV and Mycobacterium avium-intracellulare (MAI)
- Protein electrophoresis for Beta2 micro globulin, the highest levels are found in patients with AIDS the lowest levels in patients with HIV infection who are asymptomatic therefore this test has a predictive value for AIDS
- CBC with WBC differential and platelet counts
  - For total lymphocyte count
  - To detect low platelets an early consequence of HIV
  - To detect anemia a common problem in Group IV stage HIV
- Electrolytes
- Liver and kidney chemistries
- Serum albumin to determine nutritional status, often decreased in later stages
- Chest X-ray to establish baseline, assess for and monitor disease progression of PCP or tuberculosis

- Pulmonary function studies to assess lung function
- VDRL or syphilis detection test to rule out syphilis
- Tuberculin test or PPD to rule out tuberculosis
- Stool cultures and stool for ova & parasites if diarrhea is present
- Abdominal CAT scans and endoscopy for diarrhea or ascites that is undiagnosed

Treatment of HIV/AIDS infection

- Since HIV can hide in the DNA material of the immune cells themselves, it is not detected by circulating antibodies. In addition, the virus multiplies and mutates very quickly leading to a change in the antigen's appearance. When antigens change quickly or often, the antibodies the person makes does not recognize and destroy the virus. For these reasons finding a cure or vaccine for HIV is difficult.
- HIV is a chronic, life threatening illness that requires comprehensive management
- Counseling and education about the potential for spread of this infection among sexual partners or during intravenous drug use is vital
- Counseling is also important to help the patient meet and verbalize fears and concerns
- It has been recommended that since AIDS patients with CD4+ Tcell counts < 200 cells/mircroliter often are unable to make their own treatment decisions that durable power of attorney be assigned or discussed as advanced stages of the disease approach
- Treatment also involves prevention of spread of HIV-1, steps to avoid exposure as a health care worker include:
  - Good skin care to prevent dry cracked skin that is more susceptible to infections
  - Wear gloves whenever you anticipate contact with any body fluids, such as urine, feces, saliva, pus or blood
  - Wear gowns when contact with blood, urine, feces, saliva or pus may occur to clothing
  - Wear goggles and a mask if blood or body fluids are likely to splash into eyes or mouth or for coughing patients who do not cover their mouth
  - Wear gloves when starting intravenous infusions
  - Never recap needles
  - Dispose of all syringes in a suitable container in the patient's room

- Cleanse thoroughly and report any needle sticks to your supervisor (verbally and in written form) as soon as they occur
- Wear gloves to clean any blood or body fluid spills using a household bleach solution or other disinfectant approved by the CDC
- Any articles contaminated with blood or body secretions should be double bagged and labeled
- Dietary therapy involves a high calorie, high-protein diet served in small frequent meals
    - Total parental nutrition may be required in end-stage critically ill patients
- Management of respiratory condition to include:
    - Oxygen administration as needed
    - Positioning (semi-Fowler's)
    - Chest physiotherapy (CPT)
    - Postural drainage
    - Incentive spirometry
- Administration of Blood products to include:
    - Fresh frozen plasma (FFP)
    - Platelets
    - Packed red blood cells (PRBC)

Medications for HIV/AIDS infection

- The primary treatment at present is antiretroviral therapy with Zidovudine (AZT), Didanosine (ddI), Zalcitabine (ddC), Stavudine (d4T)
- Interferon-a is also used as a antiretroviral drug
- Vaccinations with pneumoccal polysaccharide and H. influenzae type b vaccines as HIV-1 positive patients are at increased risk for infections
- Prophylaxis against infections often is ordered as the patients CD4+ Tcell count drops below 200 cells/microliter, medications may include:
    - Prophylaxis against PCP
        trimethoprim/sulfamethoxazole
        atovoquone and clindamycin/pyrimethamine
        aerosolized pentamidine
    - Prophylaxis against MAC infection
        Rifabutin

- Prophylaxis against Tuberculosis
  Isoniazid
- Prophylaxis against cryptococcal and candidal infections
  fluconazole

Section VI — DIETS

- Diet is important in the treatment of immune and hematologic system disorders
- Many individuals with disorders of these systems suffer from anorexia and weight loss this may be due to:
  - Protein-calorie malnutrition
  - Hypermetabolic states associated with chronic infections which leads to a greater need for calories
  - Altered taste sensations (may be medication related)
  - Oral lesions which lead to pain
  - Dysphagia (difficulty swallowing) from esophageal lesions
  - Nausea and vomiting from chemotherapeutic agents
  - Depression from diagnoses of life-threatening illness (AIDS/HIV-1, cancer)
  - Chronic diarrhea related to infections
- Diet may be comprised of one or all of the following components
  - Small frequent meals which are usually better tolerated than a large meal
  - High-protein, high calorie diet plan
  - Use of supplemental nutritional feedings
    - Transnasal feedings with polymeric formulas
    - Percutaneous endoscopic jejunostomy
- Iron-rich foods are important for those with anemia
  - Important for the synthesis of hemoglobin
- Low caffeine diet
  - Helpful for patients with chronic diarrhea

HIGH-PROTEIN, HIGH-CALORIE DIET

General description	Diet is based on body weight with 30-40 Kcal per kilogram of patient's weight ordered, a 110 pound patient would require between 1500-2000 Kcal/day while a 176 pound patient would require between 2400-3200 calories per day Protein is replaced based on weight as well with 0.8-1.5 grams of protein per kilogram ordered One of the first steps is to determine why the patient has been unable to take in enough calories to meet body needs and to correct the problem if possible to maintain or increase current weight
Indications	Documented history of unwanted weight loss of at least 10% of original body weight Weight loss may be due to cancers, HIV/AIDS, other illnesses
Allowable foods	All foods are allowed, unless they are not tolerated by the individual. The following foods are high in protein/calories and can be easily added to the diet: Protein & calories Add 2 Tbs powdered milk to sauces, gravies, hot cereals, soups, ground meats, eggs or casseroles Substitute milk for water in recipes for cookies soups, puddings and cocoa Add meats to noodles, soups, sauces, potatoes, rice, casseroles Add cheese to noodles, vegetables, soups, sauces potatoes, rice or breads Add cottage cheese to spaghetti sauce, meat sauces, breads or use as dips Use peanut butter for vegetable dip, topping for cookies, brownies, pancakes, waffles, cakes, vegetables (celery) or fruit (apples, bananas, or pears) Add nuts to breads, cookies, cakes, ice cream, cheese or cereals Calories: Add butter or margarine to soups, vegetables, potatoes, rice, hot cereals, pancakes, waffles, breads and casseroles Add mayonnaise to sauces, eggs, sandwiches, dips sauces or milk shakes Add yogurt or sour cream to potatoes, vegetables chili, gravies, dressings and dips Add cream cheese to milkshakes Add whip cream to cocoa, pancakes, puddings, pie, fruits
Restricted Items	None, some individuals may be lactose intolerant
Nutritional Value	Diet if well-balanced should provide all of the needed nutrients
Other comments	Daily weights may be ordered to assess progress

IRON-RICH FOODS

General description	Diet is well-balanced with the addition of foods high in iron
	Average American diet has approximately 12 mg iron per 2,000 calories.
	Recommended Dietary Allowance
	    Infants 6-10 mg
	    Children 10 mg
	    Adolescent Males 12 mg
	    Adolescent Females 15 mg
	    Adult Males 10 mg
	    Adult Females 18 mg
	    Postmenopausal Females 10 mg
	    Pregnant Females 30 mg
	    Lactating Females 15 mg

Indications	Iron-deficiency anemia, pregnancy, infancy and childhood, chronic slow blood loss, disorders that interfere with iron absorption

Allowable foods	All foods are allowed, unless they are not tolerated by the individual. The following foods are high in iron:
	    Pork liver 140 mg
	    Beef liver 70 mg
	    Beef kidney 60 mg
	    Dried beans 30 mg (1 cup)
	    Beef 30 mg (1 cup)
	    Pork 30 mg (1 cup)
	    Farina cereal 90 mg (1 cup)
	    Prune juice 0 mg (1 cup)
	    Dates 30 mg (1 cup)
	    Raisins 30 mg (1 cup)
	    Spinach 30 mg (1 cup)

Restricted Items	None
Nutritional Value	Diet if well-balanced should provide all of the needed nutrients for males Female adolescents, adults, pregnant and lactating women may require iron supplements to meet RDA
Other comments	Iron supplementation is required during pregnancy Ascorbic acid aids in the absorption of iron and should be encouraged

Section VII — DRUGS

The tables supply only general information, a drug handbook or the physician's desk reference (PDR) should be consulted for details. Each classification includes detailed information about the example drug, this drug is representative of the other drugs in the classification and can be used as a model.

Every effort has been made to include the major classes of drugs used in the treatment of immune or hematologic diseases.

ANTIINFECTIVES — ANTIBIOTICS, AMINOGLYCOSIDES
Action: Inhibition of ribosomal protein synthesis, usually bactericidal

Indications: Active against serious gram-negative bacterial infections to include Citrobacter, Escherichia coli, Enterobacter, Klebsiella, Proteus, Pseudomonas aeruginosa and Serratia. Also effective against some Gram-positive organisms to include some strains of staphylococcus aureus

Example: Gentamicin sulfate (*Garamycin, Genoptic, Gentacidin*)

<u>Route:</u> IV, IM

<u>Pharmacokinetics:</u> Peak 30-90 minutes IM

<u>Contraindications:</u> sensitivity to any aminoglycoside antibiotic

<u>Common adverse effects:</u> Decreased creatinine clearance

<u>Life-threatening adverse effects:</u> nephrotoxicity

<u>Other adverse effects:</u> Ototoxicity, optic neuritis, peripheral neuritis, paresthesias, headache, lethargy, tremors, muscle cramps and twitching, convulsions, neuromuscular blockade, acute organic brain syndrome, nausea, anorexia, vomiting, weight loss, increased salivation, increased/decreased reticulocyte counts, granulocytopenia, agranulocytosis, thrombocytopenia, anemia, hepatomegaly, splenomegaly, hypotension/hypertension, local pain and irritation after IM injection

<u>Interventions:</u>

Infuse IV over 30-120 minutes, solution should be clear

Obtain cultures before first dose of medication is given

Ototoxicity may manifest itself with hearing loss 3-4 weeks after therapy

I&O should be monitored during therapy and oliguria or edema reported

Encourage fluids, patient should remain well hydrated

Peak should be 4-10 ug/ml and trough 1-2 μg/ml, Peaks above 12 and troughs above 2 are associated with toxicity

Peak should be drawn 30-60 minutes after IM and 30 minutes after

IV dose

Trough levels should be drawn just prior to next scheduled dose

Most infections respond to therapy in 24-48 hours, therapy duration 7-10 days

Examples of other drugs in this classification:

Amikacin sulfate (*Amikin*), IV/IM, used for serious infections or recurrent urinary tract infections

Kanamycin (*Kantrex*), PO/IM/IV, Used for intestinal tract infections, and also used for tuberculosis in patients resistant to conventional therapy

Neomycin sulfate (*Mycifradin, Myciguent*), PO/IM, used for severe diarrhea

Netilmicin sulfate (*Netromycin*), IV/IM, used for life-threatening or very serious infections such as septicemia or peritonitis

Paromomycin sulfate (*Humatin*), PO, Used for bacteria in patients with hepatic coma or intestinal amebiasis

Streptomycin sulfate IM, Used with other drugs to treat tuberculosis

Tobramycin sulfate (*Nebcin, Tobrex*) IV/IM, for moderate-severe infections

ANTIINFECTIVE - ANTIBIOTIC, ANTIFUNGALS

Action: Antifungals stop or kill fungal organisms causing infection

Indications: Fungal infections such as cryptococcal or candidiasis infections

Example: Fluconazole (*Diflucan*)

Route: PO, IV

Pharmacodynamics: Peak 1-2 hours

Contraindications: sensitivity to fluconazole or other antifungals

Common adverse effects: Headache, nausea, vomiting, abdominal pain, diarrhea, rash

Interventions:

Administer IV no faster than 200 mg/hr

Monitor lab values to include BUN, serum creatinine, liver function tests, bilirubin and alkaline phosphatase

Examples of other drugs in this classification:

Amphotericin B (*Fungizone*), IV, Used for potentially fatal fungal infections, wide spectrum used for aspergillosis, blastomycosis, coccidio-idomycosis, cryptococcosis disseminated candidiasis, histoplasmosis, para-coccidioidomycosis, sporotrichosis, duration 20 hours, life threatening adverse effect of nephrotoxicity may occur, administer slowly over 6 hours may be ordered on an alternate day schedule, IV site should be monitored for patency frequently, solution should be protected from light during infusion, monitor VS frequently during infusion as fever, chills, nausea, and headache are common during infusion, monitor I&O report oliguria, K+ supplements may be ordered, Also available as topical agent

Butoconazole nitrate (*Femstat*), Topical, used for vulvovaginal candidiasis

Ciclopirox olamine (*Loprox*), Topical, used for tinea cruris (jock itch)

Clioquinol (*Torofor, Vioform*), Topical, used for eczema, athlete's foot

Clotrimazole (*Lotrimin, Mycelex*), Topical, for tinea cruris, corposris, tinea versicolor and vulvovaginal and oropharyngeal candidiasis

Econazole nitrate (*Ecostatin, Spectazole*), Topical, for tinea pedis, tinea cruris, tinea corporis (ringworm of body), tinea versicolor

Flucytosine (*Ancobon, Ancotil*), PO, for serious systemic infections caused by Cryptococcus and Candida, used alone or in combination

Griseofulvin Microsize (*Fulvicin-U/F, Grifulvin V, Grisactin*), PO, for infections which have not responded to topical medications

Haloprogin (*Halotex*), Topical, used for superficial fungal infections

Itraconazole (*Sporanox*), PO, used for infections caused by blastomycosis, histophasmosis

Ketoconazole (*Nitzoral*), PO/Topical, for severe systemic fungal infections, take with food or fluids

Miconazole Nitrate (*Micatin, Monistat*), Intravaginal/IV/Bladder installation, used for vulvovaginal fungal infections, tinea cruris, tinea corporis and tinea versicolor, Administer IV slow and monitor carefully

Naftifine hydrochloride (*Naftin*), Topical, used for tinea pedis, tinea cruris and tinea corporis

Natamycin (*Natacyn*), Ophthalmic instillation, used for blepharitis, conjunctivitis, and keratitis

Nystatin (*Mycostatin, Nilstat, Nystex, O-V Statin*), PO, Vaginal, Used for Candidiasis of the oropharynx, vulvovaginal or intestinal, oral suspension is used as a mouth rinse, avoid food and drink 30 minutes after use

Oxiconazole nitrate (*Oxistat*), Topical, used for tinea pedis, tinea cruris and tinea corporis due to Trichophyton, also for candida albicans

Terbinafine cream (*Lamisil*), Topical, for superficial infections

Tolnaftate (*Aftate, Tinactin*), Topical, used for tinea pedis, tinea cruris, tinea corporis, tinea capitis and tinea unguium

ANTIINFECTIVES — ANTIBIOTIC, CEPHALOSPORINS (FIRST GENERATION)

Action: Inhibition of bacterial cell wall synthesis to stop infection
Indications: Broad-spectrum drug group, drug choice is dependent upon the infectious organism (most effective against gram-positive organisms)
Example: Cephalothin sodium (Keflin, Seffin)
Route: IV, IM
Pharmacokinetics: Peak 30 minutes after IM, 15 minutes after IV
Contraindications: sensitivity to cephalosporins
Common adverse effects: Nausea, vomiting, superinfections, diarrhea
Life-threatening effects: Anaphylactic shock
Other adverse effects: Dizziness, vertigo, headache, fatigue, malaise, dysgeusia, glossitis, anorexia, abdominal cramps, flatulence, neutropenia, leukopenia, pancytopenia, thrombocytopenia, hypoprothrombinemia, hemolytic anemia, positive Coombs test, rash, pruritus, urticaria
Interventions:
IM injection is painful, rotate IM sites, give in large muscle
IV give 1 gram over 3-5 minutes
Monitor culture and sensitivity tests
Monitor I&O, report decreased urinary output, report diarrhea or fever
Examples of other drugs in this classification:
Cefadroxil (*Duricef, Ultracef*), PO, used for urinary tract infections from E. Coli, Proteus mirabilis and Klebsiella, also for skin infections, pharyngitis and tonsillitis
Cefazolin sodium (*Ancef, Kefzol, Zolicef*), IV/IM, for severe urinary tract infections, bacteremia, endocarditis and for perioperative prophylaxis
Cephalexin (*Cefanex, Keflet, Keflex, Keftab*), PO, for respiratory and urinary tract infections, middle ear, soft tissue and bone infections
Cephapirin sodium (*Cefadyl*), IM/IV, for serious infections respiratory and urinary tracts, skin and soft tissue, ostermyelitis, septicemia and endocarditis
Cephradine (*Anspor, Velosef*), PO/IM/IV, serious infections of respiratory and urinary tracts, otitis media, skin and soft tissue infections, for perioperative prophylaxis, septicemia

ANTIINFECTIVES — ANTIBIOTICS, CEPHALOSPORINS (SECOND GENERATION)

Action & Indications: Same as first generation with broader activity against Gram-negative organisms

Example: Cefonicid sodium (*Monocid*)

Route: IV, IM

Pharmacokinetics: Peak 1 hour IM, 5 minutes IV

Contraindications: sensitivity to cephalosporins and related antibiotics, severe renal or hepatic function

Common adverse effects: Diarrhea, superinfections

Life-threatening effects: Anaphylactoid reaction

Other adverse effects: Nausea, vomiting, leukopenia, positive Coombs test, anemia, fever, rash, pruritus, erythema, myalgia, pain with IM injection, burning with IV administration, flu-like syndrome

Interventions:

If perioperative during C-section given only after umbilical cord is clamped

Administer IM injection deep into large muscle, rotate injection sites

Bolus IV administration may be given over 3-5 minutes

Monitor culture and sensitivity test results

Monitor I&O, report oliguria, report elevated temperature or diarrhea

Examples of other drugs in this classification:

Cefaclor (*Ceclor*), PO, used for otitis media and respiratory or urinary infections

Cefamandole naftate (*Mandol*), IV/IM, for serious infections of respiratory, urinary or biliary tracts, infections of skin and soft tissue, bone or joints, septicemia, peritonitis, perioperative prophylaxis

Ceforanide (*Precef*), IV/IM, for respiratory or urinary tract infections, skin, bone or joint infections, endocarditis, septicemia and perioperative prophylaxis

Cefoxitin (*Mefoxin*), IV/IM, for infections same as ceforanide plus gynecologic infections, gonorrhea, mixed aerobic-anaerobic infections

Cefprozil (*Cefzil*), PO, for respiratory tract infections, otitis media, and skin infections

Cefuroxime (*Keferox, Zinacef, Ceftin*), PO/IV/IM, used for respiratory and urinary tract infections, skin infections, meningitis, gonorrhea, otitis media and perioperative prophylaxis

ANTIINFECTIVES — CEPHALOSPORINS (THIRD GENERATION)

Action & Indications: Same as second generation except very effective against gram-negative organisms including enterobacteriaceae

Example: Cefotaxime sodium (*Claforan*)

Route: IV, IM

Pharmacokinetics: Peak 30 minutes after IM, 5 minutes after IV

Contraindications: Sensitivity to cephalosporins and other beta-lactam antibiotics

Common adverse effects: Diarrhea

Other adverse effects: Nausea, vomiting, abdominal pain, colitis, anorexia, transient leukopenia, granulocytopenia, thrombocytopenia, neutropenia, eosinophilia, positive Coombs test, rash, pruritus, fever, nocturnal perspiration, phlebitis, thrombophlebitis

Interventions:

Culture & sensitivity tests should be monitored

Monitor I&O during therapy, report diarrhea or oliguria

Examples of other drugs in this classification:

Cefixime (*Suprax*), PO, Suspension can be kept at room temperature

Cefmetazole (*Zefazone*), IV, Administer IV push or continuous infusion

Cefoperazone sodium (*Cefobid*), IV/IM, Rapid IV injection not recommended

Cefotetan disodium (*Cefotan*), IV/IM, IM injection into large muscle mass

Cefpodoxime (*Vantin*), PO, Administer with food

Ceftazidime (*Fortaz, Tazicef, Tazidime*), IV/IM, IM into large muscle mass

Ceftizoxime (*Cefizox*), IV/IM, Drug may interfere with cross-match studies

Ceftriaxone sodium (*Rocephin*), IV/IM, Single daily dose given, assess for bleeding

Moxalactam disodium (*Moxam*), IV/IM, IM injection deep into large muscle

ANTIINFECTIVES — ANTIBIOTICS, PENICILLINS (AMINO-PENICILLIN)

Action: One of the Beta-Lactams, there are three classes of penicillins, act by inhibiting bacterial cell wall synthesis

Indications: Gram-positive and gram-negative bacterial infections

Example: Ampicillin (*Amcill, Ampicin, Onmipen, Pfierpen-A, Polycillin, Principen, Totacillin*)
Route: PO, IM, IV
Pharmacokinetics: Peak 5 min IV, 1 hr IM, 2 hrs PO
Duration 6-8 hrs
Contraindications: sensitivity to penicillin
Common adverse effects: Diarrhea, rash
Life-threatening effects: Anaphylactoid reaction
Other adverse effects: Convulsive seizures, nausea, vomiting, pruritus, urticaria, eosinophilia, hemolytic anemia, thrombocytopenia, leukopenia, severe pain after IM, superinfections
Interventions:
Administer PO with full glass of fluid on empty stomach
Administer IV dose slowly over 10-15 minutes, rapid IV can cause seizures
Monitor culture and sensitivity tests
Examples of other drugs in this classification:
Amoxicillin (*Amoxil, Larotid, Moxilean, Polymox, Sumox, Trimox, Utimox, Wymox*), PO, Available chewable tablets, suspension and drops for children

Amoxicillin and clavulanate potassium (*Augmentin*), PO, two 250 mg tablets are not equivalent to one 500 mg tablet

Bacampicillin hydrochloride (*Spectrobid*), PO, Take oral suspension on empty stomach with fluids

Cylacillin (*Cyclapen-W*), PO, Take on empty stomach

ANTIINFECTIVES — ANTIBIOTICS, PENICILLINS (ANTIPSEUDOMONAL PENICILLIN)
Action: Same as other penicillins
Indications: Has the broadest spectrum of action of all the penicillins, effective against gram-positive and gram-negative organisms includes aerobic and anaerobic species, used for life-threatening illnesses
Example: Mexlocillin sodium (*Mezlin*)
Route: IM, IV
Pharmacokinetics: Peak 45 minutes IM, 5 minutes IV
Contraindications: sensitivity to penicillins or cephalosporins
Common adverse effects: Diarrhea, rash
Life threatening effects: Anaphylactic reactions
Other adverse effects: Seizures, abnormal taste sensations, nausea, vomiting, neutropenia, leukopenia, eosinophilia, thrombocytopenia, drug fever, pruritus, urticaria, superinfections, decreased Hct & Hgb

Interventions:
IM injections should be in large muscle and made slowly to reduce pain
Monitor culture and sensitivity tests
Monitor patient for anaphylactic reaction for 30 minutes with IV use
Monitor for superinfections such as vaginitis in women
Examples of other drugs in this classification:
Carbenicillin disodium (*Geopen*), IV/IM, May be reconstituted with lidocaine hydrochloride without epinephrine to reduce pain on injection if ordered

Piperacillin sodium (*Pipracil*), IV/IM, See note on Carbenicillin

Ticarcillin disodium (*Ticar*), IM/IV, Intermittent IV administration is over 30-120 minutes, can be given direct IV very slowly

Ticarcillin disodium and clavulanate potassium (*Timentin*), IV/IM, give IV slowly over at least 30 minutes, overdose may cause seizures

ANTIINFECTIVES — ANTIBIOTICS, PENICILLINS (NATURAL PENICILLIN)
Action: Same as other penicillins
Indications: Bacterial infections
Example: Penicillin G potassium (*Pfizarpen, Pentids*)
Route: PO, IV, IM
Pharmacokinetics: Peak 30-60 minutes PO, 15-30 minutes IM
Contraindications: sensitivity to any penicillin or cephalosporin, serious infections (oral administration), nausea, vomiting, gastric dilation, hypermotility, cardiospasm, sodium restricted patients
Common adverse effects: Superinfections, hypersensitivity urticaria/rash
Other adverse effects: Electrolyte imbalances, pain at injection site, abscess or phlebitis at injection site
Hypersensitivity reactions may be immediate within 2-30 minutes of drug administration with anaphylaxis (Life threatening) or occur in 1-72 hours with malaise, fever, erythema or asthma or even occur after 72 hours with serum sickness, rashes and blood changes
Interventions:
Check orders carefully for Penicillin G potassium or Penicillin G sodium
PO administer on empty stomach with full glass of water
IM injection should be deep into large muscle mass, rotate sites
IV administration should be slow to prevent electrolyte imbalances
Monitor culture and sensitivity tests

Monitor all patients for anaphylactic reaction for at least 30 minutes following IV or IM administration

Monitor I&O, report oliguria or hematuria

Monitor for immediate or delayed sensitivity reactions in patients

Examples of other drugs in this classification:

Penicillin G benzathine (*Bicillin, Permapen*), IM, Inadvertent IV use may cause cardiac arrest

Penicillin G procaine (*Crysticillin A.S., Procaine benzylpenicillin, Pfizerpen-AS, Wycillin*), IM, Inadvertent IV use may cause pulmonary infarct and death, inject drug slowly, rotate sites

Penicillin V, Penicillin V Potassium (*Beepen VK, Betapen-VK, Ledercillin VK, Penicillin VK, Pen-V, Pen-Vee K, Robicillin VK, V-Cillin, Veetids*), PO, Take after meal for best absorption, shake suspension well before use

ANTIINFECTIVES — ANTIBIOTICS, TETRACYCLINES

Action: Bacteriostatic drug, inhibits ribosomal protein synthesis

Indications: Broad spectrum of action, effective against many sexually transmitted diseases, effective against Gram-positive and Gram-negative bacterial infections. Also used as an antiacne drug.

Example: Tetracycline hydrochloride (*Achromycin, NorTet, Panmycin, Robitet, Sumycin, Tetracap, Tetracyn, Tetralan, Tetram, Topicycline*)

<u>Route:</u> PO, IM

<u>Pharmacokinetics:</u> Peak 2-4 hours

<u>Contraindications:</u> sensitivity to tetracyclines, severe renal or hepatic impairment, bile duct obstruction, children under 8, last half of pregnancy

<u>Common adverse reactions:</u> Nausea, vomiting, diarrhea, abdominal discomfort, flatulence, phototoxicity

<u>Life-threatening effects:</u> Fatty degeneration of liver, exfoliative dermatitis, anaphylaxis

<u>Other adverse effects:</u> Headache, epigastric distress, heartburn, bulky, loose stools, steatorrhea, dry mouth, dysphagia, retrosternal pain, esophagitis, esophageal ulceration, neutropenia, thrombocytopenia, toxic granulation of granulocytes, leukocytosis, decreased leukocyte ascorbic acid, atypical lymphocytes, positive antinuclear antibodies, hypokalemia, folate deficiency with megaloblastic anemia, acute hemolytic anemia, high liver function test values, decrease in cholesterol, increased BUN/serum creatinine, renal impairment, dermatitis, onycholysis, cheilosis, fixed-drug eruptions, thrombocytopenic purpura, skin irritation, dry scaly skin, super-infections, decrease in B complex vitamins, pancreatitis, pain at

injection site

Interventions:

Check expiration date on all forms of tetracycline, outdated preparations may cause Fanconi-like syndrome or LE-like syndrome, product may even be toxic

Administer oral preparation with full glass of water on empty stomach

Shake oral suspension well before administration

Prior to IM administration assess for allergy to local anesthetics such as procaine or other "caine" preparations (IM preparation contains procaine)

Administer IM injection deep into a large muscle mass, rotate sites

Monitor culture and sensitivity test results

Monitor renal and hepatic function studies when patient is on long-term therapy and monitor I&O, report oliguria or diarrhea

Monitor for superinfections such as thrush or vaginal infections

Report headache or visual disturbances (may indicate increased ICP)

Monitor for painful or difficultly swallowing may indicate esophagitis

Acne therapy may take up to 12 weeks before improvement is noted

Examples of other drugs in this classification:

Chlortetracycline hydrochloride (*Aureomycin ointment or ophthalmic*), Topical, ophthalmic and skin ointments are not interchangeable

Demeclocycline hydrochloride (*Declomycin*), PO, Administer with water on empty stomach, never with dairy products, take product while standing to help prevent esophageal irritation

Doxycycline hyclate (*Doryx, Doxy, Doxycheal, Doxy-Lemmon, SK-Doxycycline, Vibramycin, Vibra-Tabs*), PO/IV, May be taken with food or milk

Meclocycline sulfosalicylate (*Meclan*), Topical, for acne vulgaris

Minocycline hydrochloride (*Minocin*), PO/IV, Incompatible with demerol, morphine, and hydromorphone at Y-site (IV administration)

Oxytetracycline (*Terramycin*), PO/IM/IV, Do not use IM medication for IV administration as it contains lidocaine

ANTIINFECTIVES — ANTIVIRALS

Action: Reduce viral shedding and replication, interferes with DNA synthesis of specific viruses

Indications: Acyclovir is used to treat initial and recurrent herpes simplex virus types 1 and 2, varicella-zoster virus, Epstein-Barr virus and cytomegalovirus

Example: Acyclovir (*Acycloguanosine, Zovirax*)
<u>Route:</u> PO, IV
<u>Pharmacokinetics:</u> Peak 1.5-2 hrs PO
<u>Contraindications:</u> Rapid IV administration
<u>Common adverse effects:</u> Headache, nausea, vomiting, diarrhea
<u>Other adverse effects:</u> lightheadedness, lethargy, fatigue, tremors, rash, confusion, seizures, dizziness, glomerulonephritis, renal tubular damage, acute renal failure, urticaria, pruritus, burning, stinging, sloughing with IV extravasation, fever, muscle cramps, arthralgia, edema
<u>Interventions:</u>
Administer IV over 1 hour or more to patent IV site, monitor site
Check orders for "force fluids" or increased IV fluid rate to maintain hydration, monitor I&O
Apply topical preparations with gloves to prevent spread of infection
Examples of other drugs in this classification:
Amantadine hydrochloride (*Symmetrel*), PO, Used for treatment of influenza A (prophylaxis also)
Didanosine (*ddI, Videx*), PO, used for advanced HIV infection for those who are unable to take AZT, Take on empty stomach with water, do not give with fruit juice, monitor patient for abdominal pain and/or peripheral neuropathy and report
Foscarnet (*Foscavir*), IV, used for herpes zoster infections in HIV/AIDS patients and for CMV infections to include CMV retinitis
Ganciclovir (*DHPG, Cytovene*), IV, CMV infections and for prophylaxis in HIV/AIDS patients or immunocompromised patients against CMV
Idoxuridine (*Herplex Liquifilm, IDU, Stoxil*), Ophthalmic, used for herpes simplex keratitis
Ribavirin (*Virazole*), Inhalation, used for respiratory syncytial virus (RSV) infection in infants and children, Monitor VS before and during treatment, accurate I&O should be maintained
Trifluridine (*Viroptic*), Ophthalmic, used for keratoconjunctivitis from herpes simplex virus type 1 or 2 infection
Vidarabine (*Adenine arabinoside, ARA-A, Vira-A*), IV, used for herpes simplex encephalitis, herpes zoster or in Ophthalmic form for keratitis
Zalcitabine (*ddC, Hivid*), PO, for HIV/AIDS used in combination with AZT, take on empty stomach, report abdominal pain or peripheral neuropathy

Zidovudine (*Azidothymidine, AZT*), PO/IV, HIV/AIDS, administer IV over 1 hr, frequent CD4+ T cell counts should be done to monitor effectiveness

ANTIINFECTIVES — SULFONAMIDES
Action: Inhibit folic acid synthesis by susceptible bacterial organisms thereby providing a bacteriostatic effect
Indications: Infection with gram-positive or gram-negative organisms
Example: Sulfisoxazole (*Gantrisin*)
Route: PO, Vaginal
Pharmacokinetics: Peak 2-4 hrs
Contraindications: sensitivity to sulfonamides or salicylates, use for group A beta-hemolytic streptococcal infections, pregnancy, porphyria, renal or liver disease, intestinal and urinary obstruction
Common adverse effects: Nausea, vomiting, diarrhea.
Stevens–Johnson syndrome, exfoliative dermatitis may occur with hypersensitivity
Life-threatening effects: Aplastic anemia, agranulocytosis, anaphylactoid reactions
Other adverse effects: Headache, peripheral neuritis, tinnitus, hearing loss, peripheral neuropathy, hearing loss, vertigo, insomnia, drowsiness, mental depression, acute psychosis, ataxia, convulsions, abdominal pains, hepatitis, jaundice, pancreatitis, stomatitis, hemolytic anemia, thrombocytopenia, leukopenia, eosinophilia, hypoprothrombinemia, crystalluria, hematuria, proteniuria, anuria, conjunctivitis, goiter, hypoglycemia, diuresis, overgrowth of other organisms, alopecia, lymphadenopathy, fixed-drug eruptions
Interventions:
Tablet may be crushed and taken with fluids, encourage fluid intake
Monitor I&O- report oliguria, monitor temperature - fever may indicate a hypersensitivity reaction (usually develop within 10 days to 6 weeks, sore throat, malaise, unusual fatigue, joint pains, pallor, rash or bleeding tendencies, skin lesions are other signs of reaction
Pt should avoid exposure to sunlight or ultraviolet light
Examples of other drugs in this classification:
Silver sulfadiazine (*sulfisoxazole*), Topical, used in treatment of second and third degree burns to prevent sepsis

Sulfacetamide sodium (*AK-Sulf, Bleph 10, Cetamide, Isopto Cetamide, Ophthacet, Sebizone, Sodium Sulamyd*), Ophthalmic, for infections of eye

Sulfadiazine (*Microsulfon*), PO

Sulfamethoxazole (*Gamazole, Gatanol, Urobak*), PO, used frequently for urinary tract infections

Sulfasalazine (*Axulfidine*), PO, administer after meals, folic acid supplement may be prescribed for patients on long term therapy

ANTINEOPLASTICS — ALKYLATING AGENTS

Action: Treat neoplasms by interfering with DNA in new cells that are undergoing division, causes a break in the molecule blocking synthesis of DNA, RNA and protein

Indications: Malignant Neoplams

Example: Cyclophosphamide (*Cytoxan, Neosar*)

Route: PO, IV

Contraindications: Men and women in childbearing years, serious infections, myelosuppression, pregnancy, nursing mothers

Common adverse effects: Nausea, vomiting, anorexia, neutropenia, alopecia

Life-threatening effects: Sterile hemorrhagic and nonhemorrhagic cystitis, leukopenia, pulmonary emboli, interstitial pulmonary fibrosis, anaphylaxis

Other adverse effects: Mucositis, hepatotoxicity, diarrhea, bladder fibrosis, nephrotoxicity, severe hyperkalemia, SIADH, hyponatremia, weight gain, weight loss, hyperuricemia, acute myeloid leukemia, anemia, thrombophlebitis, pulmonary edema, pneumonitis, transverse ridging of nails, pigmentation of nail beds and skin, dermatitis, dizziness, fatigue, facial flushing, diaphoresis, secondary neoplasms

Interventions:

Take drug on empty stomach unless severe nausea and vomiting is present

IV administration, no faster than 100 mg over 1 minute

Monitor CBC, platelets, liver and kidney function studies, electrolytes

See also interventions for hematologic and immune problems found in this chapter, thrombocytopenia, leukopenia or pancytopenia may occur

Monitor I&O, report any hematuria, oliguria

Alopecia occurs in about 33% of patients, provide emotional support

Amenorrhea may last up to 1 year after completion of therapy in 10-30%

Examples of other drugs in this classification:

Altretamine (*Hexalen*), PO, monitor patient for neurologic symptoms to include paresthesias, hypoesthesias, muscle weakness, peripheral numbness, ataxia, decreased sensations and alterations in mood or consciousness

Busulfan (*Myleran*), PO, encourage fluids, assess for jaundice

Carboplatin (*Paraplatin*), IV, for ovarian cancer, administer over minimum of 15 minutes, premedication with an antiemetic is common, monitor for allergic reaction

Carmustine (*BCNU, BiCNU*), IV, Topical, extravasation can lead to nerve or tendon damage assess site for patency frequently, infusion given over 1-2 hours, intense flushing of skin may occur with infusion usually disappears in 2-4 hours

Chlorambucil (*Leukeran*), PO, Encourage fluid intake

Cisplatin (*CIS-DDP, CIS-platinum II, Platinol*), IV, IV hydration is begun prior to therapy and foley catheter inserted, administer infusion over 6-8 hours, premedication with an antiemetic is common, monitor patient for any sensitivity reactions

Dacarbazine (*DTIC, DTIC-Dome*), IV, Monitor carefully for extravasation which can lead to loss of mobility of limb, patient should be hospitalized during therapy, severe nausea and vomiting may develop

Estramustine phosphate sodium (*Emcyt*), PO, Administer with meals, Monitor BP and report elevations

Ifosfamide (*Ifex*), IV, Monitor urinalysis test results before giving drug

Lomustine (*CeeNU, CCNU*), PO, Administer on empty stomach, antiemetic may be given prior to therapy

Melphalan (*Alkeran, Pam, L-Pam, Phenylalanine Mustard*), PO/IV, Administer over 15 minutes, drug must be administered within 60 min of reconstitution

Pipobroman (*Vercyte*), PO, Patient usually hospitalized for therapy, assess bone marrow studies before therapy

Streptozocin (*Zanosar*), IV, Used for pancreatic cancer, Monitor carefully for extravasation as necrosis may occur, premedication with antiemetic is common

Thiotepa (*TSPA*), IV/Intratumor/Intracavitary/Intravesicular/Intrathecal, Used for lymphomas, leukemias, adenocarcinoma of breast and ovary

Uracil Mustard, PO, Administer at bedtime, alopecia is not a usual side effect (compared to other alkylating antineoplastic agents)

ANTINEOPLASTICS — ANTIBIOTICS

Action: Not used for treatment of infections due to toxicity, block DNA & RNA transcription, enhance destruction of areas that have irradiated

Indications: Malignant Neoplasms (Cancers)

Example: Doxorubicin hydrochloride (*Adriamycin, ADR*)

Route: IV

Contraindications: Myelosuppression, impaired cardiac function, patient reaching maximum total dose of 500-550 mg/m2, obstructive jaundice

Common adverse effects: Stomatitis, severe myelosuppression, complete alopecia

Life-threatening effects: Congestive heart failure, ventricular arrhythmia, left ventricular failure, leukopenia, anaphylactoid reaction

Other adverse effects: Hypertension, hypotension, esophagitis with ulcers, nausea, vomiting, anorexia, diarrhea, thrombocytopenia, anemia, hyperpigmentation of nail beds, tongue and/or buccal mucosa, rash, drowsiness, fever, hematuria, hyperuricemia

Interventions:

Medical personal who are pregnant should not prepare or administer IV drug

Administer with butterfly needle using a large vein, assess for patency

Administer into already established intravenous line of D5W or NaCl

Administer over 3-5 minutes, too rapid of administration will result in facial flushing, monitor for extravasation which can lead to severe cellulitis, vesication and tissue necrosis, plastic surgery may be required

Monitor patient for signs of hypersensitivity to include red flare around injection site, erythema, skin rash, pruritus, angioedema, urticaria, fever or chills

Obtain baseline VS and monitor VS and I&O during therapy

Assess for liver or kidney dysfunction, monitor laboratory values

CBC levels and for leukopenia, anemia and thrombocytopenia

Assess for stomatitis and dysphagia (difficulty swallowing)

See also interventions for hematologic and immune problems this chapter

Be advised that drug turns urine red for 1-2 days after administration

Complete alopecia is common, provide emotional support to patient

Examples of other drugs in this classification:

Bleomycin sulfate (*Blenoxane*), SC/IM/IV, Inject IM dose deep, rotate sites, anaphylactoid reactions can be fatal monitor for hypersensitivity to drug, monitor VS and ausculte chest frequently during first 24 hours after drug is given, reaction includes hypotension, elevated temperature, chills, confusion and wheezing

Daunorubicin hydrochloride (*Doxorubicin*), IV, Used for leukemias, monitor serum bilirubin levels, serum uric acid levels, report breathlessness

Mitomycin (*Mutamycin*), IV, Patient should be hospitalized during therapy, Encourage fluids and hydration, monitor I&O

Plicamycin (*Mithracin*), IV, Assess for purpura and report, monitor calcium levels, monitor stool pattern as drug diminishes peristalsis and can lead to impactions

ANTINEOPLASTICS — ANTIMETABOLITES

Action: Destroy normal cell function by either interfering with DNA production or function

Indications: Metastatic neoplasms (cancer)

Example: Fluorouracil (*Adrucil, Efudex, 5-Fluorouracil, 5-FU, Fluoroplex*

Route: IV

Contraindications: Poor nutritional states, myelosupression

Common adverse effects: Nausea, vomiting, stomatitis, diarrhea, alopecia

Life threatening effects: Leukopenia

Other adverse effects: Euphoria, insomnia, acute cerebellar syndrome, mild angina to crushing chest pain with ECG changes, anorexia, medicinal taste, proctitis, paralytic ileus, GI hemorrhage, anemia, thrombocytopenia, SLE-like dermatitis, photosensitivity, erythema, increased pigmentation, skin dryness, rash, dermatitis, nephrotoxicity, epistaxis, lacrimation

Interventions:

May be administered by direct IV route over 1-2 minutes, inspect site frequently, avoid extravasation which may result in local tissue damage

Monitor CBC for pancytopenia and report any abnormal values

See also interventions for hematologic and immune problems in this chapter

Obtain baseline weight, I&O, vital signs, bowel elimination patterns

Antiemetics are often ordered before and after administration

Assess for stomatitis (early sign of toxicity) and promptly report dry mouth, cracked lips, white patches or redness of mouth, other signs of toxicity include anorexia, vomiting, nausea, diarrhea and GI bleeding

Patient should avoid exposure to sunlight or ultraviolet lights

Assess for ability to ambulate and report any difficulties

Examples of other drugs in this classification:

Cytarabine (*ARA-C, Cytosar-U, Cytosine, Arabinoside*), IV/SC/Intrathecal, Administer IV 100 mg/3minutes

Floxuridine (*FUDR*), Intraarterial infusion, Administer via infusion pump

Hydrozyurea (*Hydrea*), PO, Capsule may be opened and mixed with water

Mercaptopurine (*6-MP, 6-Mercaptopurine*), PO, Increase fluid intake

Methotrexate (*Amethopterin, Mexate, MTX, Rheumatrex, Folex, Mexate*), PO/IM/IV, Administer PO dose before meals, Monitor liver and renal function studies, chest x-ray is usually ordered, monitor urine for glucosuria

Procarbazine hydrochloride (*Matulane*), PO, Patient is hospitalized during therapy to monitor for toxicity, monitor patient for paresthesias, confusion, lesions or soreness in oral cavity, diarrhea, bleeding, or signs of pancytopenia, report any signs of pleural effusion (chills, fever, shortness of breath, productive cough, weakness) jaundice

Thioguanine (*TG, 6-Thioguanine*), PO, Assess for jaundice

ANTINEOPLASTICS — MITOTIC INHIBITORS

Action: Arrest cell division during the metaphase portion of the cycle

Indications: Malignant neoplasms (cancer)

Example: Vincristine (*LCR, Oncovin, VCR*)

Route: IV

Contraindications: Obstructive jaundice, pregnancy, use in men and women of childbearing age, Charcot-Marie-Tooth syndrome

Common adverse effects: Peripheral neuropathy, paresthesias, constipation, paralytic ileus, alopecia

Life-threatening effects: Hepatotoxicity

Other adverse effects: (usually dose-related) Neuritic pain, foot and hand drop, sensory loss, athetosis, ataxia, loss of deep tendon reflexes, muscle atrophy, dysphagia, weakness in larynx, ptosis, diplopia, mental depression, optic atrophy, blindness, ptosis, diplopia, photophobia, stomatitis, pharyngitis, anorexia, nausea, vomiting, diarrhea, abdominal cramps, rectal bleeding, urinary retention, polyuria, dysuria, uric acid nephropathy, SIADH,

urticaria, rash, convulsions, malaise, fever, headache, hyperuricemia, hyperkalemia, weight loss, hypertension, hypotension
Interventions:
Administer over 1 minute into patent IV site with IV fluids running,
extravasation can cause cellulitis and phlebitis
Monitor CBC, I&O, BP, VS and weight prior to administration and
report any unusual findings
Assess deep tendon reflexes and muscle grasp for strength daily,
report loss of reflexes or change in strength, report any mental
changes, gait or motor abnormalities
Report any onset of pain or swelling, assess bowel patterns for
changes
Provide emotional support for patient with alopecia
Examples of other drugs in this classification:
Etoposide (*VePesid, VP-16*), IV/PO, Administer IV infusion slowly
    over 30-60 minutes to decrease hypotension and bronchospasm

Vinblastine sulfate (*Velban, Velbe, VLB*), IV, Administer over 1 min
    into running IV fluids

BLOOD FORMERS / COAGULATORS — ANTICOAGULANTS
Action: Prevent thrombus formation in the veins, inhibits synthesis
of blood coagulation factors II, VII, IX and X in the liver by
interfering with vitamin K
Indications: Prevention of and treatment for deep venous
thrombosis and pulmonary embolism
Example: Warfarin sodium (*Coumadin sodium, Panwarfin*)
Route: PO, IV
Pharmacokinetics: Onset 2-7 days; Peak 0.5-3 days
Contraindications: Persons with bleeding tendencies to include
Vitamin K or Vitamin C deficiency, hemophilia, coagulation factor
disorders, active bleeding, blood dyscrasias, open wounds, active
ulcers, esophageal varices or those with malabsorption syndromes,
hypertension, cerebral vascular diseases or disorders, pericarditis
with acute MI, severe liver or renal disease, subacute bacterial
endocarditis, recent surgery of CNS, recent lumbar anesthesia,
threatened abortion
Life-threatening adverse effects: Hemorrhage
Other adverse effects: Anorexia, nausea, vomiting, abdominal
cramps, diarrhea, steatorrhea, stomatitis, hepatitis, jaundice,
priapism, burning sensations in feet, transient hair loss, myalgia,
bone pain, osteoporosis
Interventions:
Tablet may be crushed and taken with fluids

Administer IV at 25 mg/minute

Have Vitamin K (phytonadione) on hand for antidote, may be given PO or IV

Warfarin has multiple drug interactions consult PDR if patient is on other medications for response

Monitor PT level for response time (usual is 12-15 seconds) therapeutic range is 1.5 - 2.5 times usual time

Assess for any bleeding and guaiac stools as ordered, monitor for skin necrosis (purple areas) on toes, nose, buttocks, thighs, calves, breast, and abdomen, may indicate overdosage

Examples of other drugs in this classification:

Enoxaparin (*Lovenox*), SC, used to prevent deep vein thrombosis after hip replacement surgery, given within 24 hrs of surgery, Patient should be supine during administration, given into abdomen

Heparin (check orders for calcium or sodium) (*Calciparine, Hep-Lock, Lipo-Hepin, Liquaemin sodium*), IV/SC, Avoid injection within 2 inches of umbilical area, Do not massage injection site, rotate SC sites, IV dose is given over 60 seconds, intermittent infusion or continuous infusion, monitor APTT times to keep between 1.5-2.5 times control value, Have protamine sulfate on hand for antidote

BLOOD FORMERS / COAGULATORS — HEMATOPOIETIC GROWTH FACTORS

Action: Stimulate specific blood growth factors to form mature cells

Indications: Patients who cannot produce enough blood growth factors on their own such as those with renal failure, cancer, anemias, or HIV/AIDS

Example: Epoetin alfa (*Human recombinant erythropoietin, Epogen, Procrit*

Route: SC, IV

Pharmacokinetics: Onset 7-14 days

Contraindications: Uncontrolled hypertension, sensitivity to mammalian cell products and/or albumin

Common adverse effects: Headache, hypertension, iron deficiency, clotting of AV fistula

Other adverse effects: Seizures, nausea, diarrhea, thrombocytosis, bone pain, sweating, arthralgias

Interventions:

Do not shake solution, use only one dose from each vial, never reenter the vial after medication is withdrawn, contains no preservatives

Do not use if discoloration or particulate is found in vial

Assess patients blood pressure prior to administration of drug, monitor CBC, serum iron levels, BUN, creatinine, phosphorus, and potassium

Monitor patient for seizures (may occur if Hct rises rapidly)

Patients with chronic renal failure require close monitoring for hypertension, MI, CVA, and TIAs

Supplemental iron may be ordered

Examples of other drugs in this classification:

Filgrastim (*Neupogen*), IV/SC, drug stimulates production of neutrophils, Administer drug at room temperature, discard after dose is removed, assess for sternal pain and report if found, monitor all patients with history of cardiac problems for MI and arrhythmias, monitor for signs of infection

Sargramostim (*Leukine, Prokine, GM-CSF*), used after bone marrow transplant and for HIV/AIDS patients to increase WBC count, Assess for dyspnea during administration

BLOOD FORMERS / COAGULATORS — IRON PREPARATIONS

Action: Iron is an essential mineral for the synthesis of hemoglobin, it stimulates the hematopoietic system and increases hemoglobin

Indications: Iron-deficiency anemia, pregnancy, lactating women

Example: Ferrous sulfate (*Feosol, Fer-in-sol, Fer-Iron, Fero-Gradumet, Ferospace, Ferralyn, Ferra-TD, Fesofor, Hemantinic, Mol-Iron, Slow-Fe*)

Route: PO

Contraindications: Peptic ulcer, regional enteritis, ulcerative colitis, hemolytic anemias, hemochromatosis, hemosiderosis, patients who have had repeated transfusions, pyridoxine-response anemia, cirrhosis of liver

Common adverse effects: Nausea, heartburn, constipation, black stools

Other adverse effects: (usually slight) Anorexia, diarrhea, epigastric pain, abdominal distress, yellow-brown discoloration of eyes and teeth

Interventions:

Administer on empty stomach with full glass of water, if liquid solution it must be administered via a straw or placed on back of tongue to prevent staining of the patient's teeth, rinse mouth with water following drug

Iron absorption is impaired if taken with milk, eggs or caffeine

Drug may cause black or green stools, constipation or diarrhea may occur

Examples of other drugs in this classification:

Ferrous fumarate (*Feco-T, Femiron, Feostat, Fersamal, Fumasorb, Fumerin, Hemocyte, Ircon-FA, Palmiron*), PO

Ferrous Gluconate (*Fergon, Ferralet, Fertinic, Novoferrogluc, Simron*), PO

Iron Dextran (*Imfed, Imferon*), IM/IV, used when oral administration is not possible, test dose is given first with epinephrine on hand for severe reaction which can include fatal cardiac arrhythmias within few minutes of injection

IMMUNOMODULATORS

Action: Inhibit the multiplication of many viruses

Indications: Neoplasms, HIV/AIDS associated Kaposi's sarcoma, Hepatitis C, Broad spectrum of activity: antiviral, cytotoxic and equips the immune system to better fight off foreign antigens and viruses

Example: Interferon Alfa-2A (*Roferon-A Injection*)

Route: SC, IM

Pharmacokinetics: Peak 15-60 minutes IV, 1-8 hours IM

Contraindications: sensitivity to alpha interferons or any component thereof or to mouse immunoglobulin

Common adverse effects: Flulike syndrome, fatigue, dizziness, nausea, diarrhea, anorexia, rash

Life-threatening adverse effects: Myelosuppression

Other adverse effects: Confusion, paresthesias, lethargy, psychosis, depression, nervousness, forgetfulness, dyspnea, edema, hypertension, palpitations, vomiting, abdominal pain, taste changes, leukopenia, neutropenia, thrombocytopenia, dry skin, pruritus, alopecia, urticaria, reactivation of herpes labialis, impotence, arthralgia, coughing

Interventions:

Administer dose at same time each day

Monitor laboratory values to include CBC, liver and renal function tests

Monitor I&O, force fluids, administer antiemetic if ordered

Caution patient that flu-like syndrome is common within 2-6 hours of dose

Monitor VS, BP changes may occur

Examples of other drugs in this classification:

Interferon Alfa-2B (*Intron A*), IM/SC, Patient is usually hospitalized for initial therapy

Section VIII — GLOSSARY OF TERMS

ABO	Blood type groups
AIDS	Acquired Immune Deficiency Syndrome caused by HIV-1 virus
Agranular leukocytes	Lymphocytes and monocytes
Alopecia	Loss of hair, may be complete or partial
Anemia	Decrease in functional RBCs or hemoglobin
Aplastic anemia	Anemia from bone marrow disease or destruction
APPT	Activated partial thromboplastin time, a laboratory test to assess the clotting ability of the blood
Basophils	Type of WBC, known to release heparin, histamine and serotonin
Blast	Immature cell
Cachexia	Malnourished condition with muscle wasting related to severe or prolonged illness
Carcinoma	Pertaining to cancerous growth
Differential count	Calculation of the percentage of each type WBC
Disseminated intravascular coagulation	(DIC) Condition where blood coagulation is altered, leading to a tendency for large scale bleeding (life-threatening condition)
Dyspnea	Difficult breathing with noted increase in work above normal respirations
Ecchymosis	A bruise, an irregular shaped area on the skin that is blue-black, green to yellow, or brown caused a hemorrhagic spot below the skin
ECF	Extracellular fluid
Embolus	Any foreign material in circulating blood
Eosinophils	Type of WBC, usually increased in allergic reactions

Epistaxis	Nose bleed
Erythrocyte	Red blood cell (RBC)
Erythropoiesis	Formation of RBCs
Extravasation	The escape of fluids and/or medications into the surrounding tissue
Erythropoietin	Hormone that stimulates erythropoiesis
Fractionated blood	Blood separated into its components
Granular luekocytes	Neutrophils. eosinophils and basophils
Hematocrit (Hct)	Value of the blood cell volume in whole blood, primarily RBCs
Hematoemesis	Vomiting with blood
Hematoma	Accumulation of blood in tissue, organ or space
Hematuria	Blood in urine
Hemoglobin(Hgb)	Iron caring red pigment found in RBCs
Hemolysis	Rupture of RBC with loss of hemoglobin
Hemophilia	Hereditary disease due to a deficiency in clotting factors in the blood
Hemoptysis	Spitting up blood
HIV-1	Human immunodeficiency virus, the virus that causes AIDS
Hypoxia	Cellular oxygen deficiency
Leukemia	Uncontrolled, unorderly multiplication of WBCs may be acute or chronic
Leukocyte	White blood cell (WBC)
Leukopenia	Decrease in number of WBCs in blood <5000
Lymphoblast	Precursor for lymphocyte
Lymphoma	Malignant growth of tissue in the lymphatic system

Megakaryoblast	Precursor for platelets
Melena	Black tarry stools
Monocytes	WBC, generally increased in chronic infections
Monoblast	Precursor for monocyte
Myeloblast	Precursor for neutrophils, eosinophils and basophils
Myelosuppression	Bone marrow suppression
Neutrophils	Most active WBC during early bacterial infections, destroy bacteria by phagocytosis
Nutritional anemia	Anemia produced by inadequate dietary intake of iron rich foods
Pancytopenia	Decrease of all elements in the blood (RBC, WBC, platelets)
Pernicious anemia	Anemia produced by inadequate intrinsic factor
Petechiae	Small pinpoint hemorrhages in skin or mucous membranes
Polycythemia	An excess of red blood cells
PTT	Partial thromboplastin time, a laboratory test used to detect clotting deficiencies
Septicemia	Disease resulting from toxins or bacteria in the blood
Serum	Plasma minus clotting proteins
Splenomegaly	Enlargement of the spleen
Syncope	Fainting, usually due to an inadequate blood flow to the brain
Thalassemia	Hereditary anemias where hemoglobin production is abnormal, more common in Mediterranean (Greek) and Southeast Asian populations
Thrombus	A clot lodged in a vessel or heart cavity
Thrombocyte	Platelet

Thrombocytopenia Decrease in number of platelets in blood

Type and hold   Blood sample is typed and screened for
                        irregular antibodies but blood is not matched
                        to specific donor units

Type and   Blood sample is typed and the patient's blood
cross-match   is matched to specific donor units

Xerostomia   Dryness of mucous membranes

Reproductive System

REPRODUCTIVE SYSTEM

Table of Contents

Section I — THE OVERVIEW

Primary Functions:
- The reproduction of the human species, the duplication and transfer of genetic information from one generation to another
- Male reproductive system functions
  - Produce and store mature sperm cells
  - To transport sperm cells to the female reproductive system where the mature sperm may fertilize the female eggs
- Female reproductive system functions
  - To produce and store ova (eggs)
  - To provide a medium for the fertilization of ova
  - To provide nutrients for, and remove waste products from, the developing fetus during the 40 week gestation period
  - To transport the developed fetus from the uterus (womb) to the external environment via the vagina

Components:
- Male and female reproductive systems

Male reproductive system (Figure 6A)
- Composed of scrotum and testes, vas deferens, seminal vesicles, prostate gland and penis

Scrotum & Testes
- The scrotum is a pouch or sac that contains the testes
- Scrotum appears longer in older males or in warm temperatures
- The two reproductive glands located in the scrotum and suspended from the body by the spermatic cord are the testes
- Each testis or testicle is about 4cm long and 2.5 cm wide
- The left testis is suspended slightly lower than the right
- Produce sperm and testosterone (male hormone)
- Testosterone is necessary for development of secondary sexual characteristics and sexual functioning

Vas deferens
- Cord-like muscular tube that transports sperm from each testis to the prostatic urethra
- Approximately 18 inches or 45.7 cm long
- Also known as the Ductus deferens or seminal duct

The Male Reproductive System

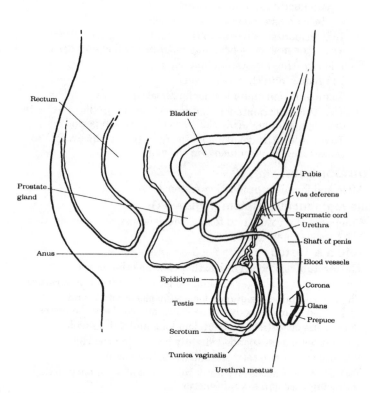

Figure 6A

- Ejaculatory duct is located at the end near where it joins the seminal vesicles

Seminal vesicles
- Two saclike structures found behind the bladder
- Connect to the vas deferens on each side
- Secrete a thick fluid that forms part of the semen
- Do not store or secrete sperm

Prostate
- A gland that surrounds the neck of the bladder and male urethra
- Gland is about 2 x 4 x 3 cm normally and weighs 20 grams
- Secretes a thin fluid that forms part of the semen
- Enlargement is common after middle age

Penis
- Cylindrical organ used for ejaculation of sperm and release of urine
- Composed of three columns of erectile tissue, two known as corpora cavernosa, the remaining column contains the urethra
- When sexual arousal occurs, the corpora cavernosa fill with blood causing the penis to become erect and more triangular in shape
- The distal end is known as the glans penis and is covered by a moveable prepuce or foreskin
- If circumcision has been performed the foreskin will not be present
- The urethral opening is located in the glans penis

Female reproductive system (Figure 6B)
- Composed of ovaries, fallopian tubes, uterus, cervix, vagina, labia and clitoris

Ovaries
- Two reproductive glands located inside the pelvic cavity, one on either side of the uterus
- Each ovary is about 4 cm long and 2 cm wide
- Contain a fixed number (100,000-400,000) of primary oocytes (undeveloped eggs) present since birth
- At puberty these oocytes will develop into ova
- Produce the hormones estrogen & progesterone

Fallopian tubes
- Tube that transports ova from the ovaries to the uterus

The Female Reproductive System

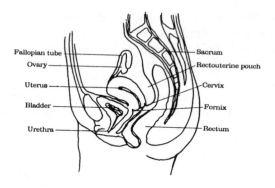

Fallopian tube
Ovary
Uterus
Bladder
Urethra

Sacrum
Rectouterine pouch
Cervix
Fornix
Rectum

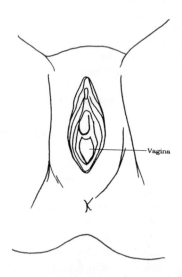

Vagina

Figure 6B

- Distal end of each tube opens into the peritoneal cavity near each ovary and is funnel-shaped with fringed projections
- The other end opens into the uterus (fundal side)
- Tubes are lined with cilia which propel the ova toward the uterus
- Approximately 4.5 inches or 11.25 cm long
- Also known as the oviduct or uterine tube

Uterus
- Hollow, muscular, pear-shaped organ located mid pelvis
- The fallopian tube enter into the fundus (top) of the uterus
- The lower end is narrow and ends in the cervix
- Has the ability to enlarge to contain and nourish an embryo/fetus
- The innermost layer of the uterus is shed during menstruation

Cervix
- Rounded and conical neck of the uterus that projects into vagina
- Usually about 1 inch long
- The os (opening) dilates and effaces (thins) during labor to allow for a passage for the fetus from the uterus to the vagina
- The os when non-pregnant is firm; in pregnancy it softens

Vagina
- A muscular tube lined with a mucous membrane between the cervix and the vulva
- Provides a passage for menstrual fluids and fetus to leave the body and for sperm to enter the body

Labia
- Folds of tissue lying on either side of the vagina
- Two sets of labia; the outer labia majora and the inner labia minora

Clitoris
- Formed where the two labia minora join anteriorly
- Similar to the male penis, becomes engorged with sexual arousal

Concepts:
Spermatogenesis (production of sperm)
- Occurs in the male testes because it requires a temperature a few degrees lower than normal body temperature
- Each sperm cell begins as a primary spermatocyte with 46 chromosomes

- The primary spermatocyte divides into two secondary spermatocytes each with 23 chromosomes
- The secondary spermatocytes divide again into two spermatids with 23 chromosomes each that develop into mature sperm
- In summary, each primary spermatocyte develops into four sperm
- About 300 million sperm are produced every day
- Each sperm has a head, middle piece and tail
  - The head contains the nucleus with the genetic material
  - The middle provides the energy for movement
  - The flagellated tail provides propulsion for movements

Oogenesis
- Occurs in the female ovary
- Primary oocytes have been prepared and stored since before birth
- At puberty the rising level of FSH (follicle stimulating hormone) stimulates the oocyte to divide into a secondary oocyte and a polar body, each with 23 chromosomes
- The oocyte is larger than the polar body which will be discarded
- Ovulation then occurs and the secondary oocyte is released into the fallopian tube
- Another division occurs and the secondary oocyte produces two cells each with 23 chromosomes
- The cells are again unequal in size the larger cell is the ootid which will develop into the ovum
- The smaller cell is another polar body which will disintegrate
- One primary oocyte forms only one ovum

Fertilization and fetal development
- During ejaculation mature sperm are propelled from the ductus epididymis into the urethra where they are mixed with emissions from the prostate and Cowper's glands to form semen
- The semen exit out of the penis through the meatal opening and into the vagina where they make their way up the female reproductive tract
- Sperm have a life expectancy of 48-72 hours once inside the female reproductive system
- Fertilization usually occurs in the upper third of the fallopian tube during the ovum's transport to the uterus
- Once ovulation occurs, the ovum has about 24 hrs to be fertilized by the male sperm

- One sperm fertilizes one ovum, after this fertilization the ovum is impermeable to other sperm
- The fertilized ovum (zygote) contains 46 chromosomes
- Sex of the offspring is determined at fertilization by the male sex chromosome
- All oocytes are X, if the sperm which fertilizes the ovum bears the X chromosome the offspring will be female (XX), if it bears the Y chromosome it will be male (XY)
- Rapid cell division follows, and the blastocyst moves down the tube into the waiting uterus
- The blastocyst will attach to the inner wall of the uterus (the endometrium) 7-8 days after fertilization
- The embryonic period lasts 2 months, during which the embryonic membranes (support fetal life) and primary adult organs develop
- At the end of the embryonic period the embryo is called a fetus
- During the last 7 months of uterine captivity the fetus will continue to grow, develop and mature

Menstruation

- Occurs if ovum is not fertilized
- Disposal by the body of it's preparations for pregnancy
- Menstruation begins at puberty (12-13 years) and continues monthly until menopause
- Composed of four phases:
    1. Menstrual phase
       Lasts about 5 days
       Lining of the uterus (endometrium) which had been prepared to support the embryo is shed
       Consists of a discharge of mucus, epithelial cells, blood and tissue (total fluid lost is about 25-100 ml)

    2. Proliferative phase
       Lasts about 10-13 days
       At onset the endometrium is very thin
       The ovarian follicles are stimulated by FSH and LH to produce more estrogen which repairs and thickens the endometrium to prepare for possible fertilized ovum

During this time the ovary prepares one oocyte for release
Phase ends when the mature ovum is released at ovulation

3. Luteal phase
    Lasts about 10-14 days
    Begins with the release of the ovum at ovulation
    The lining of the uterus continues to thicken and increases
    in vascularization
    Progesterone secretion increases and is dominant
    If no fertilization occurs, implantation will not occur and the
    uterine lining will not be maintained

4. Premenstrual phase
    Lasts about 1-2 days
    Without fertilization the lining begins to degenerate
    The cycle is complete and the menstrual phase begins

Section II — ASSESSMENT

- It is often difficult for someone to discuss problems of this system, a supportive, non-judgmental manner is important
- Some individuals may find it more comfortable to discuss sexual concerns with a health care worker of the same sex

MALE HEALTH HISTORY

Chief complaint

- Common chief complaints for this system include:
  Discharge from penis
  Itching, rash or sore in the genital area
  Inability to retract the foreskin
  A change in sexual desire or performance
  Inability to have children (infertility)

Family and personal history

- A through personal history is important, a variety of disorders may disrupt normal sexual and reproductive functioning in men
- Assess for any medication use which may disrupt sexual function:
  Antihypertensives
  Anticholinergics
  Antidepressants
  Antipsychotics
  Alcohol use
  Central nervous system depressants (sedatives & antianxiety)
  Histamine blockers
  Street drug use (Heroin)
  Tobacco use
- Obtain specific diagnoses and age at diagnosis when known
- Obtain ages and cause of death in immediate family members
- History of sexual activity to include number of partners and use of birth control (include type)
- Knowledge and practice of self-testicular examination to detect testicular cancer
- Presence of any known fertility problems
- Assess for presence and past treatment of the following:
  Sexually transmitted diseases
  Impotence
  Testicular cancer
  Prostrate problems

- If above conditions exist assess for required life-style changes and current treatment of condition

Impotence

- Includes a variety of complaints to include
    Loss of sexual desire (libido)
    Inability to initiate or maintain an erection
    Ejaculatory failure
    Premature ejaculation
    Inability to achieve an orgasm
- May be caused by a variety of problems to include, medications, history of trauma to the penis, spinal cord disorder, brain lesion, prostatectomy, diabetes, vascular disease or psychological disorder

Infertility

- Sexual activity is present without birth control and no conception has occurred
- Over one third of all infertility problems are related to the male, problems may result from:
    Decreased sperm production
    Ductal obstruction (congenital or postinfection)
    Impotence
    Ejaculatory disturbances
    Abnormal semen
    Immature reproductive development
    Infection
    Endocrine dysfunction

Male reproductive system testing

- Assess for tests completed or ordered and patient's knowledge and understanding of any test procedures or results

FEMALE HEALTH HISTORY

Chief complaint

- Common chief complaints for this system include:
    - Painful menstrual cramps
    - Premenstrual syndrome
    - Abnormal uterine bleeding
    - Cessation of menstruation (pregnancy or menopause)
    - Unusual vaginal discharge
    - Itching, burning or rash in genital area
    - A sore that will not heal in the genital area
    - A lump in breast tissue

- A lump or cyst on the side of the vagina
- A change in sexual desire or performance
- Inability to conceive or bear children

Family and personal history

- Family history is a significant factor in some reproductive disorders, cancer of the breast or reproductive tract
- Assess for use of the drug diethylstilbestrol in patient's mother which may lead to vaginal neoplasms (DES syndrome)
- Obtain specific diagnoses and age at diagnosis when known
- Obtain ages and causes of death in immediate family members
- Age of menstrual period (MP) onset
- Date of last menstrual period (LMP)
- Date of last pap smear and results if known
- Total number of pregnancies (Gravida), includes abortions, miscarriages, stillbirths and children born live
- Total number of pregnancies that produced viable children (Para)
- Total number of abortions (includes miscarriages)
- Total number of living children
- Assess for any problems during pregnancies/ deliveries to include bleeding during pregnancy, pre-term labor, elevated blood pressure, abruptio placenta, placenta previa, gestational diabetes, dysfunctional labor, cephalopelvic disproportion, use of forceps for delivery or cesarean section delivery
- Presence of any known fertility problems
- History of sexual activity to include number of partners as risk of sexually transmitted diseases (STDs) increase as partners increase
- Use of birth control to include type and frequency of use
- Knowledge and practice of self-breast examination
- Assess for presence and past treatment of the following:
  - Abnormal pap smear
  - Breast lump
  - Fibrocystic breast disease
  - Breast cancer
  - Cancer of female reproductive tract (Cervical, Uterine)
  - Endometriosis
  - Pelvic inflammatory disease
  - Sexually transmitted disease

- If above condition exists assess for required life-style changes and current treatment of condition to include medications

Premenstrual syndrome (PMS)

- Most women with PMS do not seek help until their 30's after about 10 years of symptoms
- Common physical symptoms include:

  Abdominal bloating   Constipation or diarrhea
  Acne   Headache
  Breast engorgement/tenderness   Peripheral edema
  Weight gain

- Common emotional symptoms include:

  Anxiety   Irritability
  Depression   Insomnia
  Fatigue   Mood swings
  Food cravings   Panic attacks
  Hostility   Paranoia

Infertility

- Sexual activity is present without birth control and no conception has occurred
- Problems may be related to:

  Fallopian tube dysfunction (infection or anomaly)
  Endometriosis
  Amenorrhea
  Thyroid disorders
  Diabetes
  Severe nutritional deficiencies
  Immature reproductive development
  Infection
  Endocrine dysfunction

MALE REPRODUCTIVE SYSTEM ASSESSMENT

Chief Complaint

Patient's statement_____   Onset_____

Frequency_____   Duration_____   Other areas affected_____

Have you had this before?_____   Date?_____

What treatment was given?_____

What do you think caused this?_____

What lifestyle changes have you had to make?_____

_____

Personal and Family History

	Patient Only			Patient Only	
	Current	Past		Current	Past
Fertility problem	____	____	STDs	____	____
Penile discharge?	____	____	Genital sores?	____	____
Lumps in testes?	____	____	Pain in testes?	____	____
Burning on urination?	____	____	Difficult urinating?	____	____
Testicular self-examinations?____			Frequency of exams?____		

Problems related to sexual intercourse?_____

Sexually active?_____   Birth control/protection used?_____

Number of partners?_____

	Patient	Family
Prostrate problem	____	____
Testicular Cancer	____	____

Reproductive System Testing

Sperm studies_____   Blood tests_____

Current Treatments/Medications:

Medication_____   Dose_____   Frequency_____   Route_____

Medication_____   Dose_____   Frequency_____   Route_____

Is there anything else you want me to know?_____

_____

_____

FEMALE REPRODUCTIVE SYSTEM ASSESSMENT

Chief Complaint

Patient's statement_____ Onset_____

Frequency_____ Duration_____ Other areas affected_____

Have you had this before?_____ Date?_____

What treatment was given?_____

What do you think caused this?_____

What lifestyle changes have you had to make?_____

Personal and Family History

	Patient			Patient	
	Current	Past		Current	Past
Fertility problems	_____	_____	STD's	_____	_____
Unusual discharge	_____	_____	Genital sores	_____	_____
Lumps in breast	_____	_____	Fibrocystic		
Burning on urination?	_____	_____	breast disease	_____	_____
Any surgeries?_____			Other	_____	_____

Age at MP onset?_____ LMP?_____ Heavy MP?_____

Premenstrual syndrome?_____ Gravida_____ Para_____ Abortions_____

Children living?_____ Problems with pregnancies/deliveries?_____

Problems related to sexual intercourse?_____

Sexually active?_____ Birth control/protection used?_____

Number of sexual partners?_____ Breast self exam?_____

	Patient	Family
CA of Breast	_____	_____
CA of Uterus	_____	_____
CA of Cervix	_____	_____

Reproductive System Testing

Papanicolaou smear_____ Pregnancy tests_____ Blood tests_____

Mammogram_____ Vaginal/Cervical cultures_____ VDRL/RPR_____

Breast biopsy_____ Colposcopy_____ Culdoscopy_____

Current Treatments/Medications:

Medication_____ Dose_____ Frequency_____ Route_____

Medication_____ Dose_____ Frequency_____ Route_____

Is there anything else you want me to know?_____

Physical Assessment

- Reproductive assessment is done in the following order:
  1. Inspection
  2. Palpation
- Assessment of this system may be embarrassing for some patients, a supportive non-judgmental attitude is important
- Explain what you will be doing prior to the examination
- Patient should be undressed completely and gowned
- Patients of either sex should empty bladder prior to exam
- Warm hands and equipment prior to examination
- Wear gloves when performing reproductive examinations
- Always expose only the area needed for the examination, use sheets or gowns to drape patient properly

MALE PHYSICAL EXAMINATION

- Completed with patient standing facing seated examiner

INSPECTION

General appearance

- Assess appearance of skin, hair, penis and scrotum for any gross abnormalities

Breast

- Should be symmetrical without dimpling or discharge

Penis

- Assess for location of the urethral meatus, should be located centrally on the glans penis
  Hypospadias is when the meatus is located on the underside
- Assess for any lesions, nodules, swelling or inflammation
- Cancer of the penis is usually found on the glans penis or the inner lip of the prepuce, it may appear dry and scaly, ulcerated or nodular and is painless
- Assess for discharge which is always abnormal, if found assess for color and amount, smear and/or culture should be obtained
- If uncircumcised, ask the patient to retract foreskin for visual inspection of glans penis
  - White cheesy discharge (smegma) is found under foreskin
  - Prepuce should be easily retractable from the glans, phimosis exists when glans can not be retracted

Scrotum
- Ask patient to hold penis out of way for visualization of scrotum
- Assess for edema, lesions, nodules or rashes

PALPATION
- Completed with patient standing facing seated examiner

Breast
- Use fingertips to examine breast tissue for masses

Penis
- Palpate shaft with thumb and two fingers for swelling or nodules

Scrotum/Testes
- Spread rugated surface and palpate for nodules or cysts
- Use thumb and two fingers and palpate each testes, should be smooth (rubbery feeling), equal in size and freely moveable
- Palpate the epididymis (softer than testes) and spermatic cord to the inguinal canal for any swelling, irregularity or nodules, if found assess size, location, shape, consistency and tenderness and report to primary health care provider

FEMALE PHYSICAL EXAMINATION
- Examination of breasts is usually completed first followed by examination of genitalia

INSPECTION
Breast
- Patient should be sitting, bare to the waist with arms at sides
- Inspect for size, may vary from right to left slightly and still be normal
- Assess for dimpling, flattening or any asymmetry in contour
- Color should be consistent with skin color, redness may indicate infection or inflammatory carcinoma
- A prominent venous pattern in one breast may be a sign of carcinoma
- Assess nipples, difference in direction may indicate mass
- Note any nipple discharge to include color and amount
- Have patient raise arms above head and repeat inspection
- Have patient place arms on hips with hands pressing firmly against hips and repeat inspection
- Position changes may bring out dimpling or flattening in one breast (may indicate mass)

External genitalia
- Patient is usually positioned in lithotomy position
- Separate the labia and inspect, note any nodules, sores, ulcers, rashes, discharge, and their location

PALPATION
Breast
- Palpate breast with patient in supine position, one arm is raised over head while you examine breast on opposite side
- Compress all areas of breast in systematic manner, include axilla, all breast tissue and areola
- If nodules, note location, size, shape, consistency, and mobility

Internal genitalia
- If cervical examination is to performed, gather equipment and provide assistance

MALE REPRODUCTIVE SYSTEM EXAMINATION

INSPECTION:

Breast for symmetry_____ dimpling_____ discharge_____ ulcers_____

Genitalia for level of sexual maturity_____

Circumcision_____ Descended testicles_____ Abnormalities_____

Penis: ulcers_____ sores_____ nodules_____ discharge_____ rash_____

PALPATION:

Penal shaft: Foreskin retraction_____ Masses_____ Tenderness_____

Scrotum: Nodules_____ Ulcers_____ Tenderness_____ Masses_____

Testes: Size_____ Shape_____ Symmetry_____ Tenderness_____

Spermatic cord: Intactness_____ Course_____

Assessment Notes_____

_____

_____

_____

FEMALE REPRODUCTIVE SYSTEM EXAMINATION

INSPECTION

Breast for symmetry_____ dimpling_____ discharge_____ ulcers_____

External genitalia for nodules_____ ulcers_____ sores_____ rash_____

inflammation_____ discharge_____ Pediculosis pubis_____ other_____

Internal genitalia, cervix: color_____ nodules_____ masses_____

ulcerations_____ discharge_____ position_____ other_____

Vaginal mucosa for color_____ inflammation_____ ulcers_____

PALPATION

Breasts for tenderness_____

Lumps/masses: Location_____ size_____ shape_____

Mobility_____ consistency_____ nipple discharge_____

Axilla for enlarged nodes_____

Bimanual examination: tenderness_____ nodules_____ pain_____

Cervix for position_____ shape_____ mobility_____ tenderness_____

Ovaries for size_____ shape_____ mobility_____ tenderness_____

Assessment Notes_____

_____

_____

_____

Section III — LABORATORY AND DIAGNOSTIC TESTS

In the following section traditional laboratory values and SI unit values are given, it is important to recognize that "normal" values vary from laboratory to laboratory. Check the normal values at the agency or institution where a test is performed. Most labs print their normal values on the laboratory reporting slip or page.

Table of Common Laboratory Tests

Test Name	Indications	Comments
Alpha-fetoprotein (AFP) Blood test **Normal:** <40ng/ml or <40 ug/L (SI)	Pregnancy to R/O neural tube defects	**Regarding collection:** Use red-top tube collect 7-10 ml Gestational age is listed on slip Usually done between 16-18 weeks of gestation **Results:** Elevated levels occur in neural tube defects, multiple gestations, intrauterine fetal death/abortions Screening test only, ultrasound or amniocentesis should be performed Levels over 500 ng/mL usually indicates primary liver cancer
Antispermatozoal antibody Semen analysis Blood test **Normal:** Negative	Infertility Vasectomy	**Regarding collection:** Male should avoid ejaculation for 72 hours before test Semen is collected from male Use red-top tube collect 7-10 ml of blood from male and female Semen needs to be delivered to lab within 2 hours of collection **Results:** Positive indicates infertility
CA-125 tumor marker Blood test **Normal:** 0-35 U/mL	Ovarian cancer	**Regarding collection:** Use red-top tube, collect 7-10 ml **Results:** Often not available for 3-7 days Increased levels in ovarian cancer, pregnancy, GYN tumors, Menses and endometriosis
CA 15-3 tumor marker Blood test **Normal:** <22 U/mL	Breast cancer	**Regarding collection:** Use red-top tube, collect 7-10 ml **Results:** Often not available for 7-10 days Increased in metastatic breast cancer, used to monitor therapy

Test Name	Indications	Comments
Chlamydia Culture or blood test **Normal:** Negative culture <1:640 antibodies	Chlamydia infection of conjunctiva, pharnix, urethra, rectum or most common: genitalia	**Regarding collection:** For blood test use red-top tube For cervical culture patient should not douch or bathe before culture For eye lesion cotton-tipped applicator is used for collection For urethral specimen in males swab is used **Results:** If positive culture, all sexual partners should be examined
Gonorrhea culture **Normal:** Negative	Gonorrhea	**Regarding collection:** For cervical culture patient should not douch or bathe before culture Anal culture is taken by inserting swab 1 inch into rectum, repeat if stool contaminates swab For male urethral culture, patient should not void 1 hour before, a sterile swab is inserted into urethra while patient is supine Hypotension, bradycardia, pallor or syncope may result with collection Throat culture is obtained for patients who have engaged in oral sex **Results:** If positive, gonorrhea is indicated
Luteinizing hormone assay (LH assay or FSH) **Normal:** Male 7-24 ImU/ml Female >6-30ImU/ml Postmenopause >30	Determine ovulation Testicular or ovary dysfunction	**Regarding collection:** Use red-top tube, collect 7-10 ml Note date of LMP on lab slip **Results:** Increased in menopause, anorchia, hypogonadism, precious puberty Decreased in pituitary failure and hypothalamic failure
Pregnancy tests Blood or urine **Normal:** Negative, except in pregnancy	Suspected pregnancy	**Regarding collection:** Urine — first morning specimen Blood test use red-top tube **Results:** Increased in pregnancy, tumors, hydatidiform mole of uterus
Progesterone assay Blood test **Normal:** Preovulation 20-150 ng/dL Midcycle 300-2400ng/dL Pregnancy 2400 ng/dL	Determine ovulation	**Regarding collection:** Use red-top tube collect 7-10 ml Note date of LMP on lab slip **Results:** Increased in pregnancy, ovarian CA and Adrenal neoplasms Decreased in amenorrhea, abortion, fetal death and toxemia

Test Name	Indications	Comments
Rubella antibody test Blood test **Normal:** Immune	Pregnancy to R/O susceptibility to rubella which if aquired during pregnancy leads to congenital defects	**Regarding collection:** Use red-top tube collect 7 ml **Results:** Titer >1:10-1:20 shows a lack of susceptibility to rubella
Semen analysis Fluid analysis **Normal:** 2-5 ml Sperm count 50-200M/mL Sperm motility 60-80% mobile Sperm morphology 70-90% normal in shape	Infertility Vasectomy follow-up	**Regarding collection:** Patient should abstain from sex and alcohol use 2-3 days prior to test Patient maturbates in specimen cup Record on lab slip date of previous ejaculation and date/time of this specimen **Results:** Abnormal findings in infertility, testicular atrophy, failure or orchitis
Syphilis detection test (RPR/VDRL) Blood test **Normal:** Negative	Suspected syphilis Pregnancy	**Regarding collection:** Use red-top tube collect 7 ml Some laboratorys require fasting or avoidance of alcohol, see policy **Results:** Positive test may be confirmed by Treponema or FTA-ABS testing

Table of Diagnostic Tests

Test Name	Indications	Comments
Aminocentesis **Normal:** Depends upon the reason for aminocentesis & the gestational age of the fetus	Assess fetal lung maturity–L:S ratio, R/O chromosomal, sex linked or genetic problems Assess fetal affect of isoimmunization Fetal distress	**Pre-procedure:** Signed consent form required Aminotic fluid will be withdrawn Assess patient's BP and fetal heart tones for baseline Assess orders regarding bladder status needed for gestational age **Post-procedure:** Bandage is placed over site Rh-negative women recieves RhoGAM Assess fetal heart tones Observe puncture site for bleeding

Test Name	Indications	Comments
Chorionic villus sampling (CFS) Cell analysis **Normal:** No genetic anomalies noted	R/O suspected genetic disorders	**Pre-procedure:** Signed consent form required Performed between 8-12 weeks of gestation Procedure takes about 5 minutes Cannula is inserted through the cervix and extraplacental villi are aspirated for study **Post-procedure:** RhoGAM may be ordered for Rh-neg pt Assess VS and monitor for bleeding or signs of spontaneous abortion
Colposcopy **Normal:** Normal vagina and cervix	Abnormal PAP smear Cervical dysplasia Suspected cancer	**Pre-procedure:** Signed consent form may be required Procedure takes 5-10 minutes A colposcope is used to examine the cervix; biopsy is usually taken **Post-procedure:** Vaginal bleeding may occur Pt should abstain from intercourse & tampon use until healing
Contraction stress test or Oxytocin challenge test (OCT, CST) **Normal:** Negative—No late declearations with contractions	High-risk pregnancy	**Pre-procedure:** Signed informed consent is required Obtain maternal blood pressure Have patient empty bladder Uterine tone and FHTs are monitored for 20 minutes before oxytocin Administer oxytocin via IV pump, assess for contractions and FHT response **Post-procedure:** After oxytocin is discontinued, pt is assessed until no further Cx are noted, IV is discontinued
Endometrial biopsy **Normal:** No pathology	Determine ovulation Endometrial cancer Abnormal bleeding	**Pre-procedure:** Signed informed consent is required **Post-procedure:** Monitor VS, report elevated temp Vaginal bleeding may occur No intercourse, tampons, heavy lifting or douching for 72 hours
Mammography X-ray **Normal:** Normal breast tissue for age	Routine screening for breast cancer Breast lump	**Pre-procedure:** Talc powder or deodorant should not be worn X-ray of both breasts will be taken **Post-procedure:** No restrictions apply

Test Name	Indications	Comments
Non-stress test (NST) **Normal:** "Reactive," two or more FHR increases of 15 bpm for 15s or more within 10 minutes with fetal activity	High risk-pregnancy	**Pre-procedure:** Patient should eat if hungry Bladder should be empty Uterine and FHR monitor is applied and fetal movements are marked on strip FHT's are evaluated with regard to uterine movement **Post-procedure:** No restrictions apply
Papanicolaou smear (PAP smear) **Normal:** No abnormal cells	Screening test for cervical cancer	**Pre-procedure:** Pt should not douche or bathe 24 hr before test Bladder should be empty Reason for exam should be noted **Post-procedure:** No restrictions apply

Section IV — PROCEDURES

Contraception

- Contraception or birth control is used to avoid pregnancy
- Most of these forms of birth control are available at family planning clinics for low or no cost
- Pregnancy can occur at anytime after puberty
      The onset of puberty in girls is from 9-17 years
      The onset of puberty in boys is from 10-19 years
- Pregnancy can occur the very first time the individual has intercourse
- Pregnancy can occur during menstruation
- Pregnancy can occur up to two years after the last menses in menopausal women (documented cases even after this)
- Surgical contraception does not alter sexual desire

Contraception and sexually transmitted diseases (STDs)

- Condoms and some spermaticidal agents are effective against most STDs
- Oral contraceptives, IUD's and diaphragms are not effective against STDs

Methods of Contraception

- There are a variety of methods available (see table below)
- TSS stands for toxic shock syndrome
- Pregnancy rate is over a 1 year period

Table of Contraception Methods

Method	Pregnancy Rate* Contraindications	Side Effects	Comments
Abstinence	9% None	None	No risk of STD 100% effective
Surgical Contraception	Less than 1% Future desire for children	Rare: Infection	Usually permanent Includes: Tubal ligation Vasectomy

Method	Pregnancy Rate* Contraindications	Side Effects	Comments
Oral Contraception	0.3% - 2% Age over 40 Chronic illness Hypertension Liver problems Stroke Heart disease	See specific agent Nausea Headaches Heart attack Stroke Thrombo-embolism Stroke Migraine	Synthetic hormone Large variety Positive side effects: Regular periods Less cramping Prescription required
Condom &/or Foam	1-2% together Foam 4-29% Condom 2-10%	Mild vaginal irritation	Condom should be used only once Available OTC Provides protection from STDs
Sponge	5% Menstrual flow	Rare: Rash Irritation TSS	Soft polyurethane sponge in vagina Contains spermaticide Available OTC Leave in place 6 hrs after sex
Diaphragm	10-18% alone 3-5% with spermaticidal jelly Uterine prolapse Cystocele	Rare: TSS	Circular rubber device inserted into vagina Fitted device Leave in place 8 hrs after sex
Basal Body Temperature	6-10% None	None	Fertile periods are assessed and abstinence is used at this time
Withdrawal	15-25% None	None	Penis withdrawn prior to ejaculation Not recommended
Douching after sex	35-40% None	None	Unreliable Not recommended
No Method	80% None	None	Usually leads to pregnancy

Section V — Conditions

Sexually Transmitted Diseases (STDs)

Definition
* Diseases acquired by sexual contact or sexual intercourse with an infected individual
* Includes AIDS (see the hematologic & immune system chapter)

Prevalence
* Believed to be the second most common form of communicable disease in the USA, with the common cold being the first
* Center for Disease Control (CDC) estimates that 12 million in US acquire a STD each year
* Some estimate that 50% of Americans have had a STD by age 35
* The two most commonly transmitted STDs in the USA are Human papillomavirus (HPV) and Hepatitis B (HBV)

Etiology
* Transmission occurs from intimate contact with an infected partner
* STD's can be transmitted the very first time one has intercourse with an infected partner
* Pregnancy does not provide immunity from STDs
  One can become pregnant and acquire a STD at the same time
* STD's have not proven to be transmitted by toilet seats
* Immunity is not developed in most STDs, reinfection is possible, therefore treatment of both partners and their contacts is vital
* Some STD's are caused by bacteria
  Gonorrhea *(Neisseria gonorrhoeae)*
  Chlamydia *(Chlamydia trachomatis)*
  Syphilis *(Treponema pallidum)*
  Granuloma inguinale *(Calymmatobacterium granulomatis)*
* Some STDs are caused by viruses, most of which are incurable
  AIDS/HIV-1 (Human immunodeficiency virus)
  Adult T-cell leukemia (Human T lymphotropic virus type I)
  Herpes Simplex virus type 2 (HSV-2)
  Condylomata or veneral warts (Human papilloma virus)
  Hepatitis B virus
  Cytomegalovirus

- Some STDs are caused by protozoa or fungi
    Trichomonas *(Trichomonas vaginalis)*
    Pubic lice *(Phthirus pubis)*

Risk factors associated with STDs

- Multiple partners, risk increases as number of sexual partners increases
- Sexual contact with prostitutes and their sexual partners

Symptoms of STDs

- A vaginal or penile discharge IS NOT present in all STDs
- Sterility is a complication from many untreated STDs

Sexually Transmitted Diseases and Treatment

Disease	Symptoms	Treatment
Gonorrhea *Neisseria Gonorrhoeae* Also known as "The Clap" or "GC" Bacterial	Women — often asymptomatic Males — Penile discharge may be thick yellow to green 3-9 days post-contact Painful urination Lower abdominal pain Fever/chills Rare: arthritis, endocarditis Bacterial meningitis	Ceftriaxone Coxycycline Spectinomycin May lead to PID (pelvic inflammatory disease) if untreated
Chlamydia *Chlamydia trachomatis* Bacterial	Usually asymptomatic White to clear discharge from urethra or vagina Burning may occur Painful coitus Irregular menstruation Lower abdominal pain	Tetracycline HCL Doxycycline Minocycline Erythromycin Sulfonamide OlfoxacinR May lead to salipingo-oophoritis in females and Reiters syndrome in males if untreated
Syphilis *Treponema pallidum* Also known as "syph" Bacterial	Three stages of disease: 1) Painless chancre sore on genitals or mouth 10-30 days post-contact, no discharge and chancre disappears in few weeks 2) Secondary syphilis occurs 6 weeks after chancre, skin rash, fever, aches, hair loss, sore throat, clears by self 3) Tertiary syphilis, appears 5-40 years after chancre with heart, blood vessels and brain involvement	Benzathine penicillin G Aqueous procaine penicillin Tetracycline Permanent damage to major organs such as heart or nervous system occurs if untreated

Disease	Symptoms	Treatment
Granuloma inguinale *Calymmatobacterium granulomatis* Bacterial	Uncommon in USA Slowly progressive ulcerative skin disease that affects the subcutaneous tissue of the genital, inguinal area and anus	Tetracycline Sulfisoxazole
Herpes Simplex virus type II Viral	Painful blisters on genitalia appear 3-10 days after contact Swelling & inflammation may occur, general malaise May also be found on rectum, mouth, fingers Disappear & reappear, common with stress	No cure available Acyclovir — topical & Zovirax PO
Condylomata Human papilloma virus Also known as "Venereal Warts"	Pink, cauliflower shaped warts on genitals Warts appear 1-3 months after contact Increased in pregnancy	May reoccur even with tx Cauterization of warts Cryosurgery to warts Laser surgery Interferon-a injected in lesions
Hepatitis B virus	Incubation period 1-6 months Low-grade fever, anorexia, nausea, vomiting, fatigue, malaise, muscle & joint pain, headache, photophobia – Early clay colored stools, dark urine appear later prior to jaundice	Prevention: Vaccine is available & recommended Treatment depends on symptoms Untreated disease may resolve or lead to death
Trichomonas *Trichomonas vaginalis* Protozoan	Frothy vaginal discharge Profuse, malodorous discharge Burning on urination Intense itching Males are usually asymptomatic	Metronidazole

Components of initial examination for STDs

- *Complete medical history to include:*
- Assessment of patient's feelings of overall health status
- Assessment of risk factors for STDs to include sexual behaviors and number of partners
- Current use of condoms, spermicidal foams or other methods of contraception
- Any sexual problems currently experienced (painful intercourse may occur with STDs)
- Symptoms of current problem and how long symptoms have been present (See table on STDs for common symptoms)
- Any history of painful, frequent or difficult urination

- Past personal history of sexually transmitted diseases to include type and treatment
- Patient's understanding of prevention and treatment of STDs
- Patient's willingness to make lifestyle changes to prevent the spread of untreatable STDs
- *Physical examination to include:*
- General appearance, some STDs may lead to feelings of malaise or general ill health
- Assessment for temperature elevation
- Examination of the oral cavity for any lesions or sores
- Examination of the penis for sores or discharge
  Penile discharge may be white, clear or green
- Examination of the female external genitalia for any sores or discharge
  Vaginal discharge may be irritating, yellowish, malodorous, frothy, cheesy, gray or with intense itching
- Examination of the rectum for lesions or discharge
- *Laboratory and diagnostic testing:*
- Blood tests or cultures of discharges may be done depending upon patients symptoms

Prevention and Treatment of STDs

- Condoms are effective in preventing the spread of STDs if used properly
- Effective treatment involves treatment of the patient as well as treatment of all known sexual partners to stop transmission
- A vaccination is available for HBV (Hepatitis B) infection, no other vaccination is avilable to prevent STDs
- For treatment of specific disorders see table under symptoms

Section VI — DIETS

• Nutrition during pregnancy

NUTRITION DURING PREGNANCY

General description	Infant growth and development depends upon the nutritional status of the mother Weight grain is normal expectation of pregnancy A weight gain of 25-35 pounds is desired First trimester gain of 2-4 pounds Second trimester gain of 11 pounds Third trimester gain of 11 pounds
Indications	Pregnancy

Allowable Items	Nutritious foods are encouraged, all of the four basic food groups should be included
	The following should be included daily:
	   Water 4-6 glasses daily
	   Milk, 3-4 servings per day
	   Meats, 4-8 ounces per day (2-3 servings)
	   Bread, 4-8 servings per day
	   Vegetables, at least 3 servings per day
	   Fruits, 3-4 servings per day
	   Fats, used in moderation
	Total calories should be 300 more calories per day than non-pregnancy or about 2100-2400 per day

Restricted Items	Alcohol is restricted, no foods are restricted High calorie, low nutrition items are discouraged
Nutritional value	Pre-natal vitamins with iron are recommended Weight gain should be assessed weekly and any gain of over 2 lbs/week should be reported Diet if well-balanced should provide all of the needed nutrients

Section VII — DRUGS

The tables supply only general information, a drug handbook or the physicians desk reference (PDR) should be consulted for details. Each classification includes detailed information about the example drug, this drug is representative of the other drugs in the classification and can be used as a model.

Every effort has been made to include the major classes of drugs used in the treatment of reproductive disorders.

ANDROGENS

Action: Development of secondary male sexual characteristics, these are naturally occuring hormones in the body

Indications: Hypogonadism, hypopituitarism, dwarfism, eunuchism, oligospermia, cryptorchidism (males), some breast cancers in females

Example: Testosterone (*Andro 100, Histerone, Testoderm*)

Route: IM

Contraindications: Sensitivity to androgens, serious cardiac or renal disease, pregnancy, lactating mothers, breast CA in males, benign prostatic hypertrophy, elderly, hypertension

Common adverse effects: Sodium and water retention, edema, increase libido, acne, gynecomastia

Other adverse effects: Excitation, insomnia, skin flushing, nausea, vomiting, anorexia, diarrhea, gastric pain, jaundice, leukopenia, hypercalcemia, hypercholesterolemia, renal calculi, bladder irritability

Adverse effects for women: Suppression of ovulation, lactation or menses, hoarseness or deepening of voice, hirsutism, oily skin, clitoral enlargement, regression of breast tissue, male-pattern baldness

Adverse effects for men: Premature epiphyseal closure, phallic enlargement, priapism, testicular atrophy, decreased ejaculatory volume, azoopermia, oligospermia, impotence, epididymitis, priapism

Interventions:

Administer IM injections deep into large muscle

Assess for weight gain due to water retention, monitor for edema

Monitor cholesterol, calcium, and liver function studies during treatment

Monitor diabetic patients for hypoglycemia

Male patients should report priapism (sustained/painful erection) and gynecomastia to primary care provider, female patients should report pregnancy, increased libido, deepened voice, increased facial hair

Examples of other drugs in this classification:

Danazol (*Danocrine*), PO used to treat endometriosis and fibrocystic breast disease

Fluoxymesterone (*Halotestin*), PO give with meals to reduce GI distress

Methyltestosterone (*Android, Oreton-Methyl, Testred, Virilon*), PO, Buccal tablet should be placed between cheek and gum to absorb

Nandrolone (*Androlone-D, Deca-Durabolin, Hybolin decaneate, Nandrobolic*), IM, used for metastatic breast cancer

Oxymetholone (*Anadrol*), PO, Used for aplastic anemia

Stanozolol (*Winstrol*), PO, used for aplastic anemia

ESTROGENS

Action: Development of both primary and secondary female sex characteristics as well as changes produced by the female menstrual cycle. Synthetic forms are often used to treat menopause

Indications: Often used to treat menopause or for ovarian failure, primary amenorrhea, oophorectomy or hypopituitarism

Example: Estradiol (*Estrace, Estraderm*)

Route: PO, Topical, IM

Contraindications: Preganancy, estrogen dependent neoplasms, breast cancer, thromboembolic disorders, cholestatic disease, thyroid dysfunction, blood dyscrasias

Common adverse effects: Nausea

Life threatening effects: Thromboembolic disorders

Other adverse effects: Headache, migraines, dizziness, mental depression, chorea, convulsions, hypertension, worsening of myopia or astigmatism, vomiting, anorexia, increased appetitie, diarrhea, abdominal cramps, pain, constipation, bloating, colitis, acute pancreatitis, cholestatic jaundice, benign hepatoadenoma, mastodynia, breast secretion, spotting, menstrual flow changes, dysmenorrhea, amenorrhea, cervical erosion, premenstrual-like syndrome, vaginal candidiasis, endometrial hyperplasia, fibromyomata growth (if pre-existing), cystitis-like syndrome, hyperglycemia, hypercalcemia, folic acid deficiency, fluid retention, dermatitis, pruritus, seborrhea, oily skin, acne, photosensitivity, chloasma, hair loss, weight changes, changes in libido

Adverse effects for males: Gynecomastia, testicular atrophy, feminization, impotence

Interventions:
Usually administered for 3 weeks and then 1 week off medication
Administer with solid foods to reduce nausea (nausea is temporary)
Monitor weight, report any sudden weight gains
Assess for Homan's sign by dorsiflexing the foot, positive if patient
has pain with dorsiflexion, assess legs for tenderness, swelling and
redness
Monitor diabetic patients for hyperglycemia, reassure male patients
that feminization is reversiable with termination of therapy

Examples of other drugs in this classification:

Estrogen, conjugated (*Premarin, Progens*), PO/IM/Topical

Estrogens, esterified (*Estratab, Menest, Menrium*), PO

Estropipate (*Ogen*), PO, Intravaginal

Polyestradiol phosphate (*Estradurin*), IM, used for prostatic
    carcinoma

Quinestrol (*Estrovis*), PO

PROGESTINS

Action: Progestins maintain the endometrium and vaginal
epithelium and decrease uterine motility during pregnancy. It is
steroid naturally synthesized and released by testes, ovaries,
adrenal cortex and placenta.

Indications: Secondary amenorrhea, uterine bleeding,
endometriosis and PMS

Often used with estrogens to provide fertility control — oral
contraceptive

Example: Progesterone (*Gesterol 50, Progestasert*)

Route: IM, Intrauterine

Contraindications: Sensitivity to progestins, breast or genital
malignancy, thrombophlebitis, thromboembolic disorders, impaired
liver function, 1-4 months of pregnancy, missed abortion,
undiagnosed vaginal bleeding

Common adverse effects: Nausea, breakthrough bleeding, acne,
edema, weight changes

Life-threatening effects: Thromboembolic disorders, pulmonary
embolism

Other adverse effects: Migraine headache, dizziness, lethargy,
mental depression, somnolence, insomnia, visual changes, proptosis,
diplopia, papilledema, retinal vascular lesions, hepatic disease,
jaundice, vomiting, abdominal cramps, gynecomastia, galactorrhea,
vaginal candidiasis, pyrexia, chloasma, cervical erosion,
dysmenorrhea, amenorrhea, pruritis valvae, hyperglycemia,

decreased libido, pruritius, allergic rash, urticaria, photosensitivity, hirsutism, alopecia, fatigue

Interventions:

Administer IM injections deeply, rotate areas to reduce pain at site

Baseline VS and weight should be obtained before therapy is begun

Advise patient to use sunscreen and avoid exposure to UV light

Report sudden headache, vomiting, dizziness, fainting, numbness in extremity, chest pain, dyspnea, visual losses or changes

For Progestasert a secondary method of birth control needs to be used in the first two months, spotting, cramping and discomfort may be noted for first 3 months, contraceptive method must be changes after first year

Examples of other drugs in this classification:

Hydroxyprogesterone caproate (*Duralutin, Gesterol LA, Hylutin, Hyprogest 250, Pro-Depo*), IM

Medroxyprogesterone acetate (*Amen, Curretab, Depo-Provera, Provera*), PO,IM

Megestrol acetate (*Megace, Pallace*), PO, Advanced cancer of breast or endometrium, also used as appetite stimulant for AIDS patients

Norethindrone (*Micronor, Norlutin, Nor-Q-D*), PO

Norgestrel (*Ovrette*), PO, used as progestin-only contraceptive (minipill)

Section VIII — GLOSSARY OF TERMS

Ab	Abortion
Abortion	Pregnancy termination may occur spontaneously or be planned and induced
Abruptio placenta	Premature separation of the placenta
Afterbirth	The Placenta
Amniocentesis	Removal of amniotic fluid via the abdomen of a pregnant women to detect abnormalities or genetic problems
Amenorrhea	Lack of menses
Apgar	Assessment of color, heart rate, reflex irritability, muscle tone, and respirations of new born infant at 1 and 5 minutes
C-Section	Cesarean Section
Cervix	Rounded structure at the neck of uterus
Cesarean section	Surgical removal of fetus via an abdominal incision
Circumcision	Surgical removal of the prepuce of the penis
Coitus	Sexual intercourse
Condoms	Commercial device for prevention of pregnancy and venereal disease, consists of a thin flexible sheath that fits over the penis to collect semen
Contraception	Methods employed to prevent pregnancy
Cryptorchisim	Undesended testes
D & C	Dilation & Curettage
Dilation & Curettage	A surgical procedure where the cervix is dilated and inner wall of the uterus is scraped
Dysmenorrhea	Difficult and/or painful menstruation
Dyspareunia	Difficult or painful intercourse for women

Ectopic Pregnancy	Pregnancy where implantation occurs outside of the uterus may be in the fallopian tube, abdomen or ovary
EDC	Estimated Date of Confinement, expected due date of the pregnant woman
Embryo	Term for the product of contraception from 2nd to 8th week of gestation
Endometritis	Inflammation of the uterine lining
Estrogen	Hormone produced by the female ovary that is needed for the development of secondary sexual characteristics and menstrual cycle
Fetus	Unborn infant from the 8th to 40th week of gestation
FSH	Follicle Stimulating Hormone, secreted by the anterior pituitary gland responsible for the maturation of the follicle (oocyte and surrounding cells) prior to ovulation in the monthly menstrual cycle
G	Gravida or pregnancy, total number of pregnancies
GC	Gonorrhea, one of the sexually transmitted diseases
GU	Genitourinary, referring to the genitals and urinary organs
Genitalia	The organs of reproduction
Gravida	Pregnancy, the total number of pregnancies
Gynecomastia	Enlargement of the male breast tissue
hCG	Human Chorionic Gonadotropin
Hysterectomy	Removal of the uterus
Human Chorionic Gonadotropin	hCG, a hormone secreted by cells that surround the developing embryo, a positive hCG indicates pregnancy

LH	Luteinizing Hormone, secreted by the anterior pituitary just prior to ovulation
LMP	Last Menstrual Period
Leukorrhea	White discharge from the vagina
Menarche	Onset of menstruation in females
Menorrhea	Normal menses or normal menstrual flow
MP	Menstrual period
Mastectomy	Removal of all or part of the breast tissue
Menopause	Cessation of menses
Neonate	Newborn
OB	Obstetrics
P	Para, number of viable pregnancies
PAP smear	Papanicolaou Smear, a screening test for the detection of cervical cancer
Para	Number of viable pregnancies
Pediculosis pubis	"Crabs," a lice infestation of the hair in the genital region
PID	Pelvic Inflammatory Disease
Placenta previa	Placenta is implanted low in the uterus often called "low lying placenta", placenta may completely cover the cervix or just be implanted low
Primagravida	Women pregnant for first time
SGA	Small for gestational age
Sterility	Inability to conceive
Testosterone	One of the male sex hormones produced by the testicles, it aids in the development of secondary sexual characteristics, is needed for libido and erection of the male penis

Tubal ligation   Surgical method of contraception where the
                       fallopian tubes are blocked to prevent
                       fertilization

Venereal disease   Sexually transmitted infections that include
                       gonorrhea, syphilis, chancroid, trichomonas,
                       genital herpes, venereal warts, etc.

Endocrine System

ENDOCRINE SYSTEM

Table of Contents

Section I — THE OVERVIEW

- The response of man to the environment is controlled in a large part by the interaction of two body systems, the endocrine and the neurological system
  - Endocrine system is centrally controlled by nervous system
  - Nervous system function is negotiated by the endocrine system through hormones

Primary Functions

- Synthesis and release of hormones into the bloodstream
  - A hormone is any substance which originates in an organ or gland and then is transported in the blood to another site to stimulate function or leads to the secretion of additional hormone(s) or substance(s)
  - Hormones may produce a generalized or local effect
  - Hormones are needed:
    To control water and electrolyte metabolism
    To control gastrointestinal function
    To regulate growth
    To regulate metabolism and energy
    For reproductive function
    To control stress
    For the inflammatory process
- Controls neurotransmitters (acetylcholine and catecholamine) which are chemical mediators synthesized by nerve cells and released from nerve endings in the adrenal medulla and central nervous system
- Production of hormonal peptides such as endorphins and enkephlins involved with pain and emotions

Components and function

- The endocrine system is involved in the control and integration of many body functions via the secretion of hormones to include the hypothalamus, pituitary gland, thyroid gland, parathyroid glands, adrenal glands and the pancreas

Hypothalamus and pituitary gland

- Hypothalamus is located in the diencephalon, one of the four principal parts of the brain
- Hypothalamus is the control center: it integrates and maintains many body functions

- The pituitary gland is a small (1.3 X 1.0 X 0.5 cm) gray structure attached to the base of the brain
- The pituitary gland is an endocrine gland that secretes a number of hormones
- Pituitary is often referred to as the master gland of the body
- Hypothalamus receives input from all areas of the central nervous system (CNS) and synthesizes the following neurohormones which either stimulate or inhibit pituitary hormones

  1. Thyrotropin releasing hormone (TRH)
      Stimulates the production of thyroid stimulating hormone (TSH) and prolactin (PRL) within the pituitary
      - TSH needed for synthesis of T4 and T3 used in metabolism
      - PRL with estrogen and progesterone stimulates breast development and milk production during pregnancy

  2. Gonadotropin releasing hormone (GnRH)
      - Also called luteinizing-hormone releasing hormone (LHRH). Stimulates secretion of luteinizing hormone (LH) and follicle-stimulating hormone (FSH) from the pituitary
      - LH and FSH are involved with development of ovarian follicles, spermatogenesis, secretion of estrogens, ovulation and the development of the corpus luteum

  3. Dopamine
      - Inhibits the release of PRL, can also inhibit the release of LH, FSH and TSH under certain circumstances

  4. Corticotropin releasing hormone (CRH)
      - Stimulates the release of adrenocorticotropic hormone (ACTH) from the pituitary
      - ACTH stimulates the adrenal cortex to secrete cortisol as well as some weak androgens

  5. Growth hormone-releasing hormone (GRH)
      - Stimulates growth hormone (GH) release from the pituitary
      - Disorders associated with GH include acromegaly, dwarfism and gigantism

6.   Somatostatin
   • Inhibits the synthesis and secretion of GH and TSH 7.
   Pro-opiomelanocorticotropin (POMC)
   • Found in the hypothalamus and pituitary, this hormone
   gives rise to ACTH, B-lipotropin, B-melanocyte
   stimulating hormone, enkephalins, and endorphins
   • Enkephalins and endorphins are morphine-like peptides
   that bind and activate opioid receptors throughout the
   CNS
• These hormones are also produced in the posterior lobe of the
   pituitary gland
   1.   Antidiuretic hormone (ADH)
   Acts on the smooth muscles of the blood vessels to prevent
   excessive loss of water through the kidneys
   2.   Oxytocin
   Acts on the smooth muscle of the uterus to produce contractions

Thyroid gland
• Located below the larynx in the middle portion of the neck
• Synthesizes these thyroid hormones
   1.   Thyroxine (T4)
   Major hormone secreted by thyroid
   T4 serum levels are used to measure thyroid function
   2.   Triioddothyronine (T3)
   Secreted in smaller amounts than T4
   Its effect is more potent than T4
• Thyroid hormones are secreted in response to thyroid-stimulating
   hormone (TSH) produced in the pituitary gland and thyroid
   releasing hormone (TRH) from the hypothalamus
• Thyroid hormones have several major effects:
   • Increase metabolism (affecting all major organs)
   • Necessary for physical and mental growth and development in
   children
   • Necessary for the attainment of sexual maturity
• Endocrine disorders related to this gland include hyperthyroidism
   and hypothyroidism

Parathyroid glands
• Located on the lower edge of the thyroid gland

- Secrete parathyroid hormone (PTH) which regulates calcium-phosphorus metabolism (requires vitamin D)

Adrenal glands

- Located on the apex of each kidney
- Secretes three major types of hormones:
    1. Glucocorticoids
       Active in protecting against stress and maintaining normal metabolism
       Hydrocortisone or cortisol is the most abundant
       Corticosterone and cortisone are others
    2. Mineralocorticoids
       Help maintain water and electrolyte (Na+, K+) balance
       Aldosterone is the primary mineralocorticoid
    3. Adrenal sex hormones
       Both male (androgens) and female (estrogens) gonadocorticoids or sex hormones in small amounts
       Estrogens are also produced by the ovaries and placenta
       Testosterone (androgen) is produced by the testes
- The adrenal cortex secretes epinephrine and norepinephrine which are sympathomimetic
  Involved in the "flight or fight" response with increased blood pressure, heart rate, respirations, and decreased blood to the digestive tract during times of stress

Pancreas

- A digestive accessory gland located behind the stomach in front of the 1st and 2nd lumbar vertebrae
- Secretes the following hormones:
    1. Insulin
       Secreted by the beta cells of the islets of Langerhans
       Essential for metabolism
       Provides for glucose storage
       Prevents fat breakdown and increases protein synthesis
       Only hormone known to have a direct effect in lowering blood sugar by facilitating its transport into skeletal muscle and adipose tissue
    2. Glucagon
       Secreted by the alpha cells
       Stimulates the breakdown of glycogen and the release of glucose by the liver
       Opposite effects of insulin

3. Somatostatin
   Secreted by the delta cells
   Inhibits the secretion of insulin, glucagon and growth hormone
4. Gastrin, secretin, cholecystokinin, and gastric inhibitory peptide
   Aid in gastric control

Section II — ASSESSMENT

Assessment of the endocrine system will involve looking at the body in general for signs of endocrine system failure

HEALTH HISTORY

Chief complaint

- Common chief complaints for this system include:
  - Fatigue or weakness
  - Weight changes
  - Mood changes
  - Bowel pattern changes
  - Poor wound healing
  - Changes in hair distribution
  - Temperature tolerance changes

Family and personal history

- Obtain specific diagnoses and age of diagnosis when known
- Obtain ages and causes of death in immediate family members
- Assess for present and past treatment of the following:
  - Acromegaly
  - Addison's disease
  - Cushing's syndrome
  - Diabetes mellitus
  - Hyperthyroidism
  - Hypothyroidism
  - Hyperparathyroidism
  - Hypoparathyroidism
  - Simmond's disease
- If condition exists assess for required life style changes and current treatment of condition to include medications
- Good history is vital, family history is important as some endocrine disorders may be genetic in origin to include: Hyperthyroidism, goiter, diabetes, and growth disorders
- Symptoms of disorders for this system can be vary widely dependent upon the hormone(s) affected:

Growth hormone excess
Acromegaly
  Coarse facial features
  Thick skin and nails
  Wide hands and feet
  Weakness

Growth hormone deficiency
  Simmond's disease
  Pallor, dry skin
  Weight loss, emaciation
  Recurrent infections
  Lethargy, decreased strength

Impotence, infertility
Diplopia
Joint deformities
Joint pain
Deep voice
Diaphoresis
Hirsutism

Impotence, decreased libido
Intolerance to cold
Hypotension
Atrophy of gonads and thyroid
Amenorrhea
Decreased perspiration
Decreased pubic hair

Thyroid-excess:
Hyperthyroidism
  Anxiety, mood swings
  Heat intolerance
  Tachycardia, palpitations
  Exophthalmos
  Diarrhea
  Weight loss
  Diaphoresis
  Increased hunger

Thyroid-deficiency:
Hypothyroidism
  Mental sluggishness, fatigue
  Cold intolerance, hypothermia
  Edema
  Alopecia, coarse hair
  Constipation
  Weight gain
  Decreased diaphoresis
  Anorexia

Hyperparathyroidism:
  Renal colic or calculi
  Dysrhythmias
  Constipation, obstruction
  Anorexia, weight loss
  Nausea and vomiting
  Depression, mental dullness
  Fatigue, mood swings
  Osteoporosis, deep bone pain
  Pathologic fractures
  Muscle weakness

Hypoparathyroidism:
  Convulsions
  Dysrhythmias
  Abdominal spasms
  Dyspnea, laryngeal stridor
  Positive Trousseau's sign
  Lethargy, personality changes
  Visual disturbances
  Tingling of fingers
  Calcification of ocular lens
  Muscle spasms

Adrenal-hypercortisolism:
Cushing's syndrome
  Weight gain
  Hirsutism
  Amenorrhea
  Weakness and fatigue
  Pain in joints
  Ecchymosis
  Edema
  Hypertension

Adrenal-hypocortisolism:
Addison's disease
  Weight loss, anorexia
  Decreased pubic hair
  Depression
  Weakness and lethargy
  Hypoglycemia
  Bronzed skin pigmentation
  Dehydration, thirst
  Orthostatic hypotension

Purple striae on abdomen
Buffalo hump
Moon face
Poor wound healing
Recurrent infections
Muscle wasting

Diarrhea
Nausea

Diabetes mellitus

Weight loss, anorexia
Polydipsia, polyphagia
Acetone breath
Weakness, fatigue
Dehydration, polyuria
Increased thirst
Frequent infections
Poor wound healing
Retinopathy, blurred vision
Sexual dysfunction

Fatigue and weakness

- Assess for ability to complete activities of daily living
- Weakness and fatigue may occur with acromegaly, Simmond's disease, hypothyroidism, hypoparathyroidism, hyperparathyroidism, Cushing's syndrome, Addis's disease and diabetes mellitus

Weight changes

- Assess for any recent weight changes and patient's perception of why change occurred, may be related to hormonal imbalance or depression
- Increased weight may occur with hypothyroidism and Cushing's syndrome
- Decreased weight may occur with Addison's, growth hormone deficiency, hyperthyroidism, hyperparathyroidism, and diabetes
- Increased thirst and appetite are classic signs of diabetes

Mood changes

- Assess current mood and inquire about any mood changes
- Depression and decreased self-esteem are common
- Changes in body image may occur from changes in facial features, voice changes, changes in body hair distribution, fat pattern distribution, skin color changes or scarring

- Libido may be affected by mood — sexual dysfunction, atrophy of sexual organs, impotence and infertility may occur

Bowel pattern changes

- Assess for any changes in usual bowel pattern and patient's perception of why change occurred
- Constipation is common in hypothyroidism and hyperparathyroidism
- Diarrhea may occur with Addison's and hyperthyroidism

Frequent infections/poor wound healing

- Assess for number of infections in last six months
- Assess for any sores or wounds that are not healing well
- May occur with diabetes, growth hormone deficiency and Cushing's

Changes in hair distribution

- Decreased pubic and axillary hair may occur with growth hormone decrease and Addison's
- Hirsutism may occur with growth hormone excess and Cushing's
- Alopecia may occur with hypothyroidism

Temperature intolerance

- Assess for any history of temperature intolerance
- Heat intolerance may be related to hyperthyroidism
- Cold intolerance is common with growth hormone deficiency and hypothyroidism

Endocrine system testing

- Assess for tests completed or ordered and patient's knowledge and understanding of any test procedures or results

ENDOCRINE SYSTEM ASSESSMENT FORM

Chief Complaint

Patient's statement_____   Onset_____

Frequency_____   Duration_____   Other areas affected_____

Have you had this before?_____   Date_____

What treatment was given?_____

What do you think caused this?_____

What lifestyle changes have you had to make?_____

_____

Personal and Family History

Disorders with:	Patient	Family member		Patient only Current	Past
Thyroid	___	___	Weight change	___	___
Pituitary	___	___	Fatigue/weakness	___	___
Diabetes	___	___	Mood changes	___	___
Cushing's	___	___	Appetite changes	___	___
Addison's	___	___	Bowel changes	___	___
Growth	___	___	Infections	___	___
Parathyroid	___	___	Wound healing	___	___
			Excessive thirst	___	___
			Excessive hunger	___	___
			Excessive urination	___	___

Endocrine system testing

Cortisol_____ Sodium_____ Calcium_____ Phosphorus_____ Ketones_____

ACTH stimulation_____ T3_____ T4_____ Protein-bound iodine_____

17-ketosteroids_____ 17-hydroxycorticosteriods_ _____ Glucose_____

Glucose_____ Gl ucose tolerance testing_____ Basal metabolic rate_____

Biopsy_____ Scans_____ Ultrasonography_____ Other_____

Current treatments/medications

Medication_____ Dose _____ Frequency_____ Route_____

Is there anything else you want me to know?_____

_____

_____

_____

PHYSICAL ASSESSMENT

- Physical assessment is done in the following order:
  1. Inspection
  2. Palpation
- The primary task of this examination is to assess the body for signs of endocrine system failure
- Patient should be undressed, gowned and covered with a sheet
- Expose each area as it's examined and then re-drape

INSPECTION
General Appearance/Mood

- Appearance and mood may or may not be affected depending upon the endocrine disorder and the severity of the problem
- Descriptive terms for appearance may include: anorexic, frail, healthy, masculine, obese, physically fit, robust, stuporous, well nourished
- Persons with growth hormone deficiency may appear emaciated and pale
- A characteristic "buffalo hump" and moon face may occur with Cushing's syndrome
- Descriptive terms for mood may include attentive, anxious, cooperative, depressed, drowsy, emotionally liable, excited, inattentive, lethargic, mentally dull or slow,
- Coarse features can occur with growth hormone excess
- Deep voice may occur with growth hormone excess
- An individual with heat or cold intolerance may be dressed inappropriately for room temperature
  - Intolerance to cold may occur with growth hormone deficiency, hypothyroidism
  - Intolerance to heat may occur with thyroid excess

Skin

- Color — May be normal, bronze, pale or yellow
  - Pallor is common in growth hormone deficiency
  - Bronze skin color occurs with Addison's disease
- Temperature — may be cool, warm or hot
- Texture — May be diaphoretic, dry, elastic, leathery or thick
- Thick skin and nails are common in acromegaly
- Turgor — May be good, fair or poor

- Hair distribution — Hirsutism (abnormal hairiness) or sparse hair distribution especially pubic or axillary may be present
  - Hirsutism may occur with Acromegaly and Cushing's syndrome
  - Decreased pubic hair occurs in Simmond's disease and Addison's disease
  - Alopecia may occur with hypothyroidism
- Lesions, assess color, location, size, and temperature
- Purple striae on abdomen may occur in Cushing's syndrome
- Poor wound healing and recurrent infections occur with both Cushing's syndrome and Diabetes mellitus
- Diabetics are more susceptible to infection and usually have decreased microcirculation leading to skin disorders such as:
  - Bullosis diabeticorum — Formation of a large lesion that is filled with fluid generally on the forearm, fingers or feet
  - Diabetic dermopathy — Multiple hyperpigmented circular or oval areas on the legs ranging in size from 0.5-2 cm
  - Eruptive xanthomas — Firm, yellow, 4-6 mm lesions with a red base that appear suddenly on elbows, knees, buttocks or any site of trauma
  - Necrobiosis lipoidica diabeticorum — Red to red-brown plaques that may be yellow in the center, accompanied by shiny transparent skin, usually found on the shin, lesions may ulcerate
  - Necrolytic migratory erythema — Bright red patches found on the lower abdomen, groin, buttocks and thighs, blisters are present and quickly break leaving crusts

PALPATION

- Warm hands to avoid startling patient
- Palpate any areas where masses appear, document location size and tenderness if present
- Thickening of the skin due to deposits in the dermis which may not be visible on the surface may be related to scleredema
- Assess vital signs
  - Temperature elevation, frequent infections may occur with several types of endocrine disorders to include growth hormone deficiency, diabetes, and Cushing's syndrome
  - Pulse, rapid pulse may occur with hyperthyroidism

- Blood pressure, hypotension may occur with growth hormone deficiency and Addison's disease, hypertension may occur with Cushing's syndrome

ENDROCRINE PHYSICAL EXAMINATION

INSPECTION:

General appearance_____   Mood_____

Features_____

Visual acuity_____   Retinal changes_____

Skin color_____   Skin turgor_____   Hair distribution_____

Wounds/infected areas_____

Lesions/rashes on skin_____

Nutritional status_____   Fat distribution_____

Palpation:

Temperature_____   Pulse_____   Respirations_____   B/P_____/_____

Skin texture abnormalities_____   Reflex testing_____

Response to pinprick_____   Proprioception_____

Thyroid_____   Muscle mass_____

Auscultation

B/P: lying_____/_____   sitting_____/_____   standing_____/_____

Assessment Notes

_____

_____

_____

_____

Section III — LABORATORY & DIAGNOSTIC TESTS

In the following section traditional laboratory values and SI unit values are given, it is important to recognize that "normal" values vary from laboratory to laboratory. Check the normal values at the agency or institution where a test is performed. Most labs print their normal values on the laboratory reporting slip or page.

See also Aldosterone, antidiuretic hormone and calcium

Table of Common Laboratory Tests

Test Name	Indications	Comments
Adrenocorticot-ropic hormone (ACTH) **Normal:** 15-100 pg/ml or 10-80 ng/L (SI) between 8-10 am	Cushing's syndrome Adrenal gland CA Steroid use Pituitary cancer Addison's disease	**Regarding collection:** NPO 8-12 hrs before testing Use green top tube; collect 15-20 ml Place tube on ice for transport **Results:** Increased in Addison's disease Decreased in Cushing's syndrome, adrenal cancer and steroid use
Androstenedione Blood test **Normal:** <250 ng/dl women	Hirsutism Stein-Leventhal syndrome Adrenal tumor that has hirsutism	**Regarding collection:** Collected from women 1 wk before or after menstrual period Collect 7-10 ml in red-top tube **Results:** Elevated in Stein-Leventhal, tumor of adrenal or ovary Decreased in ovary failure
Antithyroglobu-lin antibody Blood test **Normal:** Titer <1:100	Hashimoto's thyroiditis	**Regarding collection:** Use red-top tube; collect 3-5 ml **Results:** Increased in Hashimoto's
Cortisol Blood test **Normal:** 6-28 ug/dl or 170-625 mmol/L (SI) at 8 am 2-12 ug/dl or 80-413 mmol/L (SI) 4 pm	Cushing's syndrome Addison's disease Thyroid dysfunction	**Regarding collection:** Use red or green-top tube; collect 7-10 mL, place on ice for transport May be collected in am and at 4 pm **Results:** Increased levels with Cushing's syndrome, hyperthyroidism, stress Decreased with Addison's disease, hypothyroidism, hypopituitarism

Test Name	Indications	Comments
C peptide Blood test **Normal:** 0.78-1.89 ng/ml or 0.26-0.62 mmol/L	Insulinoma Pancreatic transplants Radical pancreatectomy	**Regarding collection:** NPO except water 8-12 hrs before Use red-top tube; collect 7-10 ml **Results:** Increased in insulinoma, pancreas transplants Decreased in pancreatectomy and diabetes mellitus
Glucagon Blood test **Normal:** 30-210 pg/ml or 30-210 ng/L (SI)	Diabetes mellitus Glucagonoma Renal failure Chronic pancreatitis Pancreatectomy	**Regarding collection:** NPO for 10-12 hours prior to test Use lavender-top tube; collect 7ml Place tube on ice for transport **Results:** Increased in diabetes, glucagonoma, renal failure, pancreatitis Decreased in glucagon deficiency, chronic pancreatitis, pancreatectomy
Glucose (FBS) Blood test **Normal:** 70-105 mg/dL or 3.9-5.8 mmol/L SI	Routine test for many metabolic disorders Diabetes mellitus	**Regarding collection:** For fasting blood sugar, NPO for 8 hours before testing except water Insulin is withheld until after BS is taken unless ordered Use gray-top tube; collect 7ml **Results:** Increased in diabetes, stress, Cushing's disease, pancreatitis Decreased in insulinoma, Addison's, hypothyroidism, hypopituitarism
Glucose (2hr PPG) postprandial Blood test **Normal:** 70-140 mg/dL or <7.8 mmol/L under 50 70-150 mg/dL 50-60 yrs	Diabetes mellitus Used often as a screening test	**Regarding collection:** Patient will eat entire meal then rest for 2 hours until blood taken Use gray-top tube; collect 7-10 mls 2 hours after meal is finished **Results:** Increased in diabetes mellitus, Cushing's syndrome, malnutrition, stress and injury Decreased in hypoglycemia, adrenal gland hypofunction & hyperinsulin

Test Name	Indications	Comments
Glucose toler-ance test (GTT, OGTT) Blood and urine **Normal:** Fast 70-115 mg/dL or <6.4 mmol/L (SI) ½ hr <200 mg/dL or <11.1 mmol/L 1 hr same as ½ 2 hrs < mg/dL or <7.8 mmol/L 3 hrs 70-115 mg/dL or <6.4 mmol/L 4 hrs same as 3 hrs Urine–negative	Diabetes mellitus Gestational diabetes	**Regarding collection:** High CHO diet for 3 days prior NPO for 12 hours prior to testing Fasting blood sugar is collected Check orders if BS is >200mg Administer oral glucose solution amount based on pts weight Pt is NPO except water during testing, no tobacco is permitted Use gray-top tube; collect 5ml at ½, 1, 2, 3 and 4 hours, urine sample is collected at same time **Results:** Increased in diabetes mellitus and gestational diabetes Decreased in hypoglycemia
Glycosylated hemoglobin (Ghb, Hb A1, GHB) Blood test **Normal:** 4-8% 7% good con-trol 10% fair control 13-20% poor	To determine the effectiveness of diabetic treatment Long-term index of average blood glucose levels	**Regarding collection:** Use gray-top tube; collect 5 ml **Results:** Increased in diabetics that are new diagnoses or poorly controlled
Growth hormone Blood test **Normal:** Men <5ng/mL or <5ug/L (SI) Women <10m\ng/mL or <10ug/L	Growth disorders Dwarfism Acromegaly Gigantism Hypopituitarism H ype rpituitarism	**Regarding collection:** NPO for 8-12 hours before testing Use red-top tube; collect 7ml May be obtained during sleep Send to laboratory ASAP **Results:** Increased in gigantism, acromegaly, diabetes, anorexia, stress, surgery starvation, deep-sleep exercise Decreased in dwarfism, failure to thrive, growth hormone deficiency

Test Name	Indications	Comments
Growth hormone stimulation test (GH provocation, insulin tolerance test, ITT) Blood test **Normal:** GHL >10ng/ml or 10 ug/L (SI)	Growth hormone deficiency	**Regarding collection:** NPO for 8-10 hours except water A heparin lock is started Growth hormone, glucose & cortisol baselines are obtained Assess orders for administration of Arginine &/or insulin IV Blood glucose is monitored at 15 to 30 min intervals until BS is <40mg/dL, then growth hormone is taken Monitor patient for hypoglycemia, hypotension, nervousness Procedure takes about 2 hrs Send growth hormone samples to lab ASAP **Results:** Decreased in deficiency
17-ketosteroids (17-KS) 24 hr urine test **Normal:** Male 7-25 mg/24 hr or 24-88 umol/d SI Female 4-15 mg/24hr or 14-52 umol/d	Adrenocortical dysfunction Adrenal gland tumor Addison's disease	**Regarding collection:** Explain procedure for 24 hr urine collection to patient Keep urine on ice during collection List start time, any medications taken and end time on lab slip **Results:** Increased in pregnancy, Cushing's syndrome, adrenal tumor, ovarian testicular tumor, hyperpituitarism Decreased in Addison's, castration, hypogonadism, hypopituitarism, gout
Parathyroid hormone Blood test **Normal:** <2000 pg/mL	Hyperparathyroidism Hypercalcemia Hypoparathyroidism	**Regarding collection:** NPO for 8-12 hrs except water Specimen drawn in early morning Use red-top tube; collect 5-15 ml List time of collection on lab slip **Results:** Increased in hyperparathyroidism, carcinoma of parathyroid, vitamin D deficiency, rickets, osteomalacia Decreased in hypoparathyroidism, hypercalcemia, metastic bone tumor, vitamin D intoxication, Graves
Prolactin levels Blood test **Normal:** 0-20 ng/mL Pregnant Female 20-400 ng/mL	Pituitary tumor Hypothyroidism Polycystic ovary syndrome	**Regarding collection:** Use red-top tube; collect 5-7 ml Transport on ice to laboratory **Results:** Elevated in pituitary tumors, hypothyroidism, anorexia

Test Name	Indications	Comments
Somatomedin C Blood test **Normal:** 42-110 ng/mL	Growth hormone deficiency screening test	**Regarding collection:** NPO for 8 hours preferred Use lavender-top tube; collect 7ml **Results:** Increased in acromegaly, gigantism, hyperpituitarism Decreased in dwarfism, delayed puberty, growth hormone deficiency, pituitary tumor, hypopituitarism
(TSH) Thyroid-stimulating hormone Blood test **Normal:** 2-10 uU/mL or 2-10 mU/L (SI)	Thyroid dysfunction Congenital cretinism Pituitary dysfunction	**Regarding collection:** Use red-top tube; collect 5ml **Results:** Increased in primary hypothyroidism thyroiditis, thyroid agenesis and congenital cretinism Decreased in hypothyroidism with pituitary problems or in hyperthyroidism
Thyroxine (T4) Blood test **Normal:** 4-11 ug/dL	Thyroid dysfunction Pituitary problems	**Regarding collection:** Use red-top tube; collect 5ml List medications taken on lab slip **Results:** Increased in Grave's disease, acute thyroiditis Decreased in hypothyroidism and anterior pituitary dysfunction
Triiodothyronine (T3) Blood test **Normal:** 110-230 ng/dL or 1.2-1.5 nmol/L SI	Hyperthyroidism Thyrotoxicosis	Regarding collection: Use red-top tube; collect 5-10 ml List medications taken on lab slip **Results:** Increased in hyperthyroidism, thyrotoxicosis and thyroiditis Decreased in hypothyroidism
Triiodothyronine uptake test **Normal:** 24-34% or 24-34 AU	Thyroid dysfunction	**Regarding collection:** Use red-top tube; collect 5-7 ml List on lab slip any medications **Results:** Increased in hypothyroidism Decreased in hypothyroidism

Table of Common Diagnostic Tests

Test Name	Indications	Comments
Adrenal angiography X-ray with contrast dye **Normal** adrenal arteries	Adrenal gland tumor Adrenal hyperplasia	**Pre-procedure:** Signed consent form is required Assess patients knowledge of test A catheter is passed from femoral artery into aorta then passed into inferior adrenal artery where dye is injected and x-rays taken A burning flush will be felt when dye is passed for a few secs Assess for allergy to iodine dyes NPO after midnight before test Administer pre-medication per order Mark sites of peripheral pulses Procedure takes about 60 mins **Post-procedure:** Assess site for hemorrhage or hematoma, monitor peripheral pulses Monitor vital signs frequently Bedrest for 12-24 hrs Apply cold compresses as needed Encourage fluids
Adrenal venography X-ray with contrast dye **Normal** adrenal veins	Adrenal tumor Pheochromocytoma Cushing's syndrome	**Regarding collection:** Signed consent form is required Assess patient's knowledge of test: A catheter is passed from adrenal vein into the adrenal vein, a dye is injected and x-rays taken, blood samples are also taken Assess for allergy to iodine or seafood, report if noted Administer medications as ordered Procedure takes about 60 minutes **Post-procedure:** Monitor vital signs for hemorrhage Assess patient with suspected pheochromocytoma for hypertension if noted notify physician Assess site for redness, bleeding, pain or swelling and report
Computed tomography of the adrenals (CT) X-ray with contrast dye **Normal** adrenal gland size	Adrenal dysfunction	**Pre-procedure:** Signed consent form may be required Assess for allergy to iodine or seafood, report if noted Assess patients ability to be still during procedure NPO for 3-4 hours before scan **Post-procedure:** Assess for allergic reaction to dye No activity restrictions

Test Name	Indications	Comments
Radioactive iodine uptake ((RAIU) Nuclear scan **Normal** results: 2hr 4-12% absorbed 6hr 6-15% absorbed 24 hrs 8-30% absorbed	Thyroid tumor Thyroid dysfunction	**Pre-procedure:** Assess for allergy to iodine or seafood, report if noted NPO for 8 hours prior to testing Explain procedure to patient: Radioactive iodine capsule or drink (tasteless) will be given by mouth and X-rays will be done Patient may eat one hour after the iodine is ingested List medications on lab slip Inform patient that radioactive iodine is not harmful in this dose **Post-procedure:** Assess for signs of hyperthyroidism
Thyroid scan Nuclear scan **Normal** size, shape structure and function of gland	Thyroid dysfunction Mass in neck Thyroid nodule Thyroid cancer Hyperthyroidism	**Pre-procedure:** Assess for allergy to iodine or seafood as a radioactive technetium capsule is given by mouth before Signed consent form may be required Thyroid and cough medications are discontinued one week prior to test Procedure takes about 30 minutes **Post-procedure:** Assess for reaction to isotope
Ultrasonography Ultrasound **Normal** structure, size of thyroid, adrenals, or parathyroid depending on area scanned	Thyroid malfunction Adrenal malfunction Parathyroid malfunction	**Pre-procedure:** Procedure is non-invasive A lubricant will be applied and transducer moved over area Takes 15-30 minutes **Post-procedure:** No activity restrictions

Section IV — PROCEDURES

Insulin administration

- Insulin is required for patient with insulin dependent diabetes mellitus and those with non-insulin dependent diabetes mellitus who are severely hyperglycemic

Before drawing up medication

- Remember the five rights of medication administration
  - Right patient
  - Right medication
  - Right amount
  - Right time
  - Right route
- Assess patient's blood glucose as ordered
- Wash hands thoroughly
- Remove insulin from refrigerator (does not need to be refrigerated if kept away from heat)
- Assess orders for type and number of units of insulin, insulin needs may be calculated on sliding scale determined by patient's blood glucose levels
- Determine if more than one type of insulin will be given, regular and long-acting insulin may be mixed
- Assess insulin label(s) to be sure correct type (regular, intermediate or long-acting) and source (pork, beef, human)
- Check the expiration date on the insulin vial(s)
- Check agency policy regarding need to have two nurses check insulin prior to administration
- Warm and mix the vial(s) by gently rolling between your palms, do not shake
- Use only insulin syringes that are marked in units

Drawing up insulin

- Use an alcohol swab to cleanse rubber stopper on top of vial
- Recheck orders for correct number of units of insulin
- Inject an equal amount of air into vial(s) before drawing up insulin, this avoids creating a vacuum, if you are drawing up two types of insulin place air in long-acting (N) insulin first then into the regular insulin

- If you are administering two types of insulin draw up regular (R) insulin dose first
- Draw up required amount of insulin into syringe, if air bubbles are present tap the syringe to remove and draw up more insulin until correct number of units are present, double check to be sure the correct number of units are withdrawn
- If you are mixing insulin next withdraw the long-acting insulin into the same syringe as the regular insulin. Remember to pull the plunger back until you have the total dose, the number of units of regular insulin plus the number of units of long-acting insulin. Double check to be sure the correct number of units are withdrawn

Administering the insulin

- Recheck orders for correct type of insulin, amount and time of administration
- Check patient's identification bracelet for correct patient in correct room and bed
- Select a proper site, sites for subcutaneous injection include the abdomen, outer thighs and outer forearm. Sites should be rotated
- Pull the skin taut over site, and using alcohol swab cleanse site in a circular motion
- Pinch skin at the cleansed site between thumb and forefinger
- Plunge the syringe needle into pinched fat fold at 90 degrees until hub is at skin
- Pull back on plunger and assess for blood return, if no blood return inject insulin slowly
- If blood return, discard syringe and start procedure again
- Place an alcohol swab over site and withdraw needle
- Dispose of needle correctly, never recap

Section V — CONDITIONS

Diabetes Mellitus

Definition

- A chronic disorder
- A disorder of carbohydrate metabolism with a total or relative lack of the hormone insulin and elevated blood glucose levels
- A classification system has been developed and divides the disease into several categories
  - Type I, or insulin dependent diabetes mellitus (IDDM)
  - Type II or non-insulin dependent diabetes mellitus (NIDDM)
  - Secondary diabetes
  - Impaired glucose tolerance (IGT)
  - Gestational diabetes

Prevalence

- In the USA the prevalence of diabetes is believed to be between 2-4% of the total population with 6 million known diabetics
- Prevalence of NIDDM is difficult to assess as it may be asymptomatic, there may be 4-5 million undetected diabetics
- NIDDM is more common than IDDM
- Diabetes is the leading cause of blindness in the USA
- Approximately 20,000 amputations are done yearly secondary to complications from diabetes
- Diabetes is the causative factor in 25% of all new cases of end-stage renal failure

Etiology

- The pancreas does not produce enough insulin (total lack) or the insulin produced is not effective (relative lack), why this occurs is unknown
- Insulin is needed by the body for the transport of glucose into the cells for use as energy, if insulin is not present glucose cannot enter the cells and stays in the blood stream leading to hyperglycemia
- Obesity, pregnancy, physical and emotional stress are known contributing factors to the onset of diabetes
- Diabetes is not caused from eating too much sugar, excessive weight is a risk factor not excessive sugar intake

Classification of diabetes mellitus
- **Type I, or Insulin dependent diabetes mellitus (IDDM)**
- Formally called juvenile-onset diabetes
- May also be known as ketosis-prone diabetes
- Dependent on exogenous insulin to sustain health and life
- Accounts for 5-10% of known cases of diabetes
- Have frequent, major fluctuations in blood glucose levels
- Genetic component linked to MHC antigens (HLA) located on chromosome 6 (found in 90% of white type I diabetics), autoimmunity and viruses have also been implicated
- Family history of diabetes is minor, 10% have a parent or sibling with DM
- Onset in infancy, childhood, or young adulthood usually before age 30, peak age is 11-13 years
- Often a lean body build is present
- Usually requires a combination of intermediate-acting (NPH) and short acting (regular) insulin for control
- Ketoacidosis will develop without insulin injections
- Continuous subcutaneous insulin infusion with pumps or three or more daily insulin injections may be required
- Requires frequent blood glucose monitoring
- Self-monitoring of blood glucose (SMBG) is usually done at home, results are available quickly and the procedure can be done frequently
- Diet therapy is of major importance to maintain consistent intake of food and to synchronize food intake with insulin injection as well as exercise
- **Type II, or Non-insulin dependent diabetes mellitus (NIDDM)**
- Formally called adult-onset diabetes
- May also be known as nonketotic diabetes
- May or may not require insulin for control of hyperglycemia
- Insulin is not required for survival
- Fasting blood glucose is greater than 140 mg per dL on at least two separate occasions
- Accounts for approximately 85-90% all cases of diabetes
- Blood glucose profile is more stable in type II than in type I
- Family history is marked for diabetes

- Onset is usually after age 30, disorder develops slowly over weeks, months or years
- Includes obese (60-90% of all IDDM cases) and nonobese NIDDM
- Variable insulin production with insulin resistance
- If treated with oral agent or insulin the risk of hypoglycemia is present
- Primary dietary goal is to achieve and maintain ideal weight, this may control symptoms without medications
- **Secondary diabetes**
- Any disease process that can limit insulin secretion or impair insulin action can cause secondary diabetes
- Occurs with pancreatic disease, hormonal excess, drug induced carbohydrate metabolism changes or genetic syndromes
- **Impaired glucose tolerance (IGT)**
- Formally called borderline, chemical, latent or subclinical diabetes
- Fasting blood glucose is less than 140 mg per dL with 30, 60, or 90 minute glucose levels are greater than 200 mg dL and 2-hour plasma glucose level is between 140-200
- Microvascular damage is rare
- Most cases will not advance to overt diabetes, 2-35% will develop NIDDM over next 20 years
- **Gestational diabetes**
- Onset during pregnancy often in 2nd-3rd trimester
- Affects 2-3% of pregnant women
- The American Diabetes Association recommends that all pregnant women undergo a 1 hour oral glucose challenge test
- If glucose challenge test is 140 mg/dl or greater than a oral glucose tolerance testing (OGTT) is recommended
- Gestational DM diagnosed if more than two of the following values are met or exceeded OGTT
     1 hour OGTT of 190 mg/dl or greater
     2 hour OGTT of 165 mg/dl or greater
     3 hour OGTT of 145 mg/dl or greater
- Infants born to mothers with gestational DM are at risk for larger infants (macrosomia), delayed fetal lung maturation, neonatal hypoglycemia and even fetal demise
- Fetal well-being is monitored via fetal activity determinations (diary of fetal movement is kept), contraction stress testing, and fetal ultrasounds to rule out macrosomia

- May disappear at the end of the pregnancy
- Risk factor for the subsequent development of diabetes, therefore, postpregnancy testing should be done periodically

Symptoms
Insulin dependent diabetes mellitus
- Symptoms of diabetes are all related to hyperglycemia
- Classic symptoms of IDDM are polyuria (increased urine), polydipsia (increased thirst) and polyphagia (increased hunger)
- Onset is usually abrupt, although symptoms may have been present for several days to weeks
- Weight loss
- Fatigue
- Infection
- Ketoacidosis will develop without insulin injections

Non-insulin dependent diabetes mellitus
- No symptoms may be present
- Polyuria and polydipsia are common
- Polyphagia is less uncommon
- Onset is gradual may be several weeks or months duration
- Obesity can be a frequent feature of NIDDM
- Weight loss, weakness, fatigue are frequent

Complications of diabetes
- **Acute complications**
- **Hyperglycemia**
  - Blood glucose is abnormally high, above 110 mg/dL
  - Relative or absolute lack of insulin
  - Excess circulating stress hormones
  - Requires exogenous insulin if absolute lack of insulin is present for correction
  - If relative lack of insulin may be treated with diet alone, oral hypoglycemic agents or exogenous insulin
  - Symptoms are polyuria, polydipsia and polyphagia
  - May lead to diabetic ketoacidosis if untreated
- **Hypoglycemia**
  - Blood glucose is abnormally low
  - Most common complication of insulin treatment in IDDM

- Estimated that type I diabetics experience one episode of hypoglycemia per week
- Can occur when insulin taken is excessive, when a meal is delayed, carbohydrate intake is insufficient or gastric emptying time is delayed
- Insulin excess can occur with exercise or change of insulin injection site
- Alcohol intake or onset of menses, can lead to hypoglycemia

Signs and symptoms	Laboratory values	Management
Faintness, weakness Tremulousness Palpitations Diaphoresis, cold clammy skin Hunger Confusion Increased pulse If severe seizures or coma may result	Glucose less than 50mg/dl	Oral glucose (2-3tsp of sugar in water or fruit juice) 0.5-1mg Glucagon IV or SQ if unable to swallow If no response in 20 minutes IV glucose When patient is alert give oral carbohydrates

- **Diabetic ketoacidosis (DKA)**
  - Affects 2-5% of IDDM patients per year
  - Hyperglycemia and ketosis
  - Sepsis occurs in 1-10% of patients with up to 40% having an infection

Signs and symptoms	Laboratory values	Management

Nausea and vomiting
Abdominal pain
Dehydration
Poor skin turgor
Dry mucous membranes
Hot flushed skin
Respiratory distress
Tachypnea
Kussmaul respiration
Shock
Hypotension
Tachycardia
Fever
Possible infection
Confusion
Progressive loss of
consciousness
Coma
 	
ECG may show flat-
tened/inverted T waves
and U waves with hypoka-
lemia or tall T waves, wide
QRS and no P wave with
hyperkalemia
	Glucose elevated
	200-2000 mg/dl
	70-110 mg/dl normal
	
	Ketones 1:2-1:64
	Negative normal
	
	HCO3 4-15 meq/L
	24-28 meq/L normal
	
	Blood pH 6.8-7.30
	7.35-7.45 normal
	
	Pco2 14-30 mmHg
	35-45 normal
	
	All lab values are
	monitored frequently
		Admit to ICU
		Give insulin
		  10 U reg IV bolus
		  10 U reg/hour IV
		  If unresponsive,
		insulin is increased
		When acidosis is corrected
		1-2 U reg/hr IV
		
		Fluid replacement
		0.9% NS usually 2-3L
		within 1st hour, K+ 10-30
		meq/hour
		Then 0.45% NS at 150-300
		ml/hour until glucose is
		250 mg/dl then 5% glucose
		is added and infusion is
		slowed
		
		Weigh q 6-12 hours
		
		Monitor ECG
		Monitor output q 1-2 hrs

- **Hyperglycemic hyperosmolar coma (HHC)**
  - Usually occurs in adults over 50 years of age with NIDDM
  - In 35% of HHC cases diabetes has not yet been diagnosed
  - Onset is slower than in DKA and medical attention is usually obtained later
  - Ketosis is absent
  - Conditions that may precipitate HHC include MI, pancreatitis, sepsis, or stroke
  - Dehydration is more severe than in DKA, dehydration is due to diminished kidney function
  - May present with seizures, myoclonic jerking, or hemiparesis
  - Mortality ranges from 12-42%

Signs and symptoms	Laboratory values	Management
Same as DKA except no nausea & vomiting Also Generalized seizures Focal seizures Reversible hemiparesis Severe dehydration Severe hypotension Monitor vital signs and neurological status frequently	Glucose elevated 600-2000 mg/dl 70-110 normal Ketones not significant Osmolality elevated 280-300 normal Blood urea nitrogen elevated Creatinine elevated 0.6-1.2 normal	Admit to ICU Fluid replacement 0.9% NS, 1L in 30min; if hypotension still persists 1L in 60min 0.45% NS at 500cc/hr for 2-3 L then slowed, when glucose is 250-300 mg/dl add 5% glucose Monitor I&O and weight Insulin therapy same as DKA

- **Infections**
  - Glucosuria is associated with an increased in vaginitis
  - Minor trauma to tissues can lead to infection secondary to vascular insufficiency and decreased sensory neuropathy
  - Infections include cellulitis, soft tissue necrosis, draining wounds
  - Diabetic patients are susceptible to severe infections such as gangrene, mortality with gangrene is greater than 10%
  - Malignant otitis externa is almost exclusive for diabetics, pain and drainage from the external canal are present, infection can reach the cranial nerves, meninges or sigmoid sinus, death may occur from epidural abscess
  - Urinary tract infection is common in diabetics due to high urine glucose concentration
- **Chronic complications (usually occur after 10 years)**
- Microvascular disease
  - Capillaries are thickened
  - Renal disease or failure if the glomerular capillaries are effected, 50% of diabetics with IDDM have renal failure after 20-30 years
  - Retinal disease occurs with visual loss if retinal capillaries are affected, 50% of diabetics have some degree of problems after 10 years
- Macrovascular
  - Diabetics have an increased incidence of large vessel disease such as atherosclerosis

- Risk of death from cardiovascular disease is 3.5 times higher than that of non-diabetic
- Hypertension and diabetes is present in 2.5 million Americans
- 30% of diabetics develop peripheral vascular disease
- Diabetics require 5 times more amputations than non-diabetics
- Neuropathic diseases
  - Demyelination and degeneration of the nerves may occur with clinical neuropathy present
  - Nerve involvement may lead to pain, sensory loss, motor weakness, or loss of position sense, deep tendon reflex loss

Components of initial examination for diabetes

- *Complete medical history to include:*
- Personal history of diabetes from patient, including previous and current treatment
- History of recent weight gain or loss
- Patient's understanding of diagnosis and treatment
- Patient's willingness to make lifestyle changes
- Family history of diabetes
- Assessment of current pattern of blood sugar assessment
- Assessment of current medications, if insulin use pattern of injection rotation
- Assessment of ability to administer insulin independently
- *Physical examination to include:*
- General appearance
- Height and weight to assess for baseline
- Visual acuity, eye disease is common in diabetes
- Fundoscopic examination to detect retinopathy
- Blood pressure measurement, sitting and standing in both upper extremities
- Skin for any anomalies or lesions
- *Laboratory and diagnostic testing:*
- According to the American Diabetes Association, the diagnosis of diabetes is made when one of these criteria is met:
  1. A random blood glucose level is 200 mg/dl or greater and classic symptoms are noted
  2. A fasting blood glucose level is 140 mg/dl on at least two occasions

3. A fasting blood glucose level is less than 140 mg/dl but there are two abnormal glucose tolerance tests
- Frequent assessment of blood glucose levels, self-blood glucose monitoring is the most common laboratory test used to monitor effectiveness of treatment

Treatment of diabetes
- The goal of treatment is to maintain blood glucose as close to normal as possible to prevent complications
- Lifelong chronic disease that requires constant management of the balance between food, insulin and activity levels
- Dietary intervention is an important part of the plan for all diabetic patients (See also section—VI)
- The goals of nutrition management is to improve blood glucose, to obtain consistent nutrient intake on a day to day basis, to obtain and maintain desired weight while promoting healthy eating habits
- Individualized dietary intervention is vital for compliance
- In IDDM, patients may be underweight and maintenance of adequate nutrition is important
- In NIDDM dietary therapy may be the primary treatment, gradual weight loss is often necessary since most patients are overweight
- Exercise program, activity lowers blood glucose levels and increases circulation, both of which are desired goals for diabetes
- Exercise should be aerobic not anaerobic to produce a decrease in glucose needs
- Medical alert bracelet with name, medical condition and medications should be worn
- The diabetic should always carry a source of carbohydrate (Life Savers, orange juice, raisins) in case of hypoglycemia
- Regular medical checkups are important due to the possible need for adjustment of treatment
- Eye examinations should be performed by an ophthalmologist regularly

Medications for diabetes
- Insulin is required for IDDM and for patients with NIDDM who have severe hyperglycemia

- Insulin preparations include rapid, intermediate and long acting with regards to course of action and are available in a variety of sources beef, pork, beef-pork, or human synthetic insulins
- Oral hypoglycemic drugs are used for most NIDDM patients. Sulfonylurea drugs such as tolbutamide, tolazamide, glipizide, and glyburie may be used
- Glucosidase inhibitors are used in the treatment of hyperglycemia

Section VI — DIETS

- Diet is very important in the treatment of diabetes management . Most individuals with diabetes will require several individualized sessions with a registered dietitian familiar with diabetes management
- Some individuals with non-insulin dependent diabetes mellitus will respond to dietary treatment alone and medication will not be needed
- The goals of dietary management of diabetes include:
  - Improvement of blood glucose levels
  - Improvement of lipid levels
  - Consistent diet that is adequate in nutrients and calories to achieve and maintain ideal weight
  - Balancing exercise, insulin and diet
  - Weight management for those with IDDM

DIABETIC EXCHANGE DIET

General description	Individualized, contains enough calories to maintain ideal body weight Diet should improve blood glucose and lipid level Generally an exchange meal-planning approach is used in diabetes management Exchange plan is made up of six lists of core foods which have approximately the same amount of carbohydrates, proteins and fats within each list
Indications	Insulin dependent diabetes mellitus Non-insulin dependent diabetes mellitus Impaired glucose tolerance Gestational diabetes mellitus
Allowable Items	55-60% of the total caloric intake should be in carbohydrates, with the emphasis on unrefined carbohydrates 12-20% of the total caloric intake should be in proteins, may be modified if other conditions are present (renal disease is common in diabetes) <30% of the total caloric intake should be in fats Polyunsaturated fats up to 10% Saturated fats up to 10% Monounsaturated fats up 10-15% Fiber up to 40 grams/day unless calories are restricted then 25 grams/1000 calories See Samples of exchange lists in this section Alternative sweeteners are acceptable

Restricted items	Calories may be restricted in NIDDM to obtain and maintain ideal weight Cholesterol is limited to <300 mg/day Sodium is limited to <3000 mg/day unless another health problem exists that requires even more restriction Alcohol is limited to 1-2 equivalents per week Sucrose and refined sugars are limited based on control of blood glucose
Nutritional value	A Diabetic exchange plan diet when planned by a registered dietitian should provide all of the needed nutrients, caloric intake will vary according to patient need
Other comments	Same exchange plans are found after the six lists of core foods A very important part of diabetic meal planning is balancing the timing of the action of insulin with the composition of meals Blood glucose monitoring is used to balance the insulin intake, diet and exercise pattern

Exchange list	Carbohydrate grams (g)x4	Protein g x 4	Fat g x 9	Calories
Breads	15	3	1	80
Meats				
Lean		7	3	55
Med fat		7	5	75
High fat	5	7	8	100
Vegetables	15	2		25
Fruits				60
Milk				
Skim	12	8	1	90
Low fat	12	8	5	120
Whole	12	8	8	150
Fats			5	45

Sample exchange plans

	1300kcal	1500kcal	1800kcal	or	1800kcal
Breakfast	2 bread 1 fruit 1/2 milk* 1 fat	2 bread 1 fruit 1/2 milk* 1 fat	3 breads 1 fruit 1 milk* 1 fat		3 breads 1 meat** 1 fruit 1 milk* 1 fat
Lunch	2 bread 1 meat** 1 vegetable 1 fat	2 bread 2 meats** 1 vegetable 1 milk* 1 fruit 1 fat 1 fat	2 breads 2 meats** 1 vegetable 1 fruit		2 bread 2 meats** 1 vegetable 1 milk* 1 fruit 1 fat
Snack	1 fruit	1 bread	1 bread		1 fruit

Dinner	1 bread	1 bread	2 breads	2 breads
	3 meats**	3 meats**	3 meats**	3 meats**
	2 vegetables	2 vegetables	2 vegetables	2 vegetables
	1 milk*	1 fruit	1 fruit	1 fruit
	1 fat	1 fat	2 fats	2 fats
Snack	1 bread	1 bread	1 bread	1 bread
	1/2 milk	1/2 milk*	1 fruit	1 fruit
		1 fat	1 fat	1 fat

*   Based on low fat milk list
**   Based on medium fat meat list

DIABETIC EXCHANGE LIST

LIST 1
Starches and Breads

½ cup cold cereal
Raisin bran
40% bran flakes

1/3 cup cold cereal
All bran
Bran buds

3/4 cup cold cereal
Cheerios
Cornflakes
Grape-nut flakes
Kix
Product 19
Rice Krispies
Wheaties

1½ cups cold cereal
Puffed rice
Puffed wheat

1/2 cup hot cereal
Cream of rice
Cream of wheat
Oatmeal
Wheat bran

1/2 cup pasta
Macaroni
Egg noodles
Spaghetti

1/3 cup rice

1/2 cup beans
Kidney beans
White beans
Lentils
Black-eyed peas
Split peas

1/2 cup vegetables
Corn, whole
Corn, creamed
Lima beans
Garden peas
Mashed potatoes

LIST 2
Meats

Lean Meat Exchanges:
1 oz. broiled beef
Flank steak
Sirloin steak
Tenderloin
Top loin
1oz. roasted eye round beef
steak

1 oz. pork
Ham, fresh, cured, canned
or boiled
Canadian bacon
Roasted tenderloin

1 oz. poultry roasted
Chicken,
turkey or duck

1 oz. fish broiled
Cod, haddock,
Halibut, salmon

2 oz. clams, steamed
crab, lobster or scallops
1/4 cup tuna

1/4 cup tuna

1/4 cup cottage cheese
1 oz Lite cheese

3 egg whites
½ cup egg beaters

Med. fat exchanges:
1 oz. Beef
Ground beef – reg to
ex lean
Cubed steak
Check pot roast
Porterhouse steak
Rib roast
Rump roast
T-bone steak
Meat loaf

LIST 3
Vegetables

½ cup cooked
Asparagus
Beets
Broccoli
Brussel sprouts
Cabbage
Carrots
Cauliflower
Chinese cabbage
Greens
Green beans
Leeks
Mushrooms
Okra R Onions
Peapods
Pepper, green
Sauerkraut
Spinach
Summer squash
Tomatoes
Turnips
Zucchini

1 cup raw
Bean sprouts
Broccoli
Carrots
Cauliflower
Onions
Peppers
Tomatoes

1/2 cup juice
Tomato
Vegetable

Free foods:
1 cup of the following:
Cabbage
Celery
Cucumber
Lettuce
Mushrooms
Radishes
Spinach

LIST 1
Starches and Breads

3 oz Baked potato

1 slice bread
  White
  Whole wheat
  Rye
  Pumpernickel
  French

1/2 pita, hamburger or
frankfurter bun

2 bread sticks
  1/2 in x 4-1/2 in

1 6-in corn or wheat
  tortilla

3 Graham crackers
  2-1/2 in square
8 animal crackers
5 Melba toast
24 oyxter crackers
3 cups plain popcorn
6 saltines

LIST 2
Meats

1 oz Pork
  Center loin roast
  Center loin chop
  Pork cutlet
  Top loin chop

1 oz veal cutlet

1 oz poultry, roasted
  Chicken, turkey,
  duck or goose with
  skin

1 oz ground turkey

1/4 cup tuna canned
  in oil

1 oz cheese
  American, skim
  Mozarella
  Weight Watchers

1 egg
1/4 cup egg substitute

4 oz tofu

1 oz. liver, heart or
  kidney

High fat meats
1 oz Corned beef or
  prime rib

1 oz Ground pork or
  spareribs

1 oz Fried fish

1oz. Cheese
  American, blue,
  cheddar, monterey,
  or swiss

1 oz. Luncheon meats,
  smoked sausages,
  bratwurst, frank-
  furters

1 Tbsp Peanut butter

LIST 3
Vegetables

LIST 4
Fruits

1 2-1/2 inch
　Apple
　Nectarine
　Orange
　Peach

1/2 cup of
　Applesauce
　Cherries
　Peaches*
　Pears*
　Apple juice
　Orange juice
　Pineapple juice

3/4 cup of
　Blackberries, raw
　Blueberries, raw
　Grapefruit*
　Mandarin oranges*
　Peach, sliced
　Pineapple

1/2 cup of raw fruit
　Banana
　Grapefruit
　Mango, small
　Papaya
　Pear
　Pomegranate

1 cup of
　Cantaloupe
　Papaya
　Raspberries

1-1/4 cups of
　Strawberries
　Watermelon

Free Foods
1/2 cup of
　Cranberries, whole, raw
　Rhubarb

LIST 5
Milk

Skim/Very low fat
1 cup of
　Skim milk
　1/2% milk
　1% milk
　Buttermilk, low fat

1/3 cup nonfat dry milk

8 oz plain nonfat
　yogurt

Low-fat milk
　1 cup 2% milk

8 oz low fat yogurt

Whole milk
　1 cup whole milk
　1/2 cup evaporated
　　milk

8 oz yogurt, plain

LIST 6
Fats
Unsaturated Fats

1 tsp of
　Margarine, soft
　Margarine, hard
　Mayonnaise
　Corn oil
　Cottonseed oil
　Olive oil
　Peanut oil
　Safflower oil
　Soybean oil

1 Tbsp of
　Margaine, reduced
　　calorie
　Mayonnaise, reduced
　　calorie
　Miracle Whip,
　　reduced calorie

2 Tbsp of
　Salad dressing, reduced
　　calorie

1/8 Avacado
10 Olives

6 Almonds
10 large peanuts
2 Pecans or walnuts

Saturated Fats

1 slide bacon

1 tsp of
　Butter
　Shortening

2 Tbsp of
　Coconut
　Light cream
　Sour cream

1 Tbsp of
　Heavy whipping cream
　Cream cheese

Jam/jelly, 2 tsp*
Pancake syrup, 2 Tbsp
Whipped topping, 2 Tbs
Catsup or harseradish,
　1 Tbsp
Mustard, 1 tsp
Taco sauce, 3 Tbsp

FREE FOODS
Boullion, 8 oz
Soda, 12 oz*
Club soda, 12 oz
Coffee, 6 oz

Gelatin, 4 oz*
Equal, 1 pkg
Tea, 6 oz
Tonic water, 6 oz
Dill pickle, 1*
Hard candy*

Section VII — DRUGS

The tables supply only general information, a drug handbook or the physician's desk reference (PDR) should be consulted for details. Each classification includes detailed information about the prototype drug, this drug is representative of the other drugs in the classification and can be used as a model.

Every effort has been made to include the major classes of drugs used in the treatment of endocrine diseases

ADRENAL CORTICOSTEROIDS — CLUCOCORTICOIDS

Action: The major action is the stimulation of enzymes responsible for these three effects: antiinflammatory, immunosuppressant and catabolism of protein, fats and carbohydrates into glucagon which raises glucose levels

Indications: Replacement of missing hormones as occurs in Addison's disease (adrenal insufficiency), the most use however is the suppression of inflammation or allergic responses

Example: Prednisone (*Deltasone, Meticorten, Orasone, Panasol, Prednicen, Sterapred*)

Route: PO

Pharmacokinetics: Peak 1-2 hours

Duration 24-36 hours

Contraindications: Sensitivity to Prednisone, systemic fungal infections

Adverse effects: Euphoria, headache, insomnia, confusion, psychosis, CHF, edema, nausea, vomiting, ulcer, muscle weakness, delayed wound healing, muscle wasting, osteoporosis, fractures, moon face, growth suppression in children, carbohydrate intolerance, hyperglycemia, leukocytosis, low K+

Interventions:

Administer in am (before 9am) with food to reduce gastric irritation

Tablets may be crushed and mixed with food or fluid of choice

Assess orders carefully for daily dose scheduling, Route may be adjusted if patient is under extra stress (surgery, infection or trauma)

Drug is withdrawn slowly in increments to prevent withdrawal symptoms

Obtain baseline vital signs and I&O ratio at start of treatment

Monitor BP and compare to baseline, report significant changes

Monitor blood glucose, serum K+, 17-KS lab values as ordered

Monitor for signs of infection (slow wound healing) may be masked by drug

Caffeine should be avoided to prevent gastric upset

Patient's on long term therapy should carry medical identification card

Examples of other drugs in this classification:

Cortisone Acetate (Cortistan, Cortone), PO/IM, Sodium chloride and a mineralocorticoid are usually given at the same time

Dexamethasone (*Decaderm, Decadron, Dexameth, Dexasone, Dexone, Hexadrol, Mymethasone, Decadrol*) PO/IM/IV, Wide variety of uses including allergic states, cerebral edema, hematologic disorders, inflammation, administer IM preparation deep, IV push may be given rapidly

Methylprednisolone (*Medrol, Solu-Medrol, Depoject, DepoMedrol, Medralone*) PO/IM/IV, Also used for bronchial asthma (short term use)

Paramethasone acetate (*Haldrone*), PO, 2mg paramethasone is equal to 5mg of prednisone

Prednisolone (*Delta-Cortef, Predcor, Pred Mild, Inflamase Forte*), PO/IM/IV Give IV at rate of 10mg over 1 minute

Example: Hydrocortisone (*Cortisol*) Wide variety of trade names, also a variety of forms to include Hydrocortisone Acetate, Hydrocortisone Cypionate, Hydrocortisone Sodium Phosphate, Hydrocortisone Sodium Succinate and Hydrocortisone Valerate

Route: PO, IM, IV

Pharmacokinetics: PO onset 1-2 hours, IV immediate onset
PO peak 1 hour, IM peak 4-8 hours
PO duration 24-36 hours, IM duration 24-36 hours

Contraindications: Sensitivity to glucocorticoids, idiopathic thrombocytopenic pupura, psychoses, acute glomerulonephritis, viral disease of skin, bacterial disease of skin, infections not controlled well with antibiotics amebiasis, Cushing's syndrome, smallpox vaccination

Common adverse effects: Sodium and water retention, weight gain, nausea, impaired wound healing, acne, depend upon length of treatment and dosage

Life-threatening adverse effects: Masking of infectious process

Other adverse effects: Vertigo, headache, nystagmus, mental disturbances, aggravation of psychiatric conditions, insomnia, syncope, thrombophlebitis, thromboembolism, fat embolism, palpitations, tachycardia, angiitis, growth suppression in children, decreased glucose tolerance, hyperglycemia, hypocorticism, amenorrhea, menstrual difficulties, cataracts, glaucoma, exophthalmos, increased intraocular pressure, fungal infections of cornea, blurred vision, decreased visual acuity, hypocalcemia, hypokalemia, CHF, hypertension, increase in appetite, esophagitis, pancreatitis, abdominal distention, peptic ulcer, melena, thrombocytopenia, muscle wasting, tendon rupture, fracture, osteoporosis, aseptic necrosis, petechiae, bruising, hypopigmentation, hyperpigmentation, hirsutism, fat atrophy, dermatitis, urticaria, sweating, malaise, hiccups, hoarseness, dry mouth, sore throat, obesity, decreased sperm motility, decreased sperm counts, enuresis, urinary frequency, urinary urgency, effects related to dose and duration

Interventions:

Administer before 9am with food to reduce gastric irritation

Administer IM deep into buttocks, avoid use of deltoid muscle, rotate site

Administer IV at rate of 25 mg/ minute or slower

Inspect skin carefully before topical administrations are applied

Monitor vital signs, weight, I&O and sleep patterns, compare to baseline

Monitor plasma cortisol levels, blood glucose, K+, on patients on long-term therapy, regular eye examinations should also be performed

Monitor for changes in mood and behavior and report if noted

Monitor for signs of infection and/or delayed wound healing, report

Withdrawal syndrome may occur if drug is withdrawn quickly after long-term use, discontinue slowly per orders

Caffeine and alcohol use should be avoided while taking this drug

Medical identification bracelet or card should be carried while on drug

Examples of other drugs in this classification:

Amcinonide (*Cyclocort*) Topical, for psoriasis, eczema or dermatitis

Beclomethasone Diproprionate (*Beclovent, Beconase nasal inhaler, Vancenase nasal inhaler*), Oral or Nasal Inhaler, for bronchial asthma, rhinitis

Betamethasone (*Celestone, Benisone, Uticort, Alphatrex, Diprogen, Betameth, Betacort, Betatrex, Ectosone, Valisone, Valnac*) PO/IV/IM/ Topical, Also used for prevention of neonatal respiratory distress syndrome by injection into women in pre-term labor

Clocortolone Pivalate (*Cloderm*) Topical, Avoid application to large areas

Desonide (*DesOwen, Tridesilon*) Topical, For skin disruptions

Desoximetasone (*Topicort*), Topical, Do not apply to vulvovaginal or perianal areas

Diflorasone Diacetate (*Florone, Maxiflor, Psorcon*) Topical, Stop drug if Striae or atrophy of skin are noted

Triamcinolone (*Aristocort, Atolone, Kenacort, Azmacort, Cenocort, Kenalog, Triamonide, Tri-kort, Amcort, Articulose, Kenacort, TriamForte, Trilone, Aristospan*) PO/IM/SC/Inhaler, used in inhaler form for patients who do not respond to conventional inhalers

ANTIDIABETICS — INSULIN

Action: Stimulate carbohydrate metabolism by promoting the uptake of glucose, reduces the rate of glycogenolysis

Indications: Used to manage insulin dependent diabetes mellitus (IDDM) and for non-insulin dependent diabetes mellitus that is not responding to oral hypoglycemics and diet therapy alone or during periods of excessive stress

Example: Insulin injection (*Humulin R, Novolin R, Regular Insulin, Pork Regular Iletin II, Regular Purified Pork Insulin, Velosulin, Velosulin H*)

Insulin in general is:

Available in   short-acting (Regular, R) types listed above
                intermediate-acting (NPH or lente)
                long-acting (ultralente or protamine zinc insulin)

Available derived from cow pancreas (bovine, beef) or pig (porcine), or be commercially produced by recombinant DNA technology (human)

Route: SC, IV, IV is given by continuous infusion

Insulin therapy attempts to mimic the natural pattern of insulin secretion

Possible insulin therapies include combinations of the three types (R,NPH) therapy is individualized and determined by blood glucose response

Pharmacokinetics: Onset 0.5-1 hour R, 2 hours NPH

Peak 2-3 hours R,

Duration 5-7 hours R, 18-24 hours NPH

Contraindications: Sensitivity to insulin animal proteins

Life-threatening adverse reactions: Anaphylaxis (rare)

Other adverse effects- Hypoglycemia: profuse sweating, nausea, palpitation, tremulousness, hunger, headache, tremors, tachycardia, weakness, fatigue, nystagmus, circumoral pallor, numb sensations to mouth, tongue, visual disturbances, double vision, blurred vision, staring expressions, ataxia, confusion, apprehension, irritability, personality changes, loss of consciousness, delirium, convulsions, coma, manical behavior

Other adverse effects — sensitivity to insulin: reaction at injection site, urticaria or bullae, lymphadenopathy

Interventions:

Assess orders carefully to determine if insulins are to be mixed, mix as directed in procedure section this chapter, Assess type of insulin ordered, R, NPH, or ultra-lente, strength U-40, U-100, type beef, pork or human

Always use syringe that matches insulin strength (most insulins 100U)

Administer regular insulin 20-30 minutes prior to meals so that peak will match the hyperglycemic surge following the meal

Administer insulin as per procedure outlined in this chapter

Monitor for hypoglycemia at insulin peak, hypoglycemia may occur rapidly

With IV administration monitor blood pressure, urine glucose and ketones

Monitor blood sugar to determine insulin therapy response to treatment

The following are possible target blood sugars in young person with IDDM

Before meals 70-130 1 hour after meals 100-180

2 hours after meals 80-150 Pre-dawn (0200-0400) 70-120

ANTIDIABETICS — SULFONYLUREAS

Action: Augments insulin secretion by stimulating the release of insulin by the pancreas, thereby lowering blood glucose levels. Not for use in IDDM where no natural insulin is secreted, not an oral insulin.

Indications: NIDDM where insulin secretion is decreased or insulin action is impaired and diet alone cannot provide control.

Example: Tolcutamide (*Orinase*)

Route: PO

Pharmacokinetics: Peak 3-5 hours, Duration 6-10 hours

Contraindications: Sensitivity to sulfonylureas, IDDM, repeated episodes of ketoacidosis, severe stress, infection, trauma, severe renal, hepatic or endocrine disease

Life-threatening adverse effects: Agranulocytosis, aplastic anemia

Other adverse effects: nausea, heartburn, anorexia, constipation, diarrhea, thrombocytopenia, leukopenia, hepatic porphyria, SIADH, pruritus, erythema, urticaria, photosensitivity, taste alterations,

headache, hypoglycemia is common if overdose occurs
<u>Interventions:</u>
Tablet may be crushed and mixed with water
Monitor patient carefully until initial Route is established for signs
of hypoglycemia (see diabetes this chapter), monitor urine and blood
glucose levels as ordered, usually 2-3 hours after eating
Explain to patient that oral medications are only one part of
treatment for NIDDM and that diet, exercise and medication need to
be balanced
Alcohol use is not recommended while taking this medication
Examples of other drugs in this classification:
Acetohexamide *(Dymelor)* PO, Often used in NIDDM patients with
   gout, may have diuretic action

Chloropropamide *(Chloronase, Diabinese, Glucamide)* PO, Take with
   meals to reduce GI upset, may be given 1-3 times daily

Glipizide *(Glucotrol)*, PO, Administer 30 minutes before meals

Glyburide *(DiaBeta, Glynase, Micronase)*, PO, Administer 15-30
   minutes before meals

Tolazamide *(Tolinase)*, PO, Duration 10-20 hours, absorbed slowly
   therefore usually given in one dose before breakfast, may be
   given in divided doses

PITUITARY HORMONES — ANTIDIURETIC HORMONES
Action: Smooth muscle contraction of the digestive tract and uterus,
the contraction of smooth muscle in the vascular bed, promotion of
water reabsorption and concentration of urine
Indications: Treatment of diabetes insipidus due to posterior
pituitary hormone deficiency, also may be used for postoperative
abdominal distension
Example: Vasopressin Injection *(Pitressin)*
<u>Route:</u> IM/SC, IV
<u>Pharmacokinetics:</u> Duration 2-8 hours in aqueous solution (IM/SC)
Duration 48-72 hours in oil (IM/SC)
<u>Contraindications:</u> Chronic nephritis with nitrogen retention,
ischemic heart disease, advanced arteriosclerosis, PVCs
<u>Life-threatening adverse effects:</u> sensitivity with anaphylaxis or
cardiac arrest, peripheral vascular collapse may occur with large
doses
<u>Other adverse effects:</u> intranasal administration may lead to
congestion, runny nose, mucosal ulceration and pruritus, headache,
conjunctivitis, heartburn, abdominal cramps, increase in bowel
movements

<u>Interventions:</u>
Prior to IM administration warm vial by rolling between palms,
shake vial vigorously to mix prior to drawing up dose, IM injection is
painful
Administer only Vasopressin aqueous injection IV, never tannate solution
Monitor vital signs compare BP to baseline, monitor I&O pattern
and ratio
Water intoxication can occur with sensitivity to medication
Monitor weight and compare to baseline to assess any unusual increases

THYROID PREPARATIONS — ANTITHYROID AGENTS
Action: Inhibit the synthesis of thyroid hormones
Indications: Treatment of hyperthyroidism, iodine-induced
thyrotoxicosis
Example: Propylthiouracil (*PTU*)
<u>Route:</u> PO
<u>Pharmacokinetics:</u> Peak 1-1.5 hours
<u>Contraindications:</u> Administration with sulfonamides, aminopyrine
or antipyrine, pregnancy last trimester and lactation
<u>Adverse effects:</u> paresthesias, headache, vertigo, drowsiness,
neuritis, nausea, vomiting, diarrhea, dyspepsia, taste loss or change,
sialoadenitis, hepatitis, myelosuppression, lymphadenopathy,
periarteritis, hypoprothrombinemia, thrombocytopenia, leukopenia,
agranulocytosis, enlarged thyroid, reduce GI motility, periorbital
edema, puffy hands and feet, bradycardia, cool skin, pale skin,
sleepiness, fatigue, mental depression, dizziness, vertigo, cold
sensitivity, paresthesias, muscle cramps, menstrual changes, weight
gain, skin rash, urticaria, pruritis, hyperpigmentation, hair loss,
arthralgia, sensitivity vasculitis
<u>Interventions:</u>
Administer at the same time each day (example with morning meal)
Discontinue drug 3-4 days prior to radioactive iodine treatment per
orders
Monitor for therapeutic response to include weight gain, decreased
pulse rate, and reduced laboratory T4 levels
Monitor for hypothrombinemia to include ecchymoses, pupura,
petechiae, or bleeding, report if found
Instruct patient to avoid over the counter medications which may
contain iodides such as medications for cough or asthma

Examples of other drugs in this classification:

Methimazole *(Tapazole)* PO, 10 times more ptent than PTU

Potassium Iodide *(Pima, SSKI)*, PO/IV, IV drug used in thyroid storm/crisis

Monitor for GI bleeding, pain or vomiting, sudden withdrawal may lead to thyroid storm or crisis

THYROID PREPARATIONS — THYROID AGENTS

Action: Increases the metabolic rate, Used as replacement or substitution therapy

Indications: Used in the management of hypothyroidism, myxedema, cretinism or goiter

Example: Levothyroxine Sodium *(T4, Eltroxin, Levothroid, Noroxine, Synthroid, Synthrox, Syroxine)*

Dosage: PO, IV

Pharmacokinetics: Peak 3-4 weeks

Duration 1-3 weeks

Contraindications: Sensitivity to levothyroxine, thyrotoxicosis, severe heart disease, adrenal insufficiency, pregnancy

Common adverse effects: Insomnia

Other adverse effects: irritability, nervousness, headache, tremors, palpitations, tachycardia, arrhythmias, angina pectoris, hypertension, nausea, diarrhea, appetite changes, menstrual changes, weight loss, heat intolerance, sweating, fever, leg cramps, hair loss

Interventions:

Administer PO dose in one dose before breakfast to prevent insomnia

Shake vial until clear and administer IV dose just after reconstitution with NaCl, administer at rate of 0.1 mg/min, discard any unused portion

Monitor for therapeutic effect to include weight loss and diuresis

Monitor pulse rate to determine drug effectiveness, if rate is >100 bpm, report to primary care provider, monitor laboratory values to determine if thyroid levels are returning to normal from before treatment start

Patient should avoid over the counter drugs unless approved by physician

Trade names of medications are not interchangeable, hormone content may vary

Therapy is life-long, patient may want to discontinue therapy when symptoms of hypothyroidism subsides

Examples of other drugs in this classification:

Liothyronine Sodium (*Cytomel, T3*), PO, also used for T3
   suppression test

Liotrix (*Euthroid, Thyrolar, T3/T4*), PO, Headache should be
   reported as it may require dosage adjustment

Thyroglobulin *(Proloid)*, PO, Tablet may be crushed and mixed with
   fluids or foods

Thyroid (*Armour thryroid, Thyrar*), PO, Administer on empty
   stomach, foods high in iodine to include seafood, turnips,
   cabbage, soybeans and some breads

Section VIII — GLOSSARY

Acromegaly	Pituitary hypersecretion of growth hormone with enlargement of the hands, feet and face
Adrenalectomy	Surgical removal of adrenal glands
Adrenalitis	Inflammation of the adrenal glands
Aldosteronism	Adrenocortical hyperfunction with muscular weakness, excessive thirst and urination
Cretinism	Infantile hyperthyroidism, symptoms include growth and mental retardation
Diabetes	Metabolic disorder with polyuria and insipidus polydipsia, caused by insufficient amounts of antidiuretic hormone
Dwarfism	Growth disorder caused by anterior pituitary growth hormone hypofunction
Euthyroid	Normal function of thyroid gland
Exophthalmos	Eyes that are protruding
Giantism	Excessive growth beginning in adolescence caused by excessive secretion of growth hormone
Hirsutism	Abnormal hairiness
Hypophysectomy	Removal of the pituitary gland
Myxedema	Adult hypothyroidism
Parathyroid-ectomy	Surgical removal of parathyroid gland
Polydipsia	Excessive thirst
Polyuria	Excessive urination
Radioisotope	Isotope that is radioactive, used as a tracer to diagnose thyroid function
Thyrasthenia	Weakness caused by hypothyroidism
Thyroidectomy	Surgical removal of thyroid gland

Thyroid	Exacerbation of existing hyperthyroidism, may crisis be caused by trauma, surgery, or severe adrenocortical insufficiency
Thyroiditis	Inflammation of the thyroid gland
Thyrotoxicosis	Thyroid crisis
Virilism	Masculinity, may be secondary to hyperplasia of both adrenal glands or due to adrenal tumor
von Recklinghausen's disease	Bones are light and brittle in this disease which is due to a deficiency in calcium

Musculoskeletal System

MUSCULOSKELETAL SYSTEM

Table of Contents

Section I—THE OVERVIEW

Primary Functions
- Provides a supporting framework for the body
- Provides internal support and protection to the tissues and organs of the body
- Enables body movement and postural changes to be made and/or maintained
- Bones serve as storage receptacles for calcium, magnesium and phosphorus
- Bone marrow provides for the manufacture of blood cells

Components
The musculoskeletal system is composed of the bones, cartilages, muscles, joints, ligaments and tendons of the body.

Bones (skeletal system) (Figure 8A)
- The human skeletal system contains 206 bones
- It is grouped into two sub-sections called the axial skeleton and the appendicular skeleton
- The axial skeleton includes the bones that are found in the center axis of the body
- The appendicular skeleton contains the bones that are appendages to the axial skeleton including the shoulder and hip girdles, the arms and legs

Axial Skeleton

Bone	Location
8 Bones of the cranium	The bones that cover the brain & organs of hearing/sight
1 Frontal	Forehead
2 Parietal	Sides of the cranium
2 Temporal	Begins at temples, continues back behind the ear
1 Occipital	Back portion of the cranium
1 Sphenoid	Bottom of cranium (butterfly shaped)
1 Ethmoid	Behind the nasal bones, and above the sphenoid bone
14 Facial Bones	Bones of the face
2 Nasal	Bridge of the nose
2 Maxillae	Upper jawbone
2 Zygomatic	Cheekbones
1 Mandible	Lower jawbone
2 Lacrimal	Behind the nasal bones in the eye socket
2 Palatine	Back portion of the hard palate part of the floor/walls nasal cavity
2 Inferior nasal conchae	Located within the skull behind the nose
1 Vomer	Nasal septum
1 Hyoid	Supports the tongue

The Bones of the Body

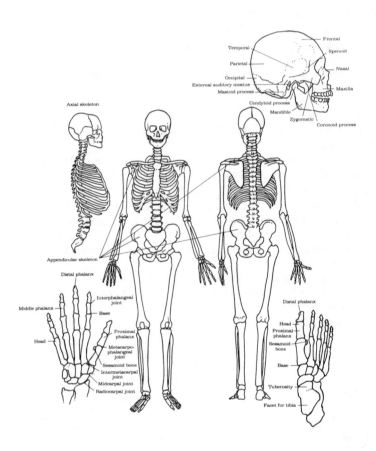

Figure 8A

Bone	Location
6 Auditory	Bones of the inner ear
2 Malleus	The hammer
2 Incus	The anvil
2 Stapes	The stirrups
51 Trunk Bones	From the skull to the end of spinal column
26 Vertebrae	The spinal column
7 Cervical	Neck
12 Thoracic	Back
5 Lumbar	Lower back
1 Sacral	Center bone of pelvic girdle
1 Coccyx	Tail bone
24 Ribs	Ribcage in front of body
14 True Ribs	1st-7th ribs attach to sternum
6 False Ribs	8th-10th ribs attach to one another
4 Floating Ribs	11 & 12 do not attach in front at all
1 Sternum	Bone over the center of the chest

Appendicular skeleton

Bone	Location
4 Bones Shoulder Girdle	Shoulders
2 Clavicles	Collarbones
2 Scapulae	Shoulderblades
60 Bones Upper extremities	Arms, wrist and hands
6 Bones in the arms	
2 Humerus	Bone between elbow & shoulder
2 Radius	Between elbow & wrist (thumb side)
2 Ulna	Between elbow & wrist (little finger side)
16 Carpus Bones	Wrist
2 Navicular (Scaphoid)	
2 Lunate	
2 Triquetrum	
2 Pisiform	
2 Trapezium	
2 Capitate	
2 Hamate	
38 Bones in the hand	
10 Metacarpals	Bones in the palm
28 Phalanges	Finger bones
2 Coxal bones	Pelvic Bones or Hips
60 Bones Lower extremities	Legs, Ankles, and Feet
8 Bones in the Legs	Thigh
2 Femurs	Inside of the lower leg
2 Tibia	Outside of the lower leg
2 Fibula	Knee cap
2 Patella	Ankle

Bone	Location
14 Tarsus Bones	
2 Talus	
2 Calcaneus	
2 Cuboid	
2 Navicular	
6 Cuneiform	
38 Bones of the feet	
10 Metatarsals	Toes
28 Phalanx	

Cartilage

* Dense connective tissue, not bone
* Found in the ribs, nasal septum, external ear, larynx, trachea, bronchi, vertebrae, and the articular surface of bone
* Capable of withstanding great pressure and tension
* Does not have a nerve or blood vessel supply of it's own like bone

Muscle (Figure 8B)

* Muscle tissue is composed of fibers which have the ability to contract or shorten (elasticity properties) and therefore cause movement of an organ or bone to occur
* There are three kinds of muscle tissue in the body
    Striated or skeletal
    Visceral or smooth
    Cardiac
* Striated muscle attaches to the bone
    * Skeletal muscle is striated and under voluntary control
    * There are more than 600 striated muscles in the body
    * Make position changes possible by the movement of the bones of the skeleton
    * Grouped by the type of movement they produce
            Flexors
            Extensor
            Abductors
            Abductors
            Internal rotators
            External rotators
            Circumflexors
* Visceral muscle (smooth muscle) is found in the blood vessels, stomach, and intestines
    * Generally under involuntary control

The Muscles of the Body

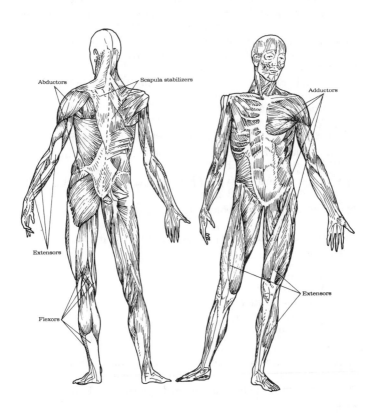

Figure 8C

- Cardiac muscle is both striated and under involuntary control
  - Found in the heart tissue

Joints

- The bones in our body are rigid and serve us as levers
- The joints connect the bones together and allow a position change of the bone so they serve as fulcrums for the levers
- The junction at which the bones and joints meet are secured by ligaments or other binding tissue, which can allow for much movement or none
- The joints in our body can be divided into three main types
  Fibrous
  Cartilaginous
  Synovial
- Fibrous joints do not move at all or only slightly (teeth)
- Cartilaginous joints are bones held together with a band of cartilage (symphysis pubis)
- Synovial joints are the typical joint adapted for movement (ankle, shoulder, elbow, hip and knee)
- The largest joint in the body is the Tibiofemoral synovial joint (knee)
- The joints move body parts in seven different patterns
  Flexion
  Extension
  Abduction
  Adduction
  Internal rotation
  External rotation
  Circumduction

Ligaments

- Bands or sheets of strong connective tissue that connect the end of the bones together to create or limit movement
- The ligaments of the body are named according to location

Tendons

- Bands or sheets of strong connective tissue that connect muscles to bones
- One of the most familiar tendons in the body is the Achilles tendon

Section II — ASSESSMENT

HEALTH HISTORY

- Assessment of the musculoskeletal system involves both the muscular and the skeletal system

Chief complaint

- Common chief complaint's for this system include:
  - Back pain or stiffness
  - Pain, stiffness and swelling of the joints
  - Bone pain
  - Reduced range of motion or reduced abilities
  - Muscle pain, cramps or weakness
  - Fractures, sprains or strains

Family and Personal History

- The family or personal history may supply clues that will aid in the diagnosis
- Obtain specific diagnoses and age at diagnosis when known
- Obtain ages and causes of death in immediate family members
- Assess for presence and past treatment of the following:
  - Arthritis or rheumatism
  - Fractures
  - Muscular dystrophy
  - Poliomyelitis
  - Systemic lupus erythematosus
- If condition exists assess for required life style changes and current treatment of condition to include medications

Low back pain

- Frequent subjective complaint in this system, assess location, severity, timing and if any event preceded the pain
- Assess ability to perform activities of daily living or vocation

Joint pain or swelling

- May indicate one of the arthritic disorders
- Arthritis is an inflammation of a joint and may describe over 25 different diseases involving one or more joints
- Rheumatoid arthritis is a syndrome with inflammation and destruction of the joints
- Systemic lupus erythematosus is an inflammatory connective tissue disorder occurring mainly in women that leads to joint pain, characteristic "butterfly" rash may be present on face

Muscle pain, cramps or weakness

- May be related to simple overuse, congenital defects, or degenerative diseases, assess location, severity, timing and any event known to precede the pain

Musculoskeletal system testing

- Assess for tests completed or ordered and patient's knowledge and understanding of any test procedures or results

MUSCULOSKELETAL ASSESSMENT

Chief Complaint

Patient's statement _____   Onset_____

Frequency_____ Duration_____ Other areas affected_____

Have you had this before?_____   When_____

What treatment was given?_____

What do you think caused this?_____

What lifestyle changes have you had to make?_____

_____

Personal and Family History

	Patient	Family member		Patient only Current	Past
Muscular dystrophy	___	___	Low back pain	___	___
Arthritis or Rheumatism	___	___	Fractures location	___	___
Poliomyelitis	___	___	Joint pain or swelling	___	___
Systemic lupus erythematosus	___	___	Amputation	___	___
			Muscle pain cramps, twitching	___	___

Difficulty in walking?_____ standing?_____ sitting?_____

Difficulty with activities of daily living?_____

Musculoskeletal system testing

X-rays_____ Bone scans_____ Muscle/bone biopsy_____

Arthroscopy_____ Arthrocentesis_____ Myelogram_____

Electromyography (EMG)_____ Blood tests_____ Other_____

Current treatments/medications

Medication_____ Dose_____ Frequency_____ Route_____

Special diet_____ Usual weight_____ Exercise routine_____

Any activity restrictions?_____

Is there anything else you want me to know?_____

PHYSICAL ASSESSMENT

* Assessment of the musculoskeletal system is done in the following order:
  1. Inspection
  2. Palpation

INSPECTION

General appearance

* Assess patient's chosen position and ease of movements
* Assess for any involuntary movements, if noted are they symmetrical
* Assess the ability to obtain, maintain, and move out of a position
* Assess current comfort level — patient with bone or joint pain may guard afflicted extremity, move slowly or refuse to make position changes
* Assess for contractures, amputations, or congenital anomalies if present describe location and affect on range of motion
* Assess for hygiene and observe dress, musculoskeletal status may affect patient's ability to maintain personal care

Skin color and characteristics

* Assess for areas of ecchymoses or other discoloration related to tissue trauma
* Assess for red or bluish discoloration over joints that may be present in arthritic disorders
* Subcutaneous nodules may occur in 20-25% of patients with rheumatoid arthritis and may be found on elbows, hands and feet
* A slight blush to red rash may cover both cheeks and the bridge of the nose in systemic lupus erythematosus known as the "butterfly rash"

Spine

* Assess for normal curvature of the spine (slight lordosis)
* An exaggerated lumbar curve may be noted in obesity, pregnancy or with hip deformities (moderate to severe lordosis)
* A rounded appearance or curve to the thoracic area of the spine is known as Kyphosis and may be seen in the elderly
* Scoliosis is a lateral curve to the spine, if suspected have the patient bend forward while assessing the symmetry of the shoulder blades and hips from behind, asymmetrical in scoliosis

Gross Motor Mobility

- Assess for any Orthotic devices to include leg or wrist braces, twister cables or prosthetic devices
- Assess for any mobility aids such as wheelchairs, walkers, crutches, overhead bars or handrails regularly used
- Is patient able to ambulate (walk), if so assess gait (normal, shuffling, stable, unstable etc.)

Fine motor skills

- Observe patients hands for deformity, flexion deformities may occur with rheumatoid arthritis
- Can the patient comb their hair, brush teeth and perform other hand motor skills needed for independent daily living
- Can patient write or sign their name

Extremities

- Assess for any length variations in extremities
- Assess for deformity of the legs such as varus deformity (bowlegs) or valgus deformity (knock-knees)
- Assess for swelling in any joint(s), if present assess whether swelling is present in only one side or both sides of the body

PALPATION

- Palpation should be gentle and never painful in patients experiencing joint or bone pain

Skin temperature

- A swollen arthritic joint will feel hot and appear red and swollen

Muscle tone

- Tension that is present in a resting muscle is noted, it may be recorded as flaccid (hypotonic), normal or spastic (hypertonic)

Range Of Motion (ROM)

- Active, have the patient perform the task while you palpate the joint
- Passive, perform the task for the patient, each joint should be taken through the normal range of movement
- When assessing the degree of movement (45, 90, 180) can be listed or the term full ROM or limited ROM recorded for each joint
- Joints are taken through a variety of movements including abduction, extension, flexion, internal rotation, external rotation, supination, dorsiflexion and plantar flexion

MUSCULOSKELETAL PHYSICAL EXAMINATION

INSPECTION

General appearance_____ Positioning_____ Comfort_____

Movement quality_____ Motor mobility type_____ Anomalies_____

Skin color/characteristics_____ Spinal curvature_____

Ability to : Roll_____ Sit_____ Stand_____ Ambulate_____

Fine motor ability_____ Extremity appearance_____

Grasp strength_____ feed self_____ comb hair_____ dress_____

PALPATION:

Skin temperature_____ Muscle tone_____ Muscle strength_____

ROM:	Right	Left		Right	Left		
Shoulder			**Hip**			**Neck**	
Adduction	____	____	Flexion	____	____	Rotation	____
Abduction	____	____	Extension	____	____	Flexion	____
Flexion	____	____	Adduction	____	____	Extension	____
Extension	____	____	Abduction	____	____		
Internal Ro	____	____	Internal Ro	____	____		
External Ro	____	____	External Ro	____	____		
Elbow			**Knee**			**Waist**	
Flexion	____	____	Flexion	____	____	Flexion	____
Extension	____	____	Extension	____	____	Extension	____
Supination	____	____				Rotation	____
Pronation	____	____				Left_____	
						Right_____	
Wrist			**Ankle**				
Flexion	____	____	Plantar Flexion	____	____		
Extension	____	____	Dorsiflexion	____	____		
Radial de	____	____	Inversion	____	____		
Ulnar de	____	____	Eversion	____	____		
Fingers			**Toes**				
Flexion	____	____	Flexion	____	____		
Extension	____	____	Extension	____	____		

Note any asymmetry of muscle strength, joint pain, swelling, redness.

Assessment Notes_____

Section III — LABORATORY & DIAGNOSTIC TESTS

In the following section traditional laboratory values and SI unit values are given, it is important to recognize that "normal" values vary from laboratory to laboratory. Check the normal values at the agency or institution where a test is performed. Most labs print their normal values on the laboratory reporting slip or page.

In addition to the test listed below, see also alkaline phosphatase (gastrointestinal system), electromyography and spinal x-rays (neurological system), lactic dehydrogenase and myoglobin (cardiovascular system), uric acid (renal system).

Table of Common Laboratory Tests

Test Name	Indications	Comments
Aldolase Blood test **Normal:** 3.0-8.2 Sibley-Lechniger U/dL or 22-59 mU (SI)	Muscular dystrophy Polymyositis Dermatomyositis Muscular trauma	**Regarding collection:** Use red-top tube; collect 7 ml **Results:** Increased with muscular diseases, muscular trauma, infections also increased in chronic liver disease Decreased: late muscular dystrophy
Calcium Blood test **Normal:** 9.0-10.5 mg/dL or 2.25-2.75 mmol/L	Bone cancer Metastic cancer Immobility Multiple fractures Burns Tetany Vitamin D excess or deficiency Sarcoidosis	**Regarding collection:** Use red-top tube; collect 7 ml **Results:** Increased in hypervitaminosis, cancer, immobility, fractures Decreased in vitamin D deficiency, burns, infections, rickets and laxative use
Human lymphocyte antigen B27 (HLA-B27) Blood test **Normal:** Negative	Ankylosing spondylitis Reiter's syndrome	**Regarding collection:** Collect 10 ml in heparinized tube **Results:** Increased in Reiter's & Ankylosing spondylitis
Rheumatoid factor Blood test **Normal:** Negative	Rheumatoid arthritis, SLE	**Regarding collection:** Use red-top tube; collect 7 mil **Results:** Increase in autoimmune diseases, rheumatoid arthritis, SLE, chronic viral infections, scleroderma

Table of Common Diagnostic Tests

Test Name	Indications	Comments
Arthrocentesis with synovial fluid analysis **Normal:** Clear or straw colored fluid with no crystals, few WBCs and good mucin clot	Joint disease Joint cancer Arthritis Synovitis	**Pre-procedure:** Signed consent form may be required NPO for 8-12 hrs before testing May be performed at bedside **Post-procedure:** Assess for joint swelling or pain Apply ice to reduce pain/swelling Maintain pressure dressing over site Activity is reduced for several days to prevent injury to joint
Arthrography X-ray **Knee-Normal** medial meniscus **Shoulder-Normal** joint capsule tendon sheath intact bursa	Abnormality of the ligaments or the cartilage Ligament tears Chronic knee pain Chronic shoulder pain Performed prior to Arthroscopy	**Pre-procedure:** Check agency policy for consent Explain procedure to patient: Needle inserted into joint space and X-rays are taken Assess for iodine/seafood allergy **Post-procedure:** Assess for joint swelling or pain Apply ice to reduce pain/swelling Administer analgesics as ordered Check orders for any joint use restrictions
Arthroscopy Endoscopy **Normal** cartilage ligaments, menisci and articulation	Joint abnormality Joint surgery Torn ligaments Arthritis Generally done on the knee	**Pre-Procedure:** Signed consent form is required Explain procedure to patient: A small arthroscope is inserted into the joint via a small incision Corrective surgery may be done NPO 8-12 hours before testing Crutch gait training by PT dept Shave joint area as ordered Procedure takes about 30 minutes **Post-procedure:** Assess extremity for circulation Monitor VS, assess site for pain, swelling, redness or drainage Apply ice, administer analgesics Rest joint for 48-72 hours

Test Name	Indications	Comments
Bone Scan Nuclear scan **Normal** no abnormality	Osteomyelitis Degenerative bone diseases Bone cancer Assess response to radiation therapy or chemotherapy	**Pre-Procedure:** Explain procedure to patient: A radionuclide will be given IV After administration a 2-3 hour waiting period before scan Imaging will take 30-60 minutes Patient will need to lie still All jewelry must be removed Assess for iodine allergy **Post-Procedure:** Encourage fluids, no restrictions
Muscles Biopsy **Normal** muscle No necrosis No variation in muscle fiber size	Muscular dystrophy Werdnig-Hoffman Myotonia	**Pre-Procedure:** Signed consent form is required Surgical incision to remove muscle fibers for examination is done **Post-Procedure:** Analgesic may be ordered Assess site for drainage or any signs of infection
Magnetic resonance imaging (MRI) Magnetic study **Normal** bones and joints	May be used for a wide variety of disorders to include tumors or joint disorders	**Pre-Procedure:** Explain procedure to patient: Lie on a platform that will move areas to be scanned into magnetic field so image can be made Assess for and remove all jewelry or other metallic items If patient has plates or metal implants MRI is contraindicated Assess patients ability to lie still Procedure takes about 30-90 min a steady rhythmic pounding will be heard, earplugs may be worn **Post-Procedure:** No activity restrictions
X-Rays **Normal** bones and joint structure	Arthritis Fractures Bone diseases Congenital anomaly	**Pre-Procedure:** Frequently ordered procedure Assess type of x-ray ordered Clothing and jewelry over area should be removed Testes should be shielded Assess for pregnancy in females; should be avoided in months 1-3 **Post-Procedure:** No limitations on activity

Section IV — PROCEDURES

EXERCISE AND EXERCISE-RELATED INJURIES
Benefits of regular exercise
- Regular exercise provides a variety of benefits to include:
1. Increase in mental well being which may be due to:
   Improved physical appearance
   Improved self-image and self-esteem
   Reduction of stress and tension
   Sleep pattern improvement
   Increased self-confidence

2. Increase in physical well being which may be due to:
   Loss of excessive weight
   Increased resting metabolic rate
   Decrease in the percentage of total body fat
   Reduction in blood pressure
   Decreased resting pulse rate
   Increased cardiopulmonary fitness
   Increase in muscle tone, strength and flexibility

3. Potential prevention of disease to include:
   Coronary heart disease, exercise may:
   > Maintain or increase oxygen supply to the heart
   > Decrease the progression of atherosclerosis
   > Enlarge coronary arteries
   > Decreases the hearts oxygen demands
   Osteoporosis, exercise may:
   > Increase bone mass and mineral content in aging women
   Some studies also cite clinical improvement in selected patient's
   with the following disease states:
   > Chronic obstructive lung disease
   > Osteoarthritis
   > Intermittent claudication

Assessment prior to selection of exercise program:
- A physical assessment should be performed by a primary care provider prior to the onset of a regular exercise program
- Every person regardless of age or medical condition can benefit from a well developed individualized exercise program

- In addition to a physical the following individuals may require a stress test prior to beginning an exercise program:
  - Males over 40 years or Females over 55
  - Anyone with a family history of heart disease
  - Anyone with cholesterol level over 220
  - Anyone with blood pressure over 160/90 mmHg
  - Heavy cigarette smokers and/or heavy drinkers
- For the following conditions, a physical or occupational therapist or dietetic consultation may also be helpful:
  - Intolerance to activity (walking or stair climbing)
  - Previous orthopedic or muscular injuries
  - Arthritis (limited range of motion or strength, pain)
  - Osteoporosis (increased risk of fractures)
  - Diabetes (monitor blood glucose, diet change)
  - Severe obesity (more stress on weight bearing joints)
  - Neurologic disorders (seizures, tremors, impaired coordination, dizziness, or impaired vision)

Guidelines for selecting an exercise program:

- Any exercise program chosen will be more successful if it:
  - Matches the physical capabilities present
  - Matches the financial capabilities present
  - Is pleasurable to the individual
  - Involves easily available equipment
- There are two basic types of exercise programs, aerobic and anaerobic
- Aerobic exercise is the most common type of program used today . Aerobic exercise has the most benefits for the whole body
  - It permits the greatest increase in energy use
  - Consists of performing rhythmic movement of large muscles
- Examples of aerobic exercises include:

Aerobic dancing	Jogging	Swimming
Bicycling	Racquetball	Tennis
Canoeing	Skiing	Walking
Ice skating	Squash	

- Anaerobic exercise provides for strength training and individual muscle toning
- An example of anaerobic exercise is weight lifting
- Once the type of exercise is chosen, the program is designed
- A good exercise program follows the following guidelines
  - Frequency

- Performed between three to five times per week
- Daily vigorous exercise can increase orthopedic injury, rest days allow for tendon and muscle repair
- Duration
  - Each session should last from 15-60 minutes
- Content
  - Exercises are executed properly, training should be given in proper performance of movements and use of any equipment by a qualified instructor
  - Each session has a 3-5 minute "warm up" to increase joint and muscle readiness for exercise
  - The exercise should allow for maximum use of large muscle groups in a rhythmic fashion
  - The individual should be able to talk during the activity
  - The target heart rate (THR) during the activity is 60-75% of the maximum heart rate (MHR)
  - Increase in activity or intensity is determined by THR and tolerance to exercise
  - Session should end with a "cool down" lasting 2-5 minutes to decrease muscle stiffness and soreness

Calculation of Target and Maximum heart rates

220 – individuals age = MHR in Beats per Minute (BPM)
60-75% of this number is the THR

Example.....Find THR for a 35 year old

220	185	185
−35	X.60	X.75
185 = MHR	111.00 Low Range	138.75 High Range

Heart Rate during exercise should be between 111 & 138 BPM

Complications of Aerobic exercise

- Injuries or other complications occur when:
  Exercise program is improperly chosen
  Equipment is defective
  Program is not followed correctly (no warm-up, over-doing)
  Improper instruction has been given
  Rubberized suits are worn (overheating)
- Some of the possible complications include:

Sudden death or myocardial infarction
Musculoskeletal injuries (shin splints, tendinitis)
Joint injuries
Inadequate hydration and/or overheating during exercise
- Signs of over doing it include chest pain, light-headedness, dizziness, pallor, and nausea
- Ways to avoid complications include:
  Wear proper clothing for activity, avoid rubberized suits
  Avoid exercise in hot stuffy rooms
  Replacement of fluids before, during and after exercise
      1-2, 8 oz glasses of cold water 15-30 minutes prior
      1-3 ounces of cold water during exercise
      4-8 oz of cold water after exercise

TRACTION

Definition

- The application of a pulling force (weight) to an extremity or other part of the body

Purpose

- To correct a variety of problems to include:
  1. Fractures
     Immobilize fracture prior to reduction
     Reduce the fracture
     Immobilize fracture after reduction
     Maintain proper skeletal alignment of the fracture
     Realign bone fragments
     Relieve pain by reducing muscular spasms

  2. Dislocated or Subluxed Joints
     Maintain proper skeletal alignment
     Prevent dislocation of subluxed joints

  3. Correction/Prevention of Skeletal Deformities
     Maintain proper skeletal alignment

  4. Treatment of Muscular Spasms/Low back pain
     Relieves pain
     Prevents muscular spasms

  5. Joint replacements
     Provides temporary immobilization of new joint
     Maintains suture position
     Provides skeletal alignment during early healing process

6.   Treatment of Diseased Joints
     Allows for rest of affected joint
     Relieves pain

Four Basic Types of Traction:

Type	Comments
Manual	Hands are used to apply force of traction Short term used for emergency treatment of fractures Used until other traction is available Should be applied firmly and smoothly

Skin	Straps/Bandages are applied to the skin
	Force of traction is on patients skin
	Specific amount of weight is applied
	Short-term form of traction
	Used to prevent muscle spasms & relieve pain
	May be continuous or intermittent
	Complications:
	   Skin breakdown due to strap/bandage pressure
	   Circulatory impairment if improperly applied
	   Nerve damage

Encircling	A form of skin traction Traction device encircles extremity or body part May be continuous or intermittent Often used for cervical or pelvic traction Complications: Same as for skin traction

Skeletal	Stainless steel pins, wires, or tongs are inserted through the bone where force of traction is applied
	Continuous form of traction
	Greater weight may be applied than with other forms of traction
	Used primarily for fractures of the long bones
	Complications:
	   Infection at pin site
	   All complications of immobility

Assessment for the Patient in Traction:

- Assess physician orders for:
    Admitting diagnosis
    Date traction was applied or will be applied
    Type and purpose of traction to include affected body part
    Frequency of traction (Continuous / Intermittent)
    Diet ordered
    Type, frequency of physical therapy if ordered
- Assess patients history for:
    Any chronic or acute illness that may affect recovery
- Assess the medication record for:
    Pain medications ordered to include type, last dosage, and
    frequency
    Any bowel elimination medications

- Assess the progress and nurses notes for:
  - Patient's response to traction, medications ordered for pain
  - Date of last bowel movement & characteristics
  - Intake and Output record for imbalances
  - Last assessment findings for comparison with current condition
- Assess the patient for:
  - Any pain or discomfort to include location
  - Patients perception of traction and treatment
  - Patients current mental status (depressed, anxious, relaxed)
  - Complaints of numbness or tingling in affected extremity/part
  - Proper alignment of body
  - Affected extremity for skin color and temperature
  - Blanching of nails on affected extremity
  - Quality of pulses on both extremities
  - Pin sites should be clean and dry, free of drainage, foul odor, swelling or redness (Skeletal Traction)
  - Any wrinkles in the slings or dressings
  - Skin for signs of breakdown, redness or discoloration
  - Skin for breakdown under pressure points (heels, coccyx, elbows, scapula)
  - Abdomen for distention and presence of bowel sounds
- Assess traction equipment for:
  - Correct amount and position of weight applied
  - Free movement of ropes through pulley and freely hanging weight
  - All ropes present for any frays
  - Assess for counter traction that prevents patient from being pulled toward the traction. Counter traction may be the person's weight or supplied by a suspended balance system

Complications of Traction:

- Bone fragment motion in fractures
  Can lead to severed blood vessels and/or severed nerves
  Prevent with proper alignment
  Avoid contact with pin surfaces or trauma site
  Assess and maintain traction frequently
- Skin breakdown from pressure of traction or immobility
  Can lead to decubitus ulcers
  Prevent by using pressure relief mattress or sheepskin
  Apply lotion via massage to pressure points
  Use clean, dry, wrinkle-free linen
- Circulatory impairment and /or nerve damage
  Can lead to increased skin breakdown and infection
  Maintain proper body alignment and assess traction equipment

Assess skin traction straps for wrinkles and correct fit
Assess for adequate circulation
- Constipation related to Immobility
Assess bowel elimination pattern and characteristics
Increase fiber and fluids in diet while immobile
Provide stool softeners and laxatives as ordered and needed

Section V—CONDITIONS

Osteoarthritis (OA)

Definition

- Also known as degenerative joint disease
- A chronic disease of the joints with breakdown of cartilage and an overgrowth of bone occurring in involved joint
- Low-grade inflammation and a thickening of synovial membranes occurs in response to cartilage breakdown
- Occurs slowly over a number of years, although the disease does not have to be progressive it may stabilize and even diminish

Prevalence

- The most common joint disease
- Leading cause of joint pain in middle-age and elderly adults
- The majority of the population over 50 years of age shows some changes consistent with osteoarthritis (OA)
- Some studies indicate that 90% of persons over age 40 show changes on x-ray consistent with OA, with only 30% symptomatic
- Under the age of 55 there is no difference noted in prevalence by sex for joint involved with OA
- Over age 55 OA of the hip is more common in men, while OA of the hands is more common in women
- 90% of the population over 80 years of age has OA in some form
- OA of knee is the leading cause of chronic disability in USA

Etiology

- Aging, genetic and environmental factors have all been cited
- Aging is the most common risk factor, in the most common form no other predisposing factor is found
- Repeated trauma from sports or repetitive activities within the work place may lead to excessive wear on joints and breakdown of cartilage, this is a predisposing factor in some cases
- Previous developmental defect or deformity such as bowlegs or knock-knees may predispose to OA
- Obesity with increased stress on weight bearing joints has been associated with OA of the knee

Symptoms of osteoarthritis

- Deep aching pain in involved joint is the most prominent characteristic

- Pain is more prominent when joint is used than when at rest
- Morning stiffness of short duration usually under 20 minutes
- Stiffness may also occur after periods of inactivity (car ride)
- Joint thickening and effusion (increased fluid in joint cavity)
- Heat over the affected joint
- Crepitus may be felt or heard when a joint is moved, more common in larger joints such as the knees
- There does not appear to be a correlation between amount of pain and amount of damage detected on X-rays, some individuals with severe joint damage have little complaints of pain

Early Stages
- Joint pain is noted most with motion or at night and responds well to anti-inflammatory medications

Late Stages
- Joint pain is noted even at rest, increased with weight bearing on joint
- Pain no longer responds well to anti-inflammatory medications
- Hands may develop disfigurement
  - Heberden's nodes are hard nodules on the last phalanges of the fingers, in chronic late stages they show bony enlargement and angular deformities of the fingers
  More common in women at menopause or late middle age
  - Involvement at the thumb base may occur with swelling, tenderness, crepitus and lead to a squared appearance of the thumb
  - Carpometacarpal joint may lead to pain in the radial side of the wrist that is intensified by physical activity
- Knees are the most common source of major disability in osteoarthritis
- Degenerative changes may lead to deformities to include varus deformity (bowlegs)
- Hips usually do not develop signs of osteoarthritis until late middle age or the elderly years, if untreated may lead to severely restricted mobility
  - Pain is often referred to the groin, buttock or thigh
  - May result in loss of internal rotation, extension, adduction and flexion limiting mobility
- Spinal involvement leads to symptoms dependent upon the area of the spine affected

- Pain may radiate to other areas of the back
- The overgrowth of bone that is common in osteoarthritis may cause a narrowing of the spinal canal leading to spinal stenosis

Components of initial examination for osteoarthritis

- *Complete medical history to include:*
- Personal and family history of arthritis and joint disorders including previous and current treatments and lifestyle changes
- Patient's understanding of diagnosis and treatment
- Patient's willingness to make lifestyle changes
- History of trauma to joints
- History of frequent repetitive movements due to work or leisure activities
- Assessment of pattern of joint pain to include onset, duration, relationship to activity
- *Physical examination to include:*
- General appearance and comfort level when sitting and ambulating (pain may be more evident with use of weight bearing joints)
- Location(s) of any joint tenderness
- Examination of joints for localized tenderness, heat, swelling or deformities
- Determination of functional ability of joint
- *Laboratory and diagnostic testing:*
- No specific laboratory tests to detect osteoarthritis
- Sedimentation rate is usually normal
- Arthrocentesis with synovial fluid analysis is normal with clear fluid and negative mucin clot tests
- X-rays may be normal initially, later may show destruction of cartilage, change in joint contour and bony cysts may be noted
- Spinal x-rays may show degeneration of intervertebral discs
- CT or MRI scans may show osteoarthritis in the shoulder, hips, knees or spine but are used infrequently due to cost and availability

Treatment

- Goal of treatment is to reduce pain, maintain or restore function to affected joints and promote optimal ability
- Medications are used to relieve pain and inflammation

- Promote rest of affected joints, daily activities may need to be revised to prevent further damage to joints
- Prolonged standing, kneeling and squatting should be avoided
- Proper fitting shoes may reduce joint stress, running shoes may be helpful to cushion the joint
- Use of splints, canes, crutches, walkers or other adaptive assistive devices to reduce weight bearing on joints and promote mobility
- A cervical collar may be required for osteoarthritis in the lumbar spine to reduce extension or flexion of the neck and decrease pain
- Diet for reduction if patient is overweight to reduce stress on weight bearing joints
- Application of moist heat or cold to reduce swelling and pain
- Physical therapy and/or exercise under the guidance of physical therapist to reduce further joint degeneration
- Surgical intervention may be required for advanced OA
  - Total joint replacement
  - Wedge osteotomy
  - Arthroplasty
  - Debridement of joint

Medications

- Analgesics used intermittently to relieve pain such as acetaminophen
- Nonsteroidal anti-inflammatory drugs such as ibuprofen may relieve pain and improve mobility
- Gastric protective agents such as antacids or histamine receptor blockers to prevent untowed effects of analgesics
- Corticosteroid injections at infrequent intervals

Section VI — DIETS

• No diets specific for this system

Section VII — DRUGS

The tables below supply only general information, a drug handbook or the physicians desk reference (PDR) should be consulted for details. Each classification includes detailed information about the prototype drug, this drug is representative of the other drugs in the classification and can be used as a model.

Every effort has been made to include the major classes of drugs used in the treatment of musculoskeletal diseases. Please see also Analgesics in the neurological section and Adrenal corticosteroids in the endocrine section.

ANTIGOUT AGENTS
Action: Decrease uric acid to relieve gouty attacks, not analgesics or anti-inflammatory agent
Indications: Confirmed or suspected gout
Example: Colchicine
Route: PO, IV
Pharmacokinetics: Peak ½ to 2 hours
Contraindications: Sensitivity to colchicine, blood dyscrasias, severe GI, renal, liver or heart disease
Life-threatening adverse effects: Bone marrow suppression, agranulocytosis, aplastic anemia
Common adverse effects: nausea, vomiting, diarrhea, abdominal pain
Other adverse effects: mental confusion, muscle weakness, anorexia, steatorrhea, pancreatitis, liver impairment, thrombocytopenia, oliguria, hematuria, proteinuria, azotemia
Interventions:
Administer PO drug with milk or food to reduce GI upset
IV administration mix with approved diluent only, assess site carefully, extravasation of IV may cause severe tissue irritation or nerve damage
Monitor serum uric acid, creatinine level, CBC, electrolytes and UA

Assess patient for toxicity to include weakness, abdominal pain,
anorexia, nausea, vomiting and diarrhea, report to primary care
provider and stop medication administration

Monitor I&O and encourage fluids to prevent urinary tract calculi

Examples of other drugs in this classification:

Allopurinol (*Lopurin, Zyloprim*), PO only, tablet may be crushed,
fluid intake of 3,000 ml per day recommended, rash is common
side effect

Probenecid (*Benemid, Probalan, SK-Probenecid*), PO, may be
prescribed with Colchicine (eg. *ColBenemid*)

Sulfinpryrazone (*Antazone, Anturan, Anturane, Apo-Sulfinpyrazone,
Aprazone, Novopyrazone, Salazopyrin, Zynol*), PO, used to
prevent gout attacks, may be taken with Colchicine

GOLD COMPOUNDS

Action: Exact action is unknown, may inhibit lysosomal activity and
antigen formation. It appears to suppress the synovitis of acute
rheumatoid disease

Indications: Adult and juvenile rheumatoid arthritis when other
drugs have not been effective

Example: Aurothioglucose (*Gold Thioglucose, Solganal*) 50% gold
compound

Route: IM

Pharmacokinetics: Peaks 4-6 hours

Contraindications: Sensitivity to gold or other heavy metals,
uncontrolled diabetes, renal dysfunction, liver impairment,
hepatitis, uncontrolled CHF, severe hypertension, tuberculosis,
severe anemia, agranulocytosis, other blood disorders, radiation
therapy, colitis, urticaria, eczema, lupus erthyematosus that is
disseminated, exfoliative dermatitis

Life-threatening adverse effects: Agranulocytosis, anaphylactic
shock, exfoliative dermatitis

Common adverse effects: pruritus, urticaria, erythema, pain with
injection

Other adverse effects: keratitis, corneal ulcer, nausea, vomiting,
cramps, anorexia, metallic taste, glossitis, gingivitis, diarrhea,
eosinophilia, thrombocytopenia, leukopenia, granulocytopenia,
aplastic anemia, syncope, bradycardia, dysphagia, dyspnea,
nephrotic syndrome, proteinuria, hematuria, Stevens-Johnson
syndrome, photosensitivity reactions, hepatitis, fever, local irritation
at injection site, vaginitis, pulmonary fibrosis

Interventions:
Shake vial vigorously before using, Administer deep IM into the gluteus muscle as this injection is painful, use 18-20 gauge needle

Patient should be lying down during injection and for 10 minutes following

Monitor for gold allergy reactions after injection

Monitor liver function studies, renal function tests, CBC and urinalysis

Report any abnormal findings before injection is given

Pregnancy is a contraindication and women should be on birth control

Gold toxicity symptoms include itching, bruising, bleeding, tenderness, metallic taste, gray-blue skin discoloration, diarrhea, fatigue, jaundice, clay-colored stools, dark urine or pruritus, report if any S&S found

Examples of other drugs in this classification:

Auranofin (*Ridaura*), PO, 29% gold compound, Administer with food or fluids less toxic than aurothioglucose

Gold sodium thiomalate (*Myochrysine*), IM, 50% gold compound, monitor while lying down after injection for 30 minutes, dimercaprol is antidote

SKELETAL MUSCLE RELAXANTS
Action: To decrease muscle tone and muscle movement without loss of voluntary motor ability, also reduce anxiety, tension and pain
Indications: Relief of musculoskeletal pain from strains, sprains, low back pain, arthritis, bursitis, cerebral palsy, neck pain and multiple sclerosis
Example: Cyclobenzaprine hydrochloride (*Cycoflex, Flexeril*)
Route: PO
Pharmacokinetics: Onset 1 hour; Peak 3-8 hours; Duration 12-24 hours
Contraindications: Myocardial infarction, cardiac arrhythmias, heart block, CHF, hyperthyroidism, use longer than 2-3 weeks
Common adverse effects: drowsiness, dizziness, dry mouth
Other adverse effects: weakness, fatigue, asthenia, paresthesias, tremors, muscle twitching, insomnia, euphoria, disorientation, mania, ataxia, syncope, tachycardia, palpitations, vasodilation, chest pain, hypotension, dyspnea, indigestion, unpleasant taste sensations, coated tongue, tongue discoloration, vomiting, anorexia, abdominal pain, flatulence, diarrhea, libido changes, impotence, sweating, myalgia, hepatitis, alopecia, itching, rash, sensitivity

reaction may lead to edema of tongue
<u>Interventions:</u>
Assess for use of MAO inhibitors and do administer if in use by patient
Monitor ambulation as dizziness and drowsiness are common, assist PRN
If rash or itching are present, discontinue drug and notify primary care provider
Exercise, diet and physical therapy are often concurrent with this drug

Examples of other drugs in this classification:
Baclofen (*Lioresal, Lioresal DS*), PO, used primarily for multiple sclerosis or spinal cord injury or disease

Carisoprodol (*Rela, Soma, Soprodol*), PO, used also for cerebral palsy, administer with food to reduce GI upset

Dantrolene sodium (*Dantrium*), PO/IV, capsule may be opened and placed in juice, IV drug is given for malignant hyperthermia

Section VIII — GLOSSARY OF TERMS

Abduction   Lateral movement of a limb away from the midline of the body or one of it's parts

Achilles tendon   Tendon located at back of heel

Active movements   Movements done by the individual without help

Adduction   Movement of a limb toward the midline of the body

Amyotrophia   Atrophy of muscle tissue

Ankylosis   Immobility of a joint

Antagonist   A muscle that acts in opposition to another

Arthralgia   Joint pain

Arthritis   Inflammation of one or more joints, that may be chronic or acute

Articulation   Meeting of two or more bones

Asymmetrical   The sides of the body are unequal

Balance   Ability to maintain a steady position

Biceps   Muscle of the upper arm

Closed fracture   Fracture with skin intact

Deltoid   Muscle at shoulder

Diarthroses   Joints with free movement

Diplegia   Legs are affected more than any other body part

Dorsiflexion   Bringing the foot up

Eversion   Turning out

Extension   Straightening of a limb or increasing the joint angle

Extensors   Muscles that are used to extend a body part

External rotation   Turning of a body part outward away from the midline

Flexion	Bending at a joint or decreasing the joint angle
Flexors	Muscles that are used to flex a joint
Hemiplegia	One side of the body affected
Internal Rotation	Turning of a body part inward toward the midline of the body
Inversion	Turning inward
Involuntary muscle	Muscle that cannot be moved at will
Ligaments	Bands of connective tissue, that connect bone and cartilage
Muscle tone	Degree of tension present in muscle tissue
Myalgia	Muscular pain
Myoclonus	Spasm in muscle tissue
Myokinesis	Movement of muscle
Myopathy	Disease of the muscles
Osteitis	Inflammation of the bone
Osteomalacia	Softening of bone
Osteomyelitis	Inflammation of bone marrow
Osteoporosis	Bones are very porous, subject to fracture
Osteosarcoma	Tumor of bone that is malignant
Sphincters	Circular muscles capable of constriction
Spondylitis	Inflammation of the spinal column
Synarthroses	Joints that are immovable
Synergists	Muscles that work together in the body
Tendon	Fibrous band that connects muscle to bone
Tetany	Spasm of muscle that is paroxysmal
Tic	Muscular twitch
Trapezius	Muscle that controls shoulder movement

Triceps	Muscle in upper arm that extends forearm
Paraplegia	Lower extremities are affected
Passive movements	Movements done for the individual without his/her help
Pectoralis	Muscles in the chest
Plantar flexion	Bringing the foot down
Pronation	Facing down (palm facing down, or on abdomen)
Supination	Face up position (palm facing up, or on back)
Voluntary muscle	Muscle tissue moved at will

Renal System

RENAL SYSTEM

Table of Contents

Section I — THE OVERVIEW

Primary functions

- Control of circulating blood volume, aid in BP regulation
- Controls the composition of blood
  - Kidneys filter the blood and reabsorb needed materials
  - Kidneys filter the blood and remove selected amounts of waste products left over from the metabolism of nutrients
- Aids in electrolyte and acid-base balance
  - Excess sodium, chloride, sulfate, phosphate, and hydrogen are removed to maintain homeostasis
- Formation and excretion of urine
  - Urine consists primarily of water (95% of content) and a small amount of waste product solids in solution
- Waste products include urea, hippuric acid, uric acid creatinine, sodium and potassium
  - Excretes about 1000-2000 ml of urine daily
- Produce the hormone erythropoietin which is essential for red blood cell production
- Convert Vitamin D to a form that the body can use

Components

- Contains the kidneys, ureters, urinary bladder and the urethra

Kidneys (Figure 9A)

- A pair of organs located just above the waist on each side of the spinal column (about T12 level) on the back wall of the abdomen
- The right kidney sits slightly lower than the left due to the location of the liver
- Bean shaped, purple-brown in color, each about 4 X 3 inches and 1 inch thick, usually not palpable in the healthy adult
- Help regulate the water, electrolyte and acid-base balance of the blood by excreting and conserving these substances based on body need
- Each kidney is composed of about 1,250,000 functional units known as nephrons which complete the major work of this system
- Nephrons have three primary functions:
  - Control blood concentration of water and solutes
  - Assist in regulation of blood pH

The Urinary System

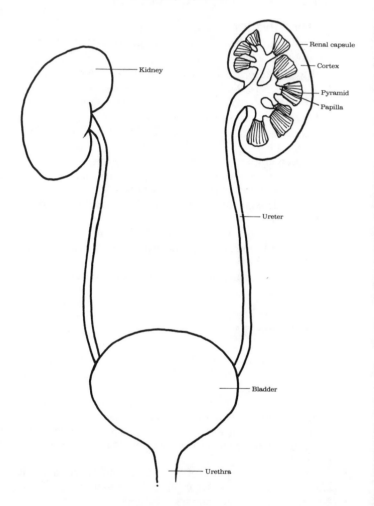

Figure 9A

- Removal of toxic wastes from the blood
- Each nephron consists of a renal tubule and a glomerulus
- The glomerulus is filled with tiny capillaries that are enclosed in a thin sac known as Bowman's capsule
  - Bowman's capsule exits into the tubules, first to the Proximal convoluted tubule then to the loop of Henle and finally to the distal convoluted tubule

Ureters
- Two tubes that provide a passageway for urine from the kidneys to the urinary bladder
- Vary in length from 28-34 cm, the right ureter is about 1 cm shorter than the left

Urinary bladder
- A muscular storage compartment for urine
- Size varies according to the amount of urine contained
- When moderately full the adult bladder holds about 500 ml, although it may hold 700-800 ml of urine
- Urge to void is generally felt when volume is between 200-400 ml

Urethra
- A single passageway for urine from the bladder to exit the body
- In males it is about 8 inches long and, as it exits the bladder, it runs vertically through the prostate; the external orifice lies on the tip of the penis
- In females it is about 1.5 inches; the external orifice lies between the vagina and the clitoris

Concepts
The formation of urine
- Involves three phases:
  - Glomerular filtration
  - Tubular reabsorption
  - Tubular secretion

Glomerular filtration
- The entire blood volume is filtered about 60 times a day
- Blood enters the glomerulus portion of the kidney's nephrons at a high pressure
- Water and plasma are forced toward Bowman's capsule to be filtered through the thin membrane walls

- Smaller materials such as water, glucose, amino acids, nitrogen wastes and electrolyte ions pass through the capsule into the tubules
- Large materials such as the formed elements of blood and larger protein's are unable to pass

Tubular reabsorption

- Occurs after glomerular filtration in the nephron tubules
- Out of the 125 ml/minute that is filtered, only 1-2 ml will be eliminated as urine, the rest is reabsorbed
- Water, glucose, amino acids, and electrolytes such as Na+, K+, Ca, Cl, and HCO3 are reabsorbed according to body need
- An example of this regulation is the reabsorption of sodium (Na+)
- If Na+ concentration in the blood is low, blood pressure will drop and the renin-angiotensinogen pathway is activated
- The kidney will release renin to convert angiotensinogen into angiotensin I which is converted to angiotensin II
- Angiotensin II stimulates the release of aldosterone which causes increased reabsorption of Na+ and water in the blood
- The increased Na+ and water raises the blood pressure
- Once the filtrate passes through the distal convoluted tubule, the remaining solution is deposited in the collecting tubules
- A single collecting tubule will contain filtrate from several nephron units

Tubular secretion

- Final phase of urine formation, the purpose is to eliminate materials and control blood pH
- Materials such as K+, H+, ammonia, creatine, and certain medications (penicillin) will be added to the filtrate from the blood
- To raise blood pH, hydrogen (H+) and ammonium (NH4+) ions are secreted into the filtrate which makes the urine pH acidic (usually around 6)

Regulation of circulating fluid volume

- The renal system aids in the regulation of blood pressure and is able to change the amount of circulating blood volume

When circulating blood volume is low

- When dehydration is present the kidneys receive less blood to filter and less nutrient's to meet their needs
- The urine is concentrated and darker in color

- To compensate the brain releases a hormone from the posterior pituitary, known as ADH or the antidiuretic hormone
- ADH increases the permeability of the collecting tubules allowing for more water to return to the vascular system

Pathophysiology of Increased ICP

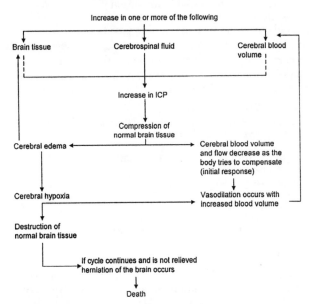

When circulating blood volume is high

- When blood volume is increased or if no ADH is released, the collecting tubules are less permeable and less water is able to move back to the vascular system
- More water is then collected for excretion and the urine is diluted in appearance

Section II — ASSESSMENT

HEALTH HISTORY
- Renal disease may occur by itself or as a manifestation of a systemic disease
- High blood pressure related to increased fluid volume often occurs with severe renal disease when the kidneys' ability to filter blood and eliminate urine is compromised
- Some individuals may find it difficult to discuss incontinence
- A supportive non-judgmental manner is important
- Some individuals find it more comfortable to discuss urinary system concerns with a health worker of the same sex

Chief complaint
- Common chief complaints for this system include:
  Increased urinary frequency
  Nocturia
  Dysuria (painful or difficult urination)
  Urinary urgency
  Incontinence
  Urinary retention
  Hematuria (blood in urine)
  Pyuria (pus in the urine)
  Oliguria (small amount of urine) or anuria (no urine)
  Excessive thirst

Family and personal history
- Renal disorders may be nonspecific, therefore, a comprehensive history, physical examination and laboratory analysis are required

Increased urinary frequency
- A urinary pattern change may accompany urinary system disorders
- Frequent urinating can be associated with diabetes, urinary tract infection (UTI), or renal failure

Nocturia (urinating at night)
- Assess the frequency patient gets up to use the bathroom
- Severe nocturia indicates the kidney's inability to concentrate the urine

Dysuria
- Dysuria (difficulty in urination) may include:

- Difficulty starting stream
- Difficulty maintaining stream
- Burning or pain with urination
- May be due to infection or stricture of urinary tract
- Urinary calculi (stones) may occur anywhere in the urinary tract causing pain, urinary obstruction and infection
- Burning on urination is usually associated with UTI or sexually transmitted disease
- Kidney infection or pyelonephritis may be acute or chronic
- Symptoms of pyelonephritis include fever, chills, flank pain, and frequent urination with burning

Incontinence
- May be related to:
  - Congenital defect
  - Urinary tract infection
  - Decreased bladder capacity
  - Urethral obstruction
- Damage to the central nervous system (stroke, spinal cord injury)
  - Some medications (diuretics, sedatives)
- Stress incontinence which is common in older women occurs when urine escapes during coughing or laughing

Hematuria/Pyuria
- Urine with frank blood (hematuria) may indicate UTI or renal calculi (stones)
- Pyuria (pus) or cloudy urine may be seen with UTI

Thirst
- Present when increased fluid volume loss is present

Urinary system testing
- Assess for tests completed or ordered and patient's knowledge and understanding of any test procedures or results

RENAL ASSESSMENT

Chief complaint

Patient's statement_____ Onset_____

Frequency_____ Duration_____ Other areas affected_____

Have you had this before?_____ When_____

What treatment was given?_____

What do you think caused this?_____

What lifestyle changes have you had to make?_____

Personal and family history

	Patient	Family member			Patient only Current	Past
High blood pressure	____	____	UTI		____	____
Dialysis Tx	____	____	Dysuria*		____	____
Kidney transplant	____	____	Urgency		____	____
Urinary system cancer	____	____	Frequency		____	____
			Incontinence		____	____
			Nocturia		____	____

*If dysuria, type_____

Urine: color_____ blood_____ pus_____ cloudy or clear_____

Urinary system testing

Urinalysis_____ Urine culture_____ 24-hour urine collection_____

Blood testing_____ Cystoscopy_____ KUB_____

IVP_____ Renal angiography_____ Renal scan_____ Biopsy_____

Cystourethrogram_____ Cystometrogram_____ Other_____

Current treatments/Medications

Medication_____ Dose_____ Frequency_____ Route_____

Special diet_____ Usual weight_____ Loss or gain?_____

Fluid restriction (type or amount)_____ How much fluid/day?_____

Is there anything else you want me to know?_____

PHYSICAL ASSESSMENT
- Assessment of this system is difficult due to the internal location of the components involved
- Includes assessment of fluid balance
- Physical assessment of this system is done in the following order:
  1. Inspection
  2. Palpation
  3. Auscultation
- Request that the patient empty bladder prior to examination
- The abdomen is generally exposed

INSPECTION

General appearance
- Assess for appearance of health, patient with renal failure may have flu-like symptoms, recent weight loss or dizziness
- Eyes appear sunken and feel soft to touch with dehydration
- Assess current comfort level, flank pain often accompanies urinary tract infections and may be severe
- Assess ability to respond to questions or simple commands, renal failure can lead to confusion, disorientation, and coma

Weight
- Obtain daily body weight on the same scale at the same time of day for any person with suspected or known renal disease
- Rapid weight changes reflect changes in body fluid volume
- A rapid weight loss indicates fluid volume deficit
  - 2% loss indicates mild fluid volume deficit
  - 5% loss indicates moderate fluid volume loss
  - 8% loss indicates severe fluid volume loss
- A rapid weight gain indicates fluid volume excess
  - 2% gain indicates mild fluid volume excess
  - 5% gain indicates moderate fluid volume excess
  - 8% gain indicates severe fluid volume excess
- 1 Kg (2.2 pounds) of body weight equals 1 liter of fluid

Comparison of intake and output (I&O)
- If a renal system disorder is suspected accurate I&O is vital
- If the total intake is substantially less than output the patient is in danger of fluid volume deficit
- If the total intake is substantially more than output the patient is in danger of fluid volume excess

- See also intake and output under procedures in this chapter

Skin

- The following may be noted in end-stage renal disease and are due to the kidneys inability to remove waste products from the blood

      Color — skin may appear yellowish brown
      Texture — Dry
      Integrity — multiple breaks or sores, record location
- Pallor and cool skin is present in fluid volume deficit

Tongue turgor

- Assess by inspecting the tongue
- Normally the tongue has one longitudinal furrow
- With fluid volume deficit the tongue will have additional longitudinal furrows and appear smaller
- With excess sodium intake the tongue may appear red and swollen

Halitosis /acetone breath

- Acetone odor to breath may occur in end-stage renal disease
- Some patients may complain of a persistent bad or metallic taste in the mouth.

Edema

- Usually starts in dependent areas and then may become generalized
- Usually not apparent until 5-10 pounds of excess fluid is present
- Note location, usually first noted in ankles, feet or hands if patient is ambulatory and in the sacral area if bedridden
- May be periorbital or anasarca (generalized edema)

Abdominal distention

- Distention with protuberant abdomen may occur in kidney disease as fluid collects in the serous cavities
- Bladder distention may occur with urinary retention

Urinary catheter

- If present list type and size and assess patency and security

Urine characteristics

- Color — may be described as colorless, straw-colored, yellow, amber, tea-colored, pale red, brown, or bloody
- Clarity — Should be clear, cloudy if infection is present, milky when alkaline and precipitated phosphates are present

- Sediment — Normal urine contains some sediment, however with disease sediment is increased

PALPATION

Skin turgor

- Assess by pinching up a small amount of skin and releasing
- Normal skin turgor, skin will immediately fall back into position after release
- Test for turgor over sternum, on forehead or inner aspects of thighs, avoid forearm where skin elasticity is often decreased with ageing
- Skin may be dry and cracked in renal failure

Buccal cavity (mouth) moisture

- Assess by running a gloved finger along where the cheek and gum meet to assess for moisture
- A dry buccal cavity indicates a true fluid volume deficit
- Dry, sticky cavity indicates sodium excess

Bladder/Kidney

- Bladder may be palpable if full
- Kidneys are not normally palpable in healthy adults
- If pain is noted on palpation note the location and severity

Edema

- Assess severity; best method is to measure the girth of an extremity to assess the effectiveness of interventions
- May be described on a scale of 1+ (barely perceptible) to 4+ (severe pitting edema)
- Pitting edema is not usually noted until a 10% increase in body weight has occurred

AUSCULTATION

- Blood pressure elevation is common in renal disease
- Assess midline of abdomen for bruits, if present may indicate renal stenosis

RENAL PHYSICAL EXAMINATION

INSPECTION

General Appearance_____ Weight_____

Intake_____ Output_____ Skin color_____ Texture_____

Breaks, lesions or sores_____ Unusual breath_____

Tongue turgor_____ Edema: location _____ severity_____

Abdominal distention_____ Body odor_____ Incontinence_____

Urinary catheter: type_____ patency_____ draininge_____

Urine: Color_____ Clarity_____ Sediment_____ Malodor ous_____

PALPATION:

Skin turgor_____ texture_____ temperatur e_____

Buccal cavity moisture_____

Bladder: distention_____ Kidney: palpable_____ tenderness_____

Pain over bladder_____ Flank pain_____ Groin pain_____

AUSCULTATION:

Blood Pressure _____/_____ Abdomen for bruit/murmur_____

Assessment Notes:

_____

_____

_____

_____

Section III — LABORATORY & DIAGNOSTIC TESTS

In the following section traditional laboratory values and SI unit values are given, it is important to recognize that "normal" values vary from laboratory to laboratory. Check the normal values at the agency or institution where a test is performed. Most labs print their normal values on the laboratory reporting slip or page.

Table of Common Laboratory Tests

Test Name	Indications	Comments
Aldosterone assay Blood or urine **Normal – Blood:** Supine 3-10 ng/dL 0.08-0.30 nmol/L Upright female 5-30 ng/dL or 0.14-0.80 nmol/L Upright male 6-22 ng/dL or 0.17-0.61 nmol/L **Normal – Urine:** 2-80 ug/24 hours 5.5-72.0 nmol/24 hr	Primary aldosteronism Renal vascular occlusion or other renal diseases 24 hour urine is considered more accurate than blood testing due to fluctuations in levels during day	**Regarding collection:** Position in supine for 1st blood Note on slip the last time that diuretics, antiyhypertensives, oral contraceptives or steroids were taken (should stop 2 weeks prior) Note on slip the last time that propranolol was taken Patient should have avoided any licorice for 2 weeks prior to test Use red-top tube collect; 5-10 ml for blood test Note: Test may be ordered again 4 hrs after patient is up and moving (2nd blood sample) Place collected blood on ice 24 hr urine specimen needs to be on ice during collection **Results:** Increased in aldosteronism and renal disease
Antidiuretic hormone (ADH) Blood test **Normal** 1.5 pg/ml or .5 ng/L (SI)	Renal diseases SIADH (Syndrome of inappropriate ADH)	**Regarding collection:** NPO for 12 hrs prior to testing Use plastic red-top tube; collect 7 ml Record on slip any medications **Results:** Sample may be sent to a regional center for processing
Blood urea nitrogen (BUN) Blood test **Normal:** 10-20 mg/dL or 3.6-7.1 mmol/L SI	Liver disease Renal diseases to include: acute tubular necrosis, glomerulonephritis, pyelonephritis, urinary obstruction	**Regarding collection:** Use red-top tube; collect 5 ml **Results:** Increased levels with renal disease urinary obstruction, hypovolemia Decreased levels with liver failure

Test Name	Indications	Comments
Chloride Blood test **Normal:** 90-110 mEg/L or 98-106 mmol/L (SI)	Kidney dysfunction Acid/base imbalance	**Regarding collection:** Use red-top tube; collect 5-10 ml **Results:** Increased with kidney dysfunction, dehydration, excessive NS IV fluid, and metabolic acidosis Decreased in over hydration, SIADH, respiratory acidosis, metabolic alkalosis and hypokalemia
Creatinine Blood test	Renal disease to include: acute tubular necrosis, glomerulonephritis, pyelonephritis, urinary obstruction or nephritis	**Regarding collection:** Use red-top tube; collect 5-10 ml **Results:** Increased in renal diseases Decreased with debilitation or diseases affecting muscle mass
Creatinine clearance Urine and blood **Normal** male: 90-139 mL/min or 0.87-1.34 mL/s/m2 female: 80-125 mL/min or 0.77-1.20 mL/s/m2	Renal dysfunction Measures the glomerular filtration rate	**Regarding collection:** Check with lab regarding any food or beverage restrictions Explain procedure for 24-hr urine collection to patient Keep urine on ice during collection List start time, patient's weight, age, height on laboratory slip Use a red-top tube to collect a blood sample during 24-hr period **Results:** Decreased levels with impaired kidney function, glomerulonephritis renal artery atherosclerosis Increased in pregnancy or exercise
Osmolality Urine test **Normal:** Random—50-1400 mOsm/kg H2O (SI) 12-14 hr fluid restricted sample >850 mOsm/kg H2O	Acute and chronic renal failure Dehydration SIADH Diabetes insipidus More exact than specific gravity	**Regarding collection:** Check order for test type; if random, no preparation is needed If fasting, assess order for a high protein diet for 3 days before test NPO for 12-14 hrs before testing For random collect, first void of day For fasting test have patient void and discard urine at 6:00 am then collect specimen at 8:00 am Indicate on lab slip type of test **Results:** Increased in SIADH, Addison's, CHF or acidosis Decreased in renal tubular necrosis, Diabetes, Aldosteronism or hypokalemia

Test Name	Indications	Comments
Potassium (K+) Blood test **Normal:** 3.5-5.0 mEq/L or 3.5-5.0 mmol/L (SI) 24-hour urine K+ may be ordered as well or instead	Diuretic use IV potassium use Trauma Surgery Suspected imbalance of electrolytes	**Regarding collection:** Use green-top tube; collect 5-10 ml Do not use tourniquet if possible to prevent hemolysis which yields a false-high result Label any drugs taken on lab slip **Results:** Increased in excessive IV potassium chronic or acute renal failure, Addison's disease, acidosis, hemolysis or excessive PO potassium Decreased in dietary K+ deficiency, diarrhea, diuretic use, alkalosis, renal tubular acidosis
Potassium Urine test **Normal:** 25-120 mEq/L/d or 25-120 mmol/d (SI)	Renal disease Adrenal disease	**Regarding collection:** Usually 24-hr urine collection Explain procedure to patient Keep specimen on ice **Results:** Increased in chronic renal failure renal tubular acidosis, Cushing's, hyperaldosteronism and alkalosis
Prostate-specific antigen (PSA) Blood test **Normal:** 136-145 mEq/L or 136-145 mmol/L SI Ordered with K+ as electrolytes 24-hr urine may be ordered as well	Suspected imbalance of sodium Fluid imbalance Dehydration Over-hydration Renal disease Trauma SIADH	**Regarding collection:** Use green or red-top tube; collect 5-10 ml, use extremity with no IV List any drugs taken on lab slip **Results:** Increased (hypernatremia) with excessive dietary or IV Na+ intake Cushing's, hyperaldosteronism, burn, diabetes insipidus Decreased (hyponatremia) with deficient intake of Na+, Addison's, diarrhea, vomiting, diuretics, CHF
Sodium (Na+) Blood test **Normal:** 136-145 mEq/L or 136-145 mmol/L SI Ordered with K+ as electrolytes 24-hr urine may be ordered as well	Suspected imbalance of sodium Fluid imbalance Dehydration Over-hydration Renal disease Trauma SIADH	**Regarding collection:** Use green or red-top tube; collect 5-10 ml; use extremity with no IV List any drugs taken on lab slip **Results:** Increased (hypernatremia) with excessive dietary or IV Na+ intake, Cushing's, hyperaldosteronism, burn, fiabetes insipidus Decreased (hyponatremia) with deficient intake of Na+, Addison's, diarrhea, vomiting, diuretics, CHF

Test Name	Indications	Comments
Sodium (Na+) Urine test **Normal:** 40-220 mEq/L/d or 40-220 mmol/L (SI)	Acute renal failure Adrenal disturbance Acid-base imbalance	**Regarding collection:** Usually 24-hr urine collection Explain procedure to patient Keep specimen on ice **Results:** Increased in SIADH, hypothyroidism, adrenocortical insufficiency Decreased in renal failure, Cushing disease, aldosteronism, diaphoresis
Uric acid Blood test **Normal** male: 2.1-8.5 mg/dL or 0.15-0.48 mmol/L female: 2.0-6.6 mg/dL or 0.09-0.36 mmol/L	Gout Renal failure	**Regarding collection:** Check agency policy regarding any food or fluid restrictions Use red-top tube to collect 5-7 ml List all drugs on lab slip **Results:** Increased levels in arthritis, gout, uric acid kidney stones, metastatic cancers, renal failure
Uric acid Urine test **Normal:** 270-750 mL/24 h or 1.48-4.43 mmol/dSI	Gout Renal calculi formation	**Regarding collection:** 24-hr urine collection Explain procedure to patient Keep specimen on ice **Results:** Increased in gout, liver disease, ulcerative colitis, toxemia of PG Decreased in urinary obstruction, kidney disease, glomerulonephritis
Urinalysis Urine test **Normal:** pH: 4.6-8.0 Appearance: Clear Color: Amber yellow Odor: Aromatic Specific gravity: 1.005-1.030 Protein: 0-8mg/dL Glucose: Negative Ketones: Negative RBCs: 1-2 RBCells WBCs: 0-4 WBCells Leukocyte esterase: Negative Bacteria: Negative Crystals: Negative	Routine screening Renal diseases Urinary tract infections Systemic diseases	**Regarding collection:** Assess order for routine or "clean catch" UA For routine: collect urine in clean specimen container, label and send to lab For "clean catch" UA: obtain sterile container and have patient clean urinary meatus well with iodine preparation, followed by cleansing wipe to remove contaminate. Have patient begin to urinate into bedpan or toilet then pause until specimen cup is in place to collect 90-120 cc or urine. Patient may then finish voiding. This is also called a "midstream" UA. **Results:** See also urinalysis later this chapter for complete listing of values and results

Test Name	Indications	Comments
Urine culture and sensitivity Urine test **Normal:** Negative	Urinary tract infection (UTI)	**Regarding collection:** "Clean catch" specimen is required; see urinalysis (above) for procedure Antibiotics should be held until specimen is collected If patient is unable to void a urinary catheterization is done Send sample to lab ASAP **Results:** Positive result indicates UTI

Table of Common Diagnostic Tests

Test Name	Indications	Comments
(CT) Computed tomography of the kidney X-ray with contrast dye **Normal:** kidney	Congenital renal anomaly Renal tumor or cyst Renal calculi Ureteral obstruction	**Pre-procedure:** Signed consent form may be required Assess orders for with or without contrast dye, assess for iodine or seafood allergy Assess patient for ability to lie still during procedure **Post-procedure:** Encourage fluids Assess for allergic reaction to dye if contrast CT was done No activity restrictions
Cystography X-ray with contrast dye **Normal** bladder structure and function	Pelvic tumor Pelvic trauma Pyelonephritis Bladder tumors Vesicoureteral reflux	**Pre-procedure:** Signed consent form may be required Explain procedure to patient: air or dye will be placed via catheter into bladder and X-rays taken Clear liquid diet morning of test Insert Foley catheter if ordered **Post-procedure:** Encourage fluids and monitor for S&S of urinary tract infection
Cystometry Manometric **Normal** bladder pressures, volumes and capacity Normal sensations of fullness	Incontinence Urinary urgency Urinary frequency Vesicoureteral reflux Spinal cord injury	**Pre-procedure:** Explain procedure to patient: measurements will be taken while they empty their bladder, then a urethral catheter is placed and residual urine volume assessed; fluid will be placed in bladder and sensations and pressures recorded Once bladder is full, the patient again empties the bladder Assess for S&S of UTI, test should not be done if UTI is present Procedure takes about 45 mins, may be repeated with medications **Post-procedure:** Monitor urine for hematuria, assess for S&S of urinary tract infection

Test Name	Indications	Comments
Cystocopy Endoscopy **Normal** urethra, bladder, ureters and prostrate	Hematuria Chronic UTI Renal cancer Renal calculi Prostatitis or hyperplasia Urethral stricture or calculi Bladder stricture	**Pre-procedure:** Signed consent form is required Explain procedure to the patient: A lighted cystoscope is passed into bladder so it can be visualized. Therapeutic procedures can be done during cystocopy Pre-medication may be ordered Check orders for increased fluids or NPO status (local or general) If NPO, assess for IV hydration orders and enema or bowel prep Procedure takes about 30-60 minutes **Post-procedure:** Assess vital signs and ability to void, urine may be pink-tinged Urine should not have clots or be bright red from fresh bleeding Monitor for dysuria; bladder spasms may occur; provide drugs as ordered Encourage fluids, monitor for S&S of infection
Intravenous pyelography (IVP, IVP, IUG) X-ray with contrast dye **Normal** kidney, ureters and bladder	Urinary calculi Urinary tumors Polycystic kidneys Recurrent UTIs	**Pre-procedure:** CT may be done with IVP procedure Signed consent form may be required Assess for allergy to iodine or seafood, report if found Check orders, clear liquid diet or NPO may be ordered, enema may be ordered; if NPO start IV per order Monitor BUN and creatinine levels, report unusual findings Procedure takes about 45 minutes **Post-procedure:** Monitor VS and compare to baseline Monitor for reaction to dye Assess urinary output Encourage fluids, maintain IV as ordered
Kidney sonogram Ultrasound **Normal** kidney size shape and position	Renal cysts Renal tumors Renal calculi Hydronephrosis	**Pre-procedure:** No special preparations are needed Procedure takes about 20 minutes **Post-procedure:** No restrictions, remove gel
Kidney, ureter and bladder (KUB) X-ray **Normal** structure, no calculi, normal GI gas pattern	Renal calculi Urethral calculi Intestinal obstruction Congenital anomaly	**Pre-procedure:** No special preparations are needed Procedure takes about 10 mins Report pregnancy in female patients **Post-procedure:** No restrictions

Test Name	Indications	Comments
Renal angiography X-ray with contrast dye **Normal** renal blood vessel patency and structure	Renal tumor Renal cyst Renal aneurysms Hypertension Renal artery stenosis Renal failure	**Pre-procedure:** Signed consent form is required Explain procedure to patient: A catheter will be inserted into femoral artery up to the renal artery for visualization of renal blood vessels Assess for allergy to iodine or seafood, report if noted Assess for recent anticoagulant use NPO for 8-12 hrs before test Mark peripheral pulses with a pen Administer pre-medication after patient voids Procedure takes 60-90 mins **Post-procedure:** Assess for bleeding, monitor VS Assess peripheral pulses compare to baseline findings Bed rest for 6-8 hrs Cold compress to puncture site Encourage fluids, monitor I&O Assess for allergic reaction to dye
Renal biopsy Microscopic exam **Normal** renal tissue	Renal failure of unknown origin Renal cancer Metastatic cancer of kidney Kidney transplant rejection	**Pre-procedure:** Signed consent form is required Explain procedure to patient: A needle is inserted through the skin into the kidney and a sample of tissue is taken NPO 8-12 hours before testing Monitor PT, PTT, Hgb & Hct; report if abnormal Check orders for need for type and cross match precautions Procedure may be done at bedside Procedure takes about 10 minutes **Post-procedure:** Pressure dressing is applied Bed rest in supine position for 24 hrs Monitor VS, puncture site and Hct for evidence of hemorrhage Report any abdominal tenderness Monitor urine for hematuria, normal for 1st 24 hrs Encourage fluids No strenuous activity for 2 wks Monitor for S&S of UTI and report
Renal Scan Nuclear scan	Tubular disease Urinary obstruction Pyelonephritis Renal vascular hypertension Renal failure	**Pre-procedure:** Explain procedure to patient: A radioactive tracer is given and its progress through the kidneys is scanned and mapped Encourage fluids before testing Have patient void before testing **Post-procedure:** Encourage fluids

Expanded Components of Urinalysis

Expected Result	Other Findings	Comments
pH: 4.6-8.0	Decreased pH<4.6 Increased pH>8.0	Average pH is 6.0 Metabolic or respiratory acidosis excessive intake of cranberries, high protein diet, starvation, diarrhea Metabolic or respiratory alkalosis, urinary tract infection (UTI), renal tubular acidosis, diuretics, vegetarian diet, gastric suction
Appearance: clear	Cloudy Milky	Infection, Pus, WBC's, RBC's, sperm or phosphates Fat, pyuria
Color: Amber yellow	Colorless Straw-colored Orange Red Red-Brown, Brown Blue, green	Diluted urine, diabetes insipidus, chronic renal disease, excessive alcohol ingestion Diluted urine Concentrated urine, fever, food coloring, increased total bilirubin Medications: Chlorzoxazone, Phenazopyridine, Phenindione, Rifampin, Sulfasalazine Menstrual blood contamination, hematuria, beets, bilirubin Medications: Anisindione, Cascara sagrada, Danthron, Dioctyl calcium sulfo succinate, Phenolphthalein, Phenothiazines, Phenytoin Rhubarb Medications: Chloroquine, Furazolidone, Iron preparations, Levodopa, Nitrofurantoin Bacterial pseudomonas infection Medications: Methylene blue, Triamterene, Amitriptyline
Odor: Aromatic	Ammonia Sweet-fruity Foul Mousey Fecal	Bacteria Diabetic ketosis Bacteria — urinary tract infection Phenylketonuria Rectal fistula
Specific gravity: 1.005-1.030	Decreased: Increased:	Usually 1.010-1.025 Inability to concentrate urine, diabetes, over-hydration, renal disease, potassium loss, diuresis Dehydration, fever, IV albumin, diabetes, SIADH, decreased renal blood flow, proteinuria
Protein: 0-8mg/dL	Increased:	Proteinuria is an indicator of renal disease, vaginal secretions may cause false-positives Complications of diabetes mellitus, glomerulonephritis, amyloidosis and multiple myeloma

Expected Result	Other Findings	Comments
Glucose: Negative	Increased: >15mg/dL	Screening for diabetes mellitus Diabetes mellitus, Cushing's, stroke, infections, anesthesia, glucose IV infusions
Ketones: Negative	Increased: 1+ - 3+	Ketoacidosis, poorly controlled diabetes mellitus, starvation High protein/low calorie diet Excessive aspirin ingestion Dehydration
Red blood cells: 1-2 RBC's	Increased RBCs	Menstrual blood contamination Traumatic urinary catheterization Trauma, renal or urinary tract disease or infection, renal tumor, renal stones, prostatitis
White blood cells: 0-4WBCs	Greater than 5 WBCs	Urinary tract infection
Leukocyte esterase: Negative	Positive False-positive	Possible urinary tract infection Contamination by vaginal secretions High levels of protein
Bacteria: Negative	Positive	Urinary tract infection
Crystals: Negative	Positive	Renal stone formation Urinary tract infection Medications: Ampicillin, Sulfonamides
Casts: Epithelial: Few Fatty: None Granular: Few Hyaline: Few Waxy: None RBC: None WBC: None	Increased Present Increased Increased PresentR Present Present	There are a variety of Cast types: Glomerulonephritis, eclampsia, heavy-metal poisoning, transplant rejection (renal) Nephrotic syndrome, renal disease Normal after exercise Renal diseases Normal after strenuous exercise Renal diseases, renal failure Chronic renal disease and failure Glomerulonephritis Acute pyelonephritis, lupus nephritis, glomerulonephritis

Section IV — PROCEDURES

INTAKE AND OUTPUT

Definition
Intake is anything that patients consume and includes:
- Oral fluids
- Foods that are liquid at room temperature
- Fluids instilled via nasogastric or gastrostomy tubes
  Also includes any irrigants
- Intravenous fluids
- Subcutaneous fluids
- Oral solids (foods)
- Blood products
- Medications
- Enemas instilled in patients who require strict I&O

Output is anything expelled from the body and includes:
- Urine
- Feces including fluid loss from diarrhea
- Emesis (vomitus)
- Blood
- Gastric secretions
- Drainage from fistulas or wounds
- Perspiration (should be noted if heavy)
- If hyperventilation is present it should be noted as it is an important route for water vapor loss

Normal intake and output
- Intake and output should balance in a healthy person
- Normal urinary output is about 1ml/Kg of body weight (adults)

Intake		Output	
Oral liquids	1300 ml	Urine	1500 ml
Water in foods	1000 ml	Stool	200 ml
Water from		Skin	600 ml
metabolism	300 ml	Lungs	300 ml
Total	2600 ml	Total	2600 ml

Measuring intake and output
- Should include time of day and type of fluid intake or output
- A patient who is experiencing a major health problem will require more frequent evaluation and hourly I&O may be needed
- Most hospitalized patients require only 8 hour I&O summaries
- All measurements should be recorded when taken, do not depend upon memory
- Measure all fluids that can be measured — do not guess
- Know the volume of glasses, cups and bowls used in your agency
- An 8 oz glass of ice chips contains only 4 ounces of fluid volume
- Parenteral fluid containers (such as IV bags) are usually overfilled to allow for clearance of tubing, record exact volume infused using a pump or run excess through tubing prior to administration
- Always ask a patient what fluids they drank, do not assume that they drank the fluids from empty containers
- Record any heavy perspiration loss, linen saturated with perspiration (requiring a bed change) may represent a liter of fluid loss
- Estimate whenever possible loss from incontinent urine or loss from emesis that is on linen or clothing
- Always include the amount used to irrigate in the input and the amount of irrigation fluid retrieved under output

Factors that affect intake and output
- Assess for balance problems, total the I&O records for several days to get a complete assessment of fluid balance status
- Monitor urine specific gravity on patients who have suspected fluid balance problems, normal range is 1.003 to 1.035
- A low urine volume with a high specific gravity indicates fluid volume deficit
- A low urine volume with a low specific gravity indicates renal dysfunction or disease
- Low urinary output usually means a fluid volume deficit although other factors may be involved to include:
  Excessive losses from skin (burns)
  Excessive losses from lungs (hyperventilation)
  Excessive losses from the GI tract (emesis or diarrhea)
  Loss of kidney's ability to concentrate urine (renal disease)
  Loss of blood volume (hemorrhage)
  Hormonal influences (ADH or aldosterone)

- High urinary output usually means a fluid volume excess
  although other factors may be involved to include:
  >   Loss of kidney's ability to excrete urine
  >   Hormonal influences (ADH or aldosterone)
- Urinary output decreases during stress and may be only 30-50ml
  per hour

COLLECTION OF 24-HOUR URINE SAMPLE
Purpose
- A 24-hour urine collection may be required for a variety of
  laboratory tests to include:
  >   Aldosterone assay
  >   Amylase, urine
  >   Calcium, urine
  >   Chloride, urine
  >   Cortisol, urine
  >   Creatinine clearance
  >   Delta-aminolevulinic acid
  >   Dexamethasone-suppression test
  >   Estriol excretion
  >   17-hydroxycorticosteroids
  >   5-hydroxy indoleacetic acid
  >   17-ketosteroids
  >   Leucine aminopeptidase
  >   Metyrapone
  >   Porphyrins and porphobilinogens
  >   Potassium
  >   Pregnanediol
  >   Schilling test (may be 24-48 hours)
  >   Sodium
  >   Tubular phosphate reabsorption
  >   Vanillylmandelic acid and catecholamines

Equipment:
- Obtain appropriate container from laboratory
- Basin for ice if specimen is to be kept on ice during collection
- Laboratory slip
- Specimen collector for toliet if patient is ambulatory

Before Collection:
- Label specimen container with patient's name and room number
- Check with laboratory for any dietary restrictions and implement
  as needed

- Have patient void into toliet, note time of this discarded voiding as start time for 24 hour urine collection
- Place start time on specimen container and laboratory slip
- Instruct ambulatory patient to always void into specimen collector and then notify staff so that urine can be placed into specimen container
- Instruct patient that no toliet tissue is to be placed in the specimen collector or container
- Instruct patient to void before defecating so that urine is not contaminated by feces
- Collect all urine voided for the next 24 hours, place in specimen container
- Post notices above toliet or on bathroom door that 24-hour urine collection is in process to prevent accidental discarding of specimen, include start and stop times
- Keep ice basin filled during the 24 hour period to keep specimen cold or refrigerate if available
- Encourage fluids as appropriate
- Last urine specimen is collected as close to the end of the 24 hour collection time as possible, this urine is added to container
- Send container to laboratory as soon as possible to maintain integrity of specimen

PERFORMING URINARY CATHETERIZATION
Purpose
Catheterization may be done for several reasons:
- To relieve urinary retention
- To obtain sterile urine specimen for testing
- To measure the amount of residual urine in the bladder
- To empty the bladder before procedures

Equipment:
- Sterile catheter of appropriate size and type
  - Size
    - 14-16 French for female adult
    - 18-20 French for male adult
    - 8-10 French for children
  - Type
    - Foley for continuous use
    - Straight for single urinary sample or single use emptying

- Sterile catheterization kit
  - Contains gloves, antiseptic solution, cotton balls, forceps, lubricant, receiving container and sterile towel
- Sterile collecting bag and syringe with sterile water if catheter is to remain in place

Steps:

- Gather equipment and wash your hands
- Prepare patient: Provide for privacy and explain the procedure
- Position the patient and expose the genitalia Female in lithotomy position, male in supine
- While maintaining sterility prepare catheterization equipment Open kit and don gloves
  Position drape — Females under buttocks, males around penis
- For continuous catheter test balloon, instill and remove fluid
- Pour antiseptic over cotton balls
- Place lubricating jelly on catheter tip
- Perform catheterization
- Using non-dominant hand expose the urinary meatus
  Females — separate labia majoria and minora
  Males — hold penis with foreskin retracted
- Holding cotton ball in forceps cleanse urinary meatus
  Females: 1 stroke with 1 cotton ball for each labia minora
              Stroke from top to bottom once then discard cotton
              1 stroke with 1 cotton ball to cleanse urinary meatus
              Stroke from top to bottom then discard cotton
  Males: 1 stroke with 1 cotton ball to encircle urinary meatus
              Discard cotton and repeat
- Insert catheter slowly, using dominant hand until urine flows
  Females: Urethra is 4 cm or 1.5 inches (approximate)
  Males: Urethra is 20cm or 8 inches (approximate)
- Stop insertion if obstruction is met, do not force catheter
- Allow urine to drain into receptacle
- For continuous drainage attach syringe to balloon port and fill
- Tug lightly on catheter to assure balloon is filled and secure
- Connect to gravity collection bag with bag positioned below bladder level and tape tubing securely to thigh

Common problems and solutions:

- Difficulty locating urinary meatus in female patients

Become familiar with the meatus location BEFORE
catheterization
A common error is insertion into the vagina, the urethra is above
the vagina
Some practitioners place a cotton ball at the vaginal opening to
prevent confusion.

- Urine on bedding or patient
  Always place the end of the catheter in a collecting basin prior to
  inserting the tip in the meatus
- Tubing detached from collection bag
  Tape all connections, tape bag to leg to prevent unnecessary
  tension on connections
- Discomfort during insertion
  Have patient take slow steady breaths with deliberate exhalation,
  this promotes relaxation and lessens feelings of helplessness

Section V — CONDITIONS

Acute Renal Failure (ARF)

Definition

- Failure of the kidneys to perform essential functions in a person who was previously healthy
- Decrease in glomerular filtration rate with impaired urine formation
- Affects both kidneys
- Acute renal failure may lead to chronic renal failure
- May range from renal impairment with no symptoms except increased BUN and creatinine levels to total renal failure
- Sudden, rapid, severe decline in glomerular filtration rate with retention of waste products leading to a uremic episode

Prevalence

- Relatively common, affects about 5% of all patients on medical and surgical units and 30% of intensive care admissions
- Most common among the elderly who have multiple system problems or preexisting renal insufficiency
- Approximately 60% of cases are related to surgery or trauma
- Acute renal failure is usually reversible
- Mortality from ARF is as high as 50-60%, mortality is highest in elderly patients with multiple system problems

Etiology

- Prerenal causes decrease the blood perfusion of the kidneys thereby leading to kidney failure, causes include:
  - Hypovolemia from blood loss (trauma, shock)
  - Fluid loss from burns, diarrhea, vomiting or diuretics
  - Congestive heart failure, dysrhythmias
  - Sepsis
  - Anaphylaxis
  - Liver failure
  - Account for about 50% of all cases of ARF
  - Rapidly reversible upon restoration of renal blood flow
- Postrenal causes are rare, they involve an obstruction of the urinary tract distal to the kidney, causes include:
  - Ureteral obstruction from calculi, cancer, or clot

- Urethral obstruction from prostatitis
- Venous occlusion from thrombosis or cancer
- Neurogenic bladder
- Accounts for about 5% of all cases of ARF
- Intra renal cause of renal failure result in primary damage to the kidney and include:
  - Malignant hypertension
  - Eclampsia
  - Scleroderma
  - Acute glomerulonephritis or pyelonephritis
  - Profound hypotension leading to renal necrosis
  - Some chemotherapeutic agents — see components initial exam

Symptoms

- Often divided into stages
- *Stage 1 — Onset*
  - May occur within hours or days of precipitating factor
  - Change in urine volume with oliguria or anuria occurring in about 50% of all cases
  - Total anuria is no urine output (rare except in postrenal ARF)
  - Anuria is <50-100 ml in 24 hours
  - Oliguria is less than 400 ml in 24 hours
- *Stage 2 — Oliguric—Anuric phase*
  - In 10-20% of cases nonoliguric failure may develop, this represents a milder renal dysfunction
  - Output is less than 400 ml in 24 hours
  - Usually output is 50-150 ml for first few days
  - Urine output gradually increases
  - May last 1 day to several weeks — average is 10-12 days
  - Electrolyte problems commonly include hyperkalemia, fluid volume excess, metabolic acidosis
  - Symptoms of hyperkalemia (potassium excess) include:
    - Muscular weakness
    - Cardiac arrhythmias, bradycardia, ECG changes
    - Paresthesias, muscle paralysis
    - Nausea, diarrhea, and ECG changes
    - One of the main causes of death in ARF

- Symptoms of fluid volume excess include edema and weight gain related to water retention
- Metabolic acidosis occurs because the body normally produces more acid than alkaline wastes and when the kidneys fail these accumulate leading to:
    - Headache, confusion, drowsiness
    - Increased respiratory rate and depth
    - Nausea and vomiting
    - Decreased cardiac output
- Calcium deficit, phosphorus excess, sodium deficits and magnesium excess may also occur
- Uremia may develop with severe ARF, symptoms include
    - Fatigue initially, very late muscle wasting
    - Insomnia
    - Anorexia, unpleasant metallic taste in mouth
    - Vomiting
    - Gastritis, hematemesis
    - Ammonia odor to breath
    - Stomatitis
    - Pale, sallow, dry, scaly, itchy skin (pruritus)
    - Bleeding tendencies (gums, nose, bruising, petechiae) related to low platelets, anemia
    - Coarse muscular twitching
    - Deep rapid respirations due to metabolic acidosis
    - Chest discomfort due to pericarditis or pleurisy
    - Peripheral neuropathy
    - Headache and visual problems related to hypertension
    - Loss of mental clarity may lead to hallucination, delusions, coma or convulsions
    - Uremic frost — urea crystals excreted through sweat glands (rarely seen)
    - Late uremia every organ system is affected
- Anemia may occur from interference with the kidneys normal ability to produce erythropoietin, from hyperkalemia or uremia
- *Stage 3 — Diuretic phase*

- Begins when daily output is greater than 400 ml in 24 hours
- Usually begins by the 10th day after onset
- Blood Urea Nitrogen (BUN), stops rising
- Urinary output usually increases in increments but may occur rapidly
- Diuresis depends upon prior treatment, if fluid volume excess was severe up to 5,000 ml/ 24 hours may be lost
- In the early diuretic phase patient's condition may not improve due to inability to concentrate urine
- Hypokalemia and hyponatremia may occur due to increased loss of potassium and sodium with increased urine output
- *Stage 4 — Recovery phase*
  - Begins with the first day BUN falls until it stabilizes
- *Stage 5 — Convalescent phase*
  - From stabilization of BUN until patient is able to resume normal activity, may take several months
  - Urine volume is normal
  - BUN is normal
  - Some patient's will develop chronic renal failure (CRF)
  - CRF results from progressive, irreversible loss of functional nephrons, occurs gradually over months or years

Components of initial examination for ARF

- *Complete medical history to include:*
- Personal and family history of renal dysfunction including previous and current treatments and lifestyle changes
- Past history of diseases that may predispose to CRF such as diabetes, analgesic abuse, recurrent UTI, nephritis or nephrotic syndrome, systemic lupus erythematous, polycystic disease, hypertension, urinary tract obstruction, calculi and hyperparathyroidism
- Patient's understanding of diagnoses and treatment
- Patient's willingness to make lifestyle changes
- Personal history should include a review of recent medications, treatments, and illnesses as a variety of conditions can lead to ARF including use of antihypertensive agents, exposure to heavy metals (arsenic, lead, mercury), x-ray contrast media, some antibiotics (cephalosporins, amino glycosides, polymyxins), antifreeze, cyclosporine, some anesthetics (methoxyflurane and enflurane)

- *Physical examination to include:*
- General appearance and current comfort level
- Vital signs, vary according to the cause of ARF, in hypovolemia low blood pressure and tachycardia is found, in hypervolemia from fluid excess high blood pressure and bounding pulse will be present, in hyperkalemia respiratory rate is increased and pulse is irregular
- Skin color - yellowish discoloration
  - Pallor with anemia
  - Itching due to uremia
  - Bruising with hematologic disorders
- Distended bladder if urinary obstruction is present
- Urine output to include volume and concentration, usually less than 400 ml/24 hours
- Baseline and daily body weight, each liter of excess fluid is equal to 1 Kg or 2.2 pounds of body weight
- Assessment for edema, usually first detected around face and in the fingers
- *Laboratory and diagnostic testing:*
- Urinalysis — see also expanded components of urinalysis
- Urinary Indices are often helpful in determining if ARF is due to prerenal or intra renal failure

Urinary Indices	Prerenal failure	Intrarenal failure
Urinary sediment	Hyaline casts	Muddy brown granular casts
Urine osmolality (mmol/kg H2O)	>500	<250
Urinary sodium (mmol/L)	<10	>20
Urine/serum creatinine	>40	<20
Urine/serum urea nitrogen	>8	<3
Urine/serum osmolarity	>1.2	<1.2
Urine specific gravity	>1.018	<1.012
Plama BUN/creatine ratio (mg/dL)	>20	<10-15
Fractional excreted sodium*	<1	>1
Renal failure index (RPFI)**	<1	>1

* Fractional excreted sodium $= \dfrac{\text{Urine/serum sodium}}{\text{Urine/serum creatinine}}$ X 100

** Renal failure index $= \dfrac{\text{Urine sodium X serum creatinine}}{\text{Urine creatinine}}$

- Serum creatine and urinary creatine clearance levels are often done serially
- Serum and urinary potassium
- Serum and urinary sodium
- Uric acid levels
- Serum and urinary osmolarity
- Blood urea nitrogen (BUN)
- Serum chloride
- Complete blood count to detect anemia and platelet anomalies
- Computed tomography of the kidney to rule out obstruction as cause of ARF
- Renal angiography for assessment of patency of renal arteries and veins if vascular obstruction is suspected
- Renal biopsy if renal failure is of unknown origin
- Renal scan to provide size and cortical thickness of kidney
- Pyelography for localization of renal calculi or other obstruction
- Serum creatinine, helpful in determining rises rapidly in ARF from renal ischemia (24-48 hours) usually peaks at 3-5 days and returns to normal in 5-7 days

Treatment
- Goal of treatment is to prevent ARF from occurring and to reverse ARF as soon as possible, if present
- Eliminate or treat the causative agent in ARF
  - Correct hypovolemia with appropriate fluids
  - Treat cardiac failure to restore renal blood flow
  - Control hypertension to restore normal renal blood flow
  - Remove calculi or other obstruction, a suprapubic catheter may be required until urinary tract flow is restored
- Medications are used to restore normal fluid, electrolyte and acid-base balance as indicated
- Diet is designed to provide enough calories to prevent starvation ketoacidosis while limiting nitrogenous waste, protein (limited to 0.7-1.0 g/Kg/day), sodium, potassium (none allowed except in food eaten) and fluids need to be adjusted according to renal function

- Fluid replacement, generally patients are allowed 500ml of fluids plus the amount of the previous days urinary output
- Continuous ECG monitoring to assess for hyperkalemia and other imbalances (widened QRS complex, AV dissociation)
- Daily weights to monitor effectiveness of treatment
- Accurate I&Os to monitor fluid status
- Ultrafiltration or dialysis may be required if more conservative methods fail and uremia, hyperkalemia (>6.5 mEq/L), severe metabolic acidosis (HCO3 < 10 mEq/L), pulmonary edema, increased urea nitrogen (>100), creatinine (> 10 mg), or encephalopathy or seizures is present
- Blood transfusions may be required with severe anemia

Medications

- Diuretics such as furosemide or bumetanide to reverse oliguria
- Polystyrene sulfonate exchange resin, insulin, glucose, sodium bicarbonate, may be ordered if hyperkalemia exists
- Fluid replacement with hypotonic solutions
- Antibiotics for any febrile patient
- A variety of medications may be ordered depending upon what the causative factor of ARF was these may include:
  - Antiarrthymic drugs or inotropic agents for cardiac failure
  - Glucocorticoids, alkylating agents with acute glomerulonephritis or vasculitis
  - ACE inhibitors for hypertension
  - Dopamine to increase renal blood flow

Section VI — DIETS

- Diet is an important part of the treatment of renal disease
- Patients who have severe renal impairment should be seen by a registered dietitian for assistance with dietary needs
- Diet may be comprised of one or all of the following components
- Potassium restriction
    - Potassium restriction is not usually required unless urine output is less than 1000 ml per day
    - Hyperkalemia (potassium excess) may occur in oliguria
    - Hyperkalemia can be life-threatening and is one of the main causes of death in acute renal failure
    - The kidney's normally excrete 80% or more of all potassium lost from the body, in renal failure they are unable to perform this function and potassium is not excreted at the previous levels leading to hyperkalemia
    - The patient with renal failure also has anorexia leading to an inadequate calorie intake; this also leads to protein breakdown with the release of more potassium
    - Another factor leading to hyperkalemia is the release of potassium with trauma or tissue death, both of these release potassium stores
    - If metabolic acidosis occurs there is a further buildup of potassium in the plasma
- Sodium restriction
    - Most renal failure patients are able to excrete sodium and do not require a sodium restricted diet unless high blood pressure is a problem
    - Sodium retention may occur when the failure of the kidneys leads to a decreased glomerular filtration rate with a loss of the ability to excrete enough sodium
    - Excessive sodium leads to water retention which leads to fluid volume excess
    - Sodium may be restricted to help avoid fluid volume excess
    - See No Extra Salt (NES) Diet in the cardiovascular system
- Protein restriction
    - Protein is restricted to limit nitrogenous waste products that the kidney is unable to handle in renal failure

- In general, the higher the protein in the diet the higher the level of serum urea concentration
- When amino acids from proteins are metabolized they form urea, reducing the amount of protein in the diet will decrease the BUN
- 0.6 grams of protein per Kg must be provided per day to prevent protein malnutrition with subsequent loss of strength, body weight and muscle mass
- A diet of 20 grams of protein per day must be supplemented with essential amino acids and alpha-ketoanalogues
- A low protein diet should also be supplemented with B vitamins, vitamin C and folic acid

POTASSIUM RESTRICTED

General description	Potassium is restricted, the amount of potassium allowed is ordered by the primary care provider
Indications	Severe renal disease, chronic renal failure the oliguric phase of acute renal failure
Allowable items	Low potassium foods: Vegetables: Green beans, Carrots, Cucumbers, Lettuce, Radishes, Romaine, Tomatoes, Green pepper Fruits: Cranberry juice, Cranberry sauce, Blueberries, Lemons, Pears, Peaches, Tangerines, Watermelon Other items: Breads, Pasta, Cottage cheese, Eggs, Chicken, Lamb, Fish, Fats, butter
Restricted items	High potassium foods: Vegetables: Artichokes, Asparagus, Lima beans, Snap beans, Broccoli, Brussel sprouts, Cauliflower, Corn, Mushrooms, Potatoes, Winter squash Fruits: Avocados, Dried apricots, Bananas, Cantaloupe, Oranges, Orange juice, Dried prunes, Raisins Other foods: Coffee, Meats, Peanut butter
Nutritional value	Diet should provide all of the needed calories

Other comments	Often ordered with sodium and protein restricted diets for the patient with oliguria Monitor for S&S of hyperkalemia to include: Nausea, diarrhea, muscle spasms, muscle weakness, cardiac arrhythmia and cardiac arrest Monitor for S&S of hypokalemia to include: Tingling in extremities, tetany, muscle twitching and convulsions Instruct patient to read labels carefully, salt substitutes may contain potassium

PROTEIN RESTRICTED

General description	Reduces the workload of the kidneys by reducing the amount of nitrogenous waste products Amount of protein allowed is specified by the primary care provider: Diet may be 20 gm, 40 gm, or 60 gm protein diet
Indications	Renal disease, Oliguric phase of acute renal failure or chronic renal failure
Allowable items	Low protein foods: Vegetables Fruits Other items Green beans Apples Fats, butter Cabbage Blackberries Margarine, oils Carrots Blueberries Sour cream Cucumbers Cherries Synthetic juices Eggplant Grapefruit Hard candies Lettuce Peaches Carbonated beverages Onions Pears Coffee Radishes Pineapple Teas Squash Prunes Tomatoes Strawberries
Restricted items	High protein foods: 20 gram diet All meats restricted except 1 egg daily 3/4 cup milk daily All protein enriched foods are restricted to include: Breads, cereals and vegetables 40-60 gram diets are individualized with the addition of a small amount of meat and more milk
Nutritional value	Diet is inadequate to meet daily nutritional requirements for protein (20 grams) Protein is needed by the body and cannot be totally eliminated for long periods of time Multi-vitamins are often prescribed to insure adequate nutrition
Other comments	Diet is often used with potassium and sodium restricted diets Compliance is difficult to obtain

Section VII — DRUGS

The tables below supply only general information, a drug handbook
or the physicians desk reference (PDR) should be consulted for details. Each classification includes detailed information about the example drug, this drug is representative of the other drugs in the
classification and can be used as a model.

Every effort has been made to include the major classes of drugs
used in the treatment of renal system disorders.

DIURETICS — LOOP

Action: Increase urine excretion by inhibiting reabsorption of
sodium and chloride in the ascending loop of Henle and in both the
proximal and distal tubules

Indications: To promote fluid loss in patients with severe edema,
may be used in congestive heart failure, cirrhosis of the liver and
renal disease

Example: Furosemide (*Lasix*)

Route: PO, IV, IM

Pharmacokinetics: Peak 60-70 minutes PO, 20-60 minutes IV
Onset 30-60 minutes PO, 5 minutes IV
Duration 2 hours

Contraindications: Sensitivity to furosemide or sulfonamides,
worsening oliguria or anuria, electrolyte imbalances (hypo),
dehydration, hepatic coma

Common adverse effects: hypokalemia, urinary urgency, frequent
urination

Life-threatening adverse effects: circulatory collapse

Other adverse effects: hypotension, dizziness, thromboembolic
episodes, fluid loss with hypovolemia, hypomagnesemia,
hypocalcemia, nausea, emesis, diarrhea, appetite loss, constipation,
abdominal cramping, pancreatitis, jaundice, flank pain, anemia,
tinnitus, hearing loss, pruritus, urticaria, photosensivity,
hyperglycemia, glycosuria, increased BUN, hyperuricemia,
weakness, pain at IM injection sites

Interventions:
Administer PO drug with food or milk to reduce stomach irritation
Administer PO drug in early am or if two doses in early am and
afternoon to prevent disruption in sleep patterns
Administer IV push at 4mg/minute, check compatibilities for
drugs/fluids
Monitor VS after IV or IM administration, monitor output, weight
daily

Monitor patient for dehydration and hypokalemia (muscle cramps, weakness)

Administer a potassium replacement as ordered (potassium depleting)

Monitor for postural hypotension and assist patient with position changes and ambulation as needed, bedside rails should be up at all times

Examples of other drugs in this classification:

Acetazolamide (*AK-Zol, Dazamide, Diamox*), PO/IM/IV, also used for seizures and glaucoma

Bumetanide (*Bumex*), PO/IM/IV, Diuretic activity is 40 times greater than furosemide, causes potassium and magnesium depletion

Ethacrynic Acid (*Edecrin*), PO/IV, IV administration must be done slowly and site changed if another IV dose is required to prevent thrombophelbitis

DIURETICS — POTASSIUM SPARING

Action: To increase urine excretion by increasing water and sodium loss while sparing potassium, binds at aldosterone receptor sites in the distal renal tubules to accomplish this

Indications: Essential hypertension, edema from systemic health problems to include cirrhosis of the liver, nephrotic syndrome, congestive heart failure and primary hyperaldosteronism

Example: Spironolactone (*Aldactone*)

Route: PO

Pharmacokinetics: Peak 2-3 days, onset is gradual and maximum affect 2 wks

Duration 2-3 days

Contraindications: Anuria, severe renal impairment, hyperkalemia

Common adverse effects: frequency of urination increased

Life-threatening adverse effects: fatal arrhythmias from hyperkalemia

Other adverse effects: lethargy, mental confusion, fatigue, headache, drowsiness, ataxia, gynecomastia, hirsutism, impotence, inability to achieve or maintain erection, amenorrhea, abdominal cramping, nausea, emesis, anorexia, diarrhea, fluid and electrolyte imbalances, hyperkalemia, hyponatremia, elevated BUN, acidosis, skin rash, urticaria, fever, hyperuricemia and gout

Interventions:

Administer with food, may be crushed and taken with foods or fluids

Assess baseline BP and weight, monitor regularly to assess effectiveness

Monitor I&O and electrolyte levels for imbalances, assess for edema

Monitor for and report if confusion, lethargy or stupor occur
Instruct patient that excessive intake of potassium should be avoided, patient may have been advised to increase potassium intake with other diuretics
Examples of other drugs in this classification:
Amiloride hydrochloride (*Midamor*), PO, usually combined with a
   thiazide or loop diuretic
Trimterene (*Dyrenium*), PO, Capsules may be emptied and mixed
   with food

DIURETIC — THIAZIDE
Action: To increase urine excretion by inhibiting the reabsorption of sodium and chloride in the ascending portion of the loop of Henle, this is the largest group of PO diuretic drugs
Indications: Edema associated with congestive heart failure, cirrhosis or renal dysfunction, also used for hypertension
Example: Hydrochlorothiazide (*Diaqua, Esidrix, HydroChlor, HydroDiuril, Hydromal, Hydro-T, Oretic, HCTZ*)
Route: PO
Pharmacokinetics: Onset 2 hours
Peak 4 hours
Duration 6-12 hours
Contraindications: sensitivity to thiazides or sulfonamides (structurally related), anuria
Common adverse effects: hyperglycemia, hyperuricemia, hypokalemia, frequent urination
Life-threatening effects: Agranulocytosis, aplastic anemia
Other adverse effects: blurred vision, mood changes, tiredness, weakness, dizziness, lightheadedness, Paresthesias, orthostatic hypotension, weak pulse, irregular heartbeats, dry mouth, increased thirst, nausea, vomiting, anorexia, diarrhea, constipation, cramping, jaundice, pancreatitis, leukopenia, glycosuria
Interventions:
Administer with food or milk to reduce gastric irritation
Administer single dose in am, if divided doses schedule to prevent nocturnal diuresis with loss of sleep
Monitor BP and I&O, assess for edema to determine drug effectiveness
Monitor electrolytes, CBC, BUN, glucose, and uric acid, report changes
Assess for hypokalemia to include fatigue, paresthesia, decreased reflexes, muscle weakness, cramps pulse irregularities, arrhythmias, hypotension and mental confusion, report if noted

Assist patient in position changes as needed, assess for orthostatic hypotension

Examples of other drugs in this classification:

Bendroflumethiazide (Naturetin), PO, Monitor for hyperglycemia which may develop slowly

Benzthiazide (*Aquatag, Exna, Hydrex, Marazide, Proaqua*), PO, used for mild hypertension

Chlorothiazide (*Diachlor, Diuril*), PO/IV, onset of 15 minutes with IV med, avoid extravasation as it is very irritating to tissues

Chlorthalidone (*Hygroton, Hylidone, Novothalidone, Thalitone, Uridon*), PO, Elderly patients are more sensitive to adverse effects, monitor carefully

Hydroflumethiazide (*Diucardin, Saluron*), PO

Methyclothiazide (*Aquatensen, Duretic, Enduron, Ethon*), PO

Polythiazide (*Renese*), PO, May be given qod

Trichlormethiazide (*Aquazide, Diurese, Metahydrin, Mono-Press, Naqua, Niazide, Trichlorex*), PO

Section VIII — GLOSSARY OF TERMS

Acetone breath	Breath with a sweet, fruity odor usually due to ketoacidosis
Anasarca	Generalized severe edema
Anuria	No urine output
Azotemia	Urea and other nitrogenous wastes in the blood, occurs in renal failure
Calculi	Stones, plural form of calculus, usually composed of mineral salts, may occur in kidney, bladder or ureters. May block urinary flow leading to pain and inflammation
Calculus	Single stone (See also calculi)
Cystitis	Inflammation of the bladder, usually due to a UTI, symptoms include dysuria and frequent voiding
Cystocele	Herniation of the bladder into the vagina, may occur due to injury during childbirth
Dialysis	The process of cleansing the blood for patients with severe renal disease. Blood is passed through a semipermeable membrane where waste products are removed
Dysuria	Difficult or painful urination
Edema	Local or general swelling of the body
Enuresis	Incontinence of urine. Involuntary urination, usually at night
Epispadias	Congenital abnormality of the urinary meatus. Meatus is not found in usual location, may occur in males or females
Filtrate	Fluid or solution that has been filtered
Halitosis	Bad breath
Hematuria	Bloody urine

Hypospadias	Male congenital abnormality of the urinary meatus where it is located on the underside of the penis
Ketones	An end-product of fat metabolism
Micturition	The act of urinating
Nephrolith	A kidney stone or calculus
Nephrectomy	Surgical removal of a kidney
Nephron	The functional unit of the kidney that filters wastes out of the blood, consists of a glomerulus and tubules
Nocturia	Urinating during the night
Oliguria	Scanty urine output, usually less than 30ml/hr
Polyuria	Excessive urination
Pyuria	Pus in the urine
Stomatitis	Inflammation of the mouth
Uremia	Azotemia, urea and other nitrogenous wastes in the blood, usually occurs in renal disease
Uresis	Normal urine output, normal urination
Urinary tract infection UTI	UTI, infection within the urinary tract
	Urinary tract infection

Gastrointestinal System

GASTROINTESTINAL SYSTEM

Table of Contents

Section I — THE OVERVIEW

Primary Functions

- Ingestion, digestion and absorption of nutrients for distribution to cells via the circulatory and lymphatic systems
- Elimination of indigestible products and waste from the body
- Assistance in maintaining fluid balance within the body
- Performance of vital metabolic functions by the liver

Components (Figure 5A and 5B)

- Gastrointestinal (GI) tract contains the pharynx, esophagus, stomach, small and large intestines, rectum and anus
- Other accessory organs include the teeth, tongue, salivary glands, liver, gallbladder and pancreas

GASTROINTESTINAL TRACT (GI tract)

Pharynx

- A 5 inch muscular tube extending from the base of the skull to the level of the 6th vertebra
- Contains the nasopharynx, oropharynx, and laryngopharynx
- Provides passageway for food from the mouth into the esophagus

Esophagus

- A hollow muscular structure about 9-10 inches in length
- Extends from the pharynx to the stomach
- Carries swallowed foods/fluids from the mouth to the stomach via peristaltic movements

Stomach

- Size and shape varies with body size, capacity is 1-2 liters
- Divided into the cardia, fundus, body, antrum and pylorus
- The wall of the stomach has four layers from inner to outer these are the mucosa, submucosa, muscle layer and serosa
- The stomach secretes several substances (gastric secretions) including mucus, pepsinogen, hydrochloric acid, intrinsic factor, and the hormone gastrin

Small intestine

- 21-23 feet in length and 1 inch in diameter
- Divided into three segments: duodenum, jejunum and ileum

The Digestive System

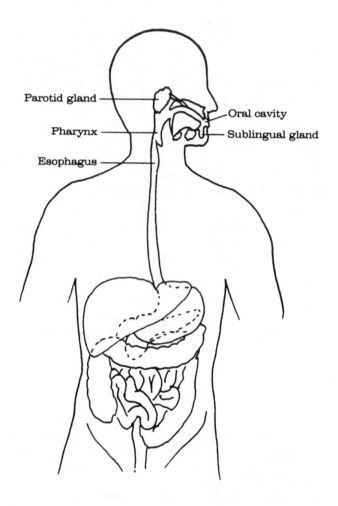

Parotid gland

Pharynx

Esophagus

Oral cavity

Sublingual gland

Figure 5A

The Digestive System

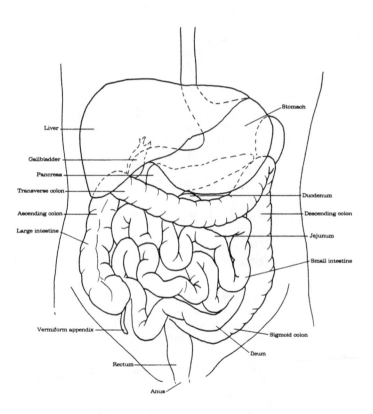

Figure 5B

- Duodenum is the shortest segment (8-10 inches) and is shaped like the letter C; it receives the food mass from the stomach, bile from the liver and gallbladder, and pancreatic juice from the pancreas
- Jejunum is about 9 feet long
- Ileum is the longest segment (13.5 feet) and is attached to the large intestine
- The small intestine is where many products of digestion are absorbed (simple sugars, amino acids, fatty acids and carbohydrates)

Large intestine
- Extends from the ileum to the anus
- Divided into three segments: cecum, colon and rectum
  - Cecum is a pouch which joins to the ascending colon
    The appendix vermiformis is attached to the cecum
  - The colon is divided into the ascending, transverse and descending colon and is 4.5-5 feet in length
  - The rectum is about 4-5 inches long and terminates at the anus
- Reabsorbs fluid and electrolytes from the intestinal contents

Anus
- The external outlet of the gastrointestinal system

ACCESSORY ORGANS

Teeth
- Adults have 32 permanent teeth
- Required for mastication (chewing) of food, healthy teeth can compress to 200 pounds of pressure per square inch, dentures provide only 25 pounds of pressure per square inch

Tongue
- Muscular organ that is required to move food into place for mastication and deglutition (swallowing)
- Contains four taste zones:
  Sweet — at the tip   Bitter — at the back
  Sour — posterior sides   Salty — anterior sides
- Required for speech production

Salivary glands
- Three pairs in mouth: parotid, sublingual and submandibular
  - Parotid secretes saliva which contains the enzyme amylase

- Sublingual secrete amylase mixed with mucous
- Submandibular secrete mostly mucous to lubricate the food
- The secretions of the salivary glands help form the masticated food into a bolus which can then be swallowed
- An adult secretes about 1,000-1,500 ml of saliva daily

Liver

- Largest and one of the most versatile organs in the body
- Located on the right side beneath the diaphragm
- Has four lobes, five ligaments and five fissures
- Performs a variety of metabolic functions to include:
  - Production of anticoagulant Heparin
  - Production of Prothrombin, fibrinogen and albumin
  - Destruction of RBC's
  - Storage of fat-soluble vitamins (ADEK), and vitamin B_{12}
  - Provides for storage of minerals (Copper, iron)
  - Manufacture of Bile (800-1000ml/day)
  - Synthesizes glycogen and stores it
  - Manufactures cholesterol and is important for lipid metabolism
  - Incorporates amino acids into proteins
  - Plays a role in blood volume regulation and is one of the main sources of body heat

Gallbladder

- Pear shaped sac located under the right lobe of the liver
- Stores and concentrates bile from the liver
- Bile exits out of gallbladder through cystic duct into the common bile duct which empties into the small intestine

Pancreas

- Located behind the stomach with it's head attached to the duodenum (lies horizontally), about 10 inches in length
- Functions as both an exocrine and endocrine gland
- Secretes pancreatic juice needed for digestion of food within the duodenum
- Important endocrine gland for its production of insulin and glucagon which are needed for carbohydrate metabolism

CONCEPTS

Digestion

- Process begins when we see or smell food, the salivary glands begin to secrete saliva in anticipation of eating
- When food enters the mouth and chewing begins the food is processed into smaller pieces, at the same time salivary amylase begins to break down polysaccharide from starches and sugars
- The food is formed into a mass by the tongue called a bolus
- The bolus is moved toward the back of the mouth by the tongue, and swallowed (deglutition)
- During swallowing the epiglottis covers the larynx so no food can enter the respiratory system instead it enters the esophagus for transport to the stomach via peristalsis
- Peristalsis is the involuntary movement of the muscles lining the GI tract by waves of contractions
- In the stomach the salivary amylase continues to breakdown the polysaccharide into monosaccharides for another 15-30 minutes
- The bolus is churned and mixed while gastric juice (secretions) are added, here proteins are broken down into peptides
- The bolus is now chyme and is thinner liquid substance
- Chyme enters the duodenum in small amounts with each peristaltic wave, the pyloric value prevents chyme from returning to the stomach
- In duodenum pancreatic, intestinal and bile are added
- Digestion continues and nutrients are absorbed by diffusion and active transport through the intestinal walls into blood capillaries for transport to body cells
- Peristalsis and absorption of nutrients is continuous
- In the large intestine the remaining products from the food will be processed even though no enzymes are secreted here
- Water will be absorbed from the chyme which now become feces
- Bacteria in large intestine does continue to breakdown proteins which may be absorbed by the mucosa
- Peristaltic movements are slower in the colon, about 3-4 times daily strong waves occur that push the contents toward the rectum for removal from the body (defecation)

Digestion

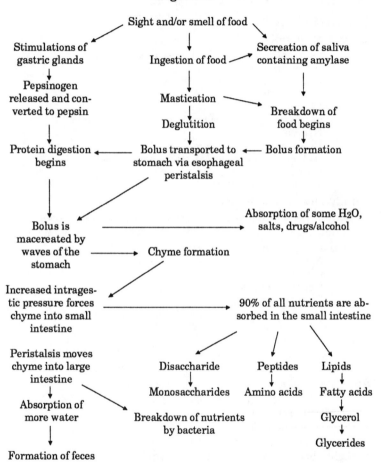

Figure 5C

Section II — ASSESSMENT

HEALTH HISTORY

Chief Complaint

- Common chief complaints for this system include:
    - Abdominal pain
    - Loss of appetite and/or weight loss
    - Constipation
    - Diarrhea
    - Flatulence (excessive gas in stomach or intestines)
    - Heartburn
    - Hematemesis (vomiting of blood)
    - Melena (blood in stools - black tarry stools)
    - Jaundice
    - Nausea and vomiting

Family and personal history

- Obtain specific diagnoses and age of diagnosis when known
- Obtain ages and causes of death in immediate family members
- Assess for present and past treatment of the following:
    - Appendicitis
    - Ulcers
    - Hepatitis or liver disease
    - Bowel obstruction
    - Bowel diseases (Crohn's, colitis, carcinoma)
    - Gallbladder disease (Cholecystitis)
    - Hiatal hernia
- If condition exists assess for required life style changes and current treatment of condition to include medications

Abdominal pain

- One of the most common chief complaints, assess location, severity and timing
- Epigastric pain (pain over the stomach) is usually related to the stomach, duodenum or pancreas
- Right upper quadrant pain is usually related to the liver, gallbladder disease or peptic ulcers within the GI system, may be cardiac (aneurysm, MI) or pulmonary (pneumonia, embolism)
- Pain around umbilicus may be small intestine in origin
- Right lower quadrant pain may be related to appendicitis, perforated peptic ulcer, Crohn's disease or gastroenteritis

- Lower abdominal pain may be related to the colon (colitis, diverticulitis, intestinal obstruction and hernias within the GI system or reproductive (pregnancy, endometriosis, ovarian) or renal
- Assess timing of pain to meals, bowel patterns and emotions, emotions may trigger digestive and bowel elimination problems

Appetite loss and weight loss

- Assess for any recent weight change and patient's perception of why change occurred, may be related to disease or depression

Bowel elimination

- Assess for frequency and consistency of bowel movements
- Assess for any change in frequency of bowel movements
- Constipation is infrequent, hard, dry stools usually with irregular bowel patterns
    - Assess activities of daily living to include fluid intake for dehydration, diet for fiber, activity for lack of exercise and for an established time for bowel elimination
    - Assess for history of laxative or narcotic use/abuse
- Diarrhea is frequent, watery, unformed stools. if acute most often related to infections (bacterial, viral, fungal, protozoan parasitic) or toxicity (food poisoning, drugs)

Gastrointestinal system testing

- Assess for tests completed or ordered and patient's knowledge and understanding of any test procedures or results

GASTROINTESTINAL ASSESSMENT

Chief Complaint

Patient's statement_____ Onset_____

Frequency_____ Duration_____ Other areas affected_____

Have you had this before?_____ Date_____

What treatment was given?_____

What do you think caused this?_____

What lifestyle changes have you had to make?_____

_____

Personal and Family History

	Patient	Family member		Patient only Current	Past
Hepatitis	_____	_____	Blood in stool	_____	_____
Ulcers	_____	_____	Vomiting blood	_____	_____
Bowel disease	_____	_____	Abdominal pain	_____	_____
Colon cancer	_____	_____	Undesired wt loss	_____	_____
			Nausea/ vomiting	_____	_____
			Jaundice	_____	_____

Surgery on esophagus, gallbladder, stomach, colon or liver?_____

Gastrointestinal System Testing

Barium enema_____ Barium swallow_____ Colonoscopy_____

CT of Abdomen_____ Paracentesis_____ Laparoscopy_____

Sigmoidoscopy_____ Stool cultures_____ Videofluoroscopy_____

Ultrasound_____ Blood tests_____

Current Treatments/Medications

Medication_____ Dose_____ Frequency_____Route_____

Special diet_____ Why_____ Usual weight_____

Cigarettes/day____/____/____yrs.   Alcoholic drinks ____/____/____yrs.

Frequency of usual bowel movements_____ Bowel problems_____

Breakfast   Lunch   Dinner

_____   _____   _____

_____   _____   _____

_____   _____   _____

Was this a typical day for you?_____

PHYSICAL ASSESSMENT

- Gastrointestinal assessment involves looking at the abdomen in the following order:
  1. Inspection
  2. Auscultation
  3. Percussion
  4. Palpation
- Request patient empty bladder prior to examination
- Patient is supine with abdomen exposed from xiphoid process to groin with genitalia covered

INSPECTION

General appearance

- Assess patient's chosen positioning — Patient with abdominal pain may draw knees up close to abdomen
- Assess current comfort level — Patient with severe abdominal pain may lie almost motionless to reduce tension or have marked restlessness

Skin

- Color — Jaundice with its yellowing of the skin, whites of eyes and mucous membranes may be present
- Shiny, tense skin over the abdomen may occur with ascites
- Striae or "stretch marks," pink or blue if recent and white if older in origin, may be due to Cushing's disease, pregnancy, abdominal tumors or obesity
- Record any scars to include location, length, width and origin

Shape or contour of abdomen

- Flat, rounded, obese or scaphoid (inverse or concave)
- Assess for umbilical hernia with umbilicus everted
- Assess for obvious separation of the rectus abdominis muscle known as diastasis recti abdominis from pregnancy or obesity
- Assess for any distention or masses within abdomen which may be due to one of the six F's: fat, feces, flatus, fetus, fluid or foreign tissue (tumor)
- Visible peristalsis may be noted in thin individual

AUSCULTATION

- Auscultate with stethoscope diaphragm prior to palpation or percussion to prevent alteration of bowel sounds

- Normal bowel sounds are high-pitched and gurgling, should occur every 5-15 seconds, listen in each quadrant
- Listen for at least 5 minutes if no bowel sounds are suspected as they may occur at irregular intervals

PERCUSSION

- The entire abdomen is percussed lightly
- Tympany will be heard over the intestines and stomach due to the presence of air
- The liver will percuss as a dull sound on the right side of the body; using percussion, boundaries can be assessed
- The spleen percusses as a dull area on the left side

PALPATION

- Warm hands before touching the patient to prevent startling
- Light and then deep palpation are performed in each quadrant
- Ask where abdomen is tender and start palpation away from and work toward this site (assists in relaxing patient)
- Light palpation is used to detect tenderness and large masses and is done with the fingertips to depth of about 1cm only
- Assess for "voluntary guarding" where the abdominal muscles are tensed to prevent actual or feared pain from palpation
- The location of tenderness on palpation gives vital clues to origin of problem

  Upper quadrant pain
  Diverticulitis or colitis
  Pneumonia

Right side	Left side
Duodenal ulcer	Gastric ulcer
Gallbladder disease	Ruptured or enlarged spleen
Pyelonephritis	Pancreatitis

  Umbilical area pain
  Acute pancreatitis
  Early appendicitis
  Aortic aneurysm

  Lower quadrant pain
  Ileitis or diverticulitis
  Incarcerated hernia
  Salpingitis, tuboovarian abscess or ectopic pregnancy
  Ureteritis
  Renal or ureteral stone

Right side	Left side
Appendicitis	Ulcerative colitis
Perforated cecum	Perforated colon

- Abdomen should be soft not rigid or boardlike (peritonitis)
- Deep palpation gives more specific information about organs and is performed with the side of the hand and the fingers
- The liver's lower edge should be palpated and when healthy should be sharp and nontender, a firm rounded or irregular edge may occur with cirrhosis and the liver may appear hard with cancer
- If abdominal mass is present, consistency, mobility, shape and size are assessed

GASTROINTESTINAL PHYSICAL EXAMINATION

INSPECTION

General appearance/posture_____

Skin color_____ Appearance_____ Scars_____

Teeth: Cavities_____ Broken teeth_____ Dentures U/L_____

Gums: Redness_____ Swelling_____ Mouth: Ulcers_____ Vesicles_____

Abdominal Shape:_____ Masses or pulsations_____

AUSCULTATION

Bowel Sounds (hypo, normal, hyper): RUQ_____ LUQ_____ LLQ_____ RLQ_____

PERCUSSION

Liver location and size_____ Spleen_____

PALPATION

Liver border, form, consistency_____ Spleen_____

Masses_____ Location_____ Size_____ Tenderness_____

Assessment Notes

_____

_____

_____

_____

Section III — LABORATORY & DIAGNOSTIC TESTS

In the following section traditional laboratory values and SI unit values are given, it is important to recognize that "normal" values vary from laboratory to laboratory. Check the normal values at the agency or institution where a test is performed. Most labs print their normal values on the laboratory reporting slip or page.

See also Aspartate aminotransferase, cholesterol and lactic dehydrogenase found under cardiovascular system laboratory tests

Table of Common Laboratory Tests

Test Name	Indications	Comments
Alanine aminotransferase (ALT) Blood test **Normal:** 5-35 IU/L 8-20 U/L (SI)	Liver disease or dysfunction	**Regarding collection:** Use red-top tube; collect 7-10ml List medications on lab slip **Results:** Increased levels in hepatic disease A variety of medications may also increase ALT levels to include aspirin, ampicillin, acetaminophen
Alkaline phosphatase (ALP) Blood test **Normal:** 30-85 ImU/mL 42-128 U/L (SI)	Liver dysfunction Intestinal infarct Bone disease	**Regarding collection:** Use red-top tube; collect 7-10ml List medications on lab slip **Results:** Increased in liver disease, healing fractures, rheumatoid arthritis Decreased in malnutrition, scurvy, pernicious anemia & celiac disease
Ammonia level Blood test **Normal:** 15-110 ug/dL or 46-65 umol/L (SI)	Severe liver dysfunction Hepatic coma or encephalopathy	**Regarding collection:** Sample may need to be placed on ice Use green-top tube; collect 5-7ml List medications on lab slip Assess site for bleeding **Results:** Increased in liver disease, renal failure and Reye's syndrome
Amylase Blood test **Normal:** 56-190 IU/L 25-125 U/L (SI)	Pancreatitis Perforated peptic ulcer Perforated or necrotic bowel Acute cholecystitis	**Regarding collection:** Use red-top tube; collect 5-7 ml List medications on lab slip **Results:** Increased levels occur within 12 hr of pancreatitis, normal levels return after 48-72 hrs

Test Name	Indications	Comments
Bilirubin Blood test **Normal Total:** 0.1-1.0 mg/dl 5.1-17.0 umol/L **Normal Indirect:** 0.2-0.8 mg/dl 3.4-12.0 umol/L **Normal Direct:** 0.1-0.3 mg/dl 1.7-5.1 umol/L	Liver dysfunction Cirrhosis Hepatitis Hemolytic jaundice Pernicious anemia Sickle cell anemia Hemolytic anemia Drug reactions	**Regarding collection:** Check agency policy re: fasting Use red-top tube collect; 5-7 ml Do not shake tube during collection Protect sample from light List medications on lab slip **Results:** Bilirubin is the by-product of Hgb breakdown; elevated levels occur with liver dysfunction Jaundice occurs when the total bilirubin levels are >2.5 mg/dl
CA 19-9 tumor marker Blood test **Normal:** <37 U/ml	Pancreatic cancer Hepatobiliary Ca	**Regarding collection:** Use red-top tube; collect 7-10 ml Sample will require processing at a central diagnostic laboratory **Results:** Available in 7-10 days CA 19-9 levels are monitored for reoccurrence or response of cancer
Gamma-glutamyl transpeptidase (GGTP, GGT) Blood test **Normal:** 8-38 U/L Female <45 yrs 5-27 U/L	Liver dysfunction Hepatitis Cirrhosis Hepatic ischemia or necrosis Jaundice Cholestasis May also be used to detect alcohol use	**Regarding collection:** Patient is NPO except for water for 8 hrs before the test Use red-top tube; collect 7-10 ml List any anti-convulsants or oral contraceptives on lab slip **Results:** Increased in liver dysfunction Rises rapidly after any alcohol
Hepatitis virus studies (HAA) Blood test **Normal:** Negative	Suspected hepatitis Hepatitis A Hepatitis B Non-A, non-B type hepatitis (C)	**Regarding collection:** Use red-top tube; collect 5-7 ml **Results:** Hepatitis profile with antigens and antibodies is usually performed to detect type of hepatitis
Lactose tolerance test Blood test **Normal:** >20 mg/dl	Lactose intolerance	**Regarding collection:** NPO except water for 8 hrs before No exercise 8 hrs before testing No smoking before testing Use gray-top tube; collect 5-7 ml Give ordered dose of lactose Use gray-top tube; collect 5-7 ml 30, 60 & 120 mins after lactose Observe for abdominal cramping, flatus, bloating and diarrhea which will occur if lactose intolerant **Results:** Decreased level with intolerance

Test Name	Indications	Comments
Lipase Blood test **Normal:** 0-110 units/L 0-417 U/L (SI)	Acute or chronic pancreatitis	**Regarding collection:** NPO except water for 12 hrs before Use red-top tube collect; 5-7 ml List medications on lab slip **Results:** Elevated in pancreatitis
Protein Blood test **Normal total:** 6.4-8.3 g/dL 64.0-83.0 g/L (SI) **Normal albumin:** 3.5-5.0 g/dL 35-50 g/L (SI) **Normal globulin:** 2.3-3.4 g/dL	Liver dysfunction Malnutrition Hepatitis Crohn's disease Sprue Whipple's disease Liver cancer Biliary obstruction	**Regarding collection:** Use red-top tube; collect 5-7 ml Observe site for bleeding **Results:** Increased in hemoconcentration Decreased in liver dysfunctions and malnutrition Albumins purpose is to maintain collidal osmotic pressure Globulins are needed to make antibodies
Stool for occult blood Stool sample **Normal:** Negative	GI tract bleeding GI tract tumors or ulcers Inflammatory bowel disease Diverticulosis	**Regarding collection:** No red meat for 3 days prior Test may be done at home & mailed List any anticoagulants on lab slip Follow instructions with test kit **Results:** Blue discoloration with GI bleeding

Table of Diagnostic Tests

Test Name	Indications	Comments
Abdominal ultra-sound Normal abdominal organs	Aortic aneurysms Gallbladder disease Liver dysfunction	**Pre-procedure:** If gallbladder disease is suspected patient may be NPO for 8 hrs prior Procedure takes about 20 minutes No activity restrictions after
Barium enema X-ray with contrast dye Normal passage of barium through the colon and appendix	Suspected colon disease Ulcerative colitis Diverticulitis Intestinal polyps Colon cancer	**Pre-procedure:** Check orders for type of bowel preparation (laxatives or enemas) NPO for 8 hours before testing except for bowel cleansing agents During procedure barium will be placed in colon with a catheter Procedure takes about 45 minutes **Post-procedure:** Bowel movements will be white Encourage fluids and rest Laxatives may be ordered to remove barium from colon

Test Name	Indications	Comments
Barium swallow X-ray with contrast dye **Normal** passage of barium through the esophagus	Esophageal anomaly Esophagael tumor, ulcers or cancer Obstruction Abnormal esophageal motility	**Pre-procedure**: NPO for 8 hours before testing Assess for adequate swallow, report if patient is at risk of aspiration During test patient will swallow contrast medium Procedure takes about 20-30 minutes **Post-procedure**: Bowel movements will be white Laxatives may be ordered to remove barium from GI tract
Colonoscopy Endoscopy **Normal** colon	Suspected colon disease Colon cancer Colon polyps Ulcerative colitis Crohn's disease Diverticulosis Colon strictures GI bleeding	**Pre-procedure:** Signed consent form is required Check orders for type of bowel preparation Pre-procedure sedative may be given A colonoscope is placed in rectum and colon visualized, biopsy may be obtained Procedure takes about 30-60 mins **Post-procedure:** Monitor VS for signs of hemorrhage Assess abdomen for distention and tenderness, notify MD if increasing Encourage fluids when allowed Assess any stools for blood
Computed tomography of the abdomen (CAT scan) X-ray with contrast dye **Normal** structures of abdominal organs	Tumors or disease of following organs: Liver Pancreas Spleen Gallbladder Kidneys Uterus, ovaries Fallopian tubes Prostate	**Pre-procedure:** Signed consent may be required Assess for allergy to iodine dye Check policy regarding intake Assess for ability to lie still Procedure takes 30-60 minutes **Post-procedure:** Encourage fluids if dye was given Assess for reaction to iodine dye
Endoscopic retrograde cholangio-pancreatography Endoscopy (ERCP) **Normal** biliary and pancreatic ducts	Jaundice Obstruction of the common bile duct Biliary sclerosis cysts or tumors of the bile ducts	**Pre-procedure**: Signed consent form is required NPO for 8 hrs prior to testing Explain procedure to patient: a local anesthetic is given and then a fiberoptic endoscope is passed through mouth, esophagus, stomach, and into duodenum for visualization Pre-procedure sedative may be given Procedure takes 1 hour, x-rays will be taken during the procedure **Post-procedure:** NPO until gag reflex returns 2-4 hrs Monitor for respiratory depression Observe for and report abdominal pain, nausea, vomiting, bleeding, fever or dysphagia

Test Name	Indications	Comments
Esophagogastro-duodenoscopy Endoscopy (EGD) **Normal** esphagus, stomach and duodenum	Esophageal tumors Esophagitis Gastroesophageal varices Gastric tumors Hiatal hernia Polyps, obstruction	**Pre-procedure:** Signed consent form may be required NPO for 8 hrs prior to testing Explain procedure to patient (same as ERCP) Procedure takes about 30 minutes **Post-procedure:** Same as for ERCP
Gallbladder scan Nuclear scan **Normal** gallbladder Also known as Cholescintigraphy Hepatobiliary imaging	Gallbladder disease Acute cholecystitis Obstruction of the bile ducts	**Pre-procedure:** NPO for 2 hrs prior to testing Explain procedure to patient: IV radionuclide will be given and then images will be obtained over 1 hour Patient may be given a fatty meal during procedure and emptying time of gallbladder is monitored Procedure takes from 1-4 hours No activity restrictions after
Liver biopsy Examination of tissue **Normal** cells and tissue	Hepatomegaly Liver tumors/abscess Hepatitis Jaundice	**Pre-procedure:** Signed consent form is required Monitor for coagulation abnormality Needle will be inserted into liver NPO for 8 hrs prior to testing Pre-procedure sedative may be given Procedure takes about 15 minutes **Post-procedure:** Send tissue to laboratory Apply dressing over insertion site Position patient on right side for 1-2 hrs to decrease hemorrhage risk Assess vital signs frequently
Liver and spleen scanning Normal liver and spleen	Suspected tumors Cirrhosis Abscesses of liver or spleen	**Pre-procedure:** Procedure takes about 1 hour Explain procedure to patient: IV radionuclide will be given and then images recorded No activity restrictions after
Paracentesis Fluid analysis **Normal:** clear or lt yellow No RBCs WBCs <300uL Protein <4.1g/dL Glucose 70-100 mg Amylase 138-404 Ammonia <50 ug/dl ALP males 90-240 females 76-196, females over 45 yr	Ascites	**Pre-procedure:** Signed consent form is required Patient should void before testing Obtain abdominal girth, weight and baseline vital signs May be performed at bedside Explain procedure to patient: a local anesthetic will be given, a sterile needle will be used to obtain a fluid sample from abdomen **Post-procedure:** Place bandaid over insertion site Send labeled specimen to lab ASAP Observe site for bleeding, drainage

Test Name	Indications	Comments
87-250 U/L No malignant cells, bacteria or fungi found		Obtain abdominal girth, weight and vital signs compare to baseline Record amount of fluid removed Administer albumin as ordered Monitor VS and laboratory values
Sigmoidoscopy Endoscopy **Normal** rectum and sigmoid colon	Suspected tumor, polyp, ulcer or hemorrhoids Ulcerative colitis Crohn's disease Intestinal ischemia Irritable bowel	**Pre-procedure:** Signed consent form is required Assess for bowel preparation order (usually enemas) Explain procedure to patient, a sidmoidoscope is inserted into anus for examination Biopsies may be performed as needed Procedure takes about 20 minutes **Post-procedure:** Patient may have flatus Monitor for abdominal distention, tenderness or rectal bleeding
Ultrasonography **Liver & Pancreato-biliary system** Ultrasound **Normal** pancreas, gallbladder and biliary ducts	Abnormalities of GI tract or in any accessory organs	**Pre-procedure:** For ultrasound of gallbladder, NPO for 8 hrs may be recommended No activity restrictions after exam
Ultrasonography **Prostate/rectum** Ultrasound **Normal** prostate gland	Prostate cancer Benign prostatic hypertrophy Prostatitis	**Pre-procedure:** Explain procedure to patient: a lubricated ultrasound probe is placed in the rectum and then ultrasound scans are performed No activity restrictions after exam
Videofluoroscopy X-ray **Normal** swallow function	Ineffective swallow	**Pre-procedure:** Explain procedure to patient: a barium containing meal or drink will be given and a video record will be made to assess the swallow No activity restrictions after exam

Section IV — Procedures

Fluid needs calculations

- Water is the most vital nutrient the body requires
- The primary functions of water in our body include:
  - Solvent to transport nutrients to cells
  - Solvent to remove waste products from cells
  - Solvent for electrolytes

Section IV — PROCEDURES

Fluid needs calculations

- Water is the most vital nutrient the body requires
- The primary functions of water in our body include:
  - Solvent to transport nutrients to cells
  - Solvent to remove waste products from cells
  - Solvent for electrolytes
  - Lubricant for movements of joints
  - Lubricant for food in mouth (saliva)
  - Aids in the breakdown of foods
    Carbohydrates to Monosaccharides
    Proteins to Amino Acids
  - Promotes digestion and elimination
  - Regulation of body temperature to prevent overheating
- The average adult has between 55-65% of body weight in water or about 42,000ml or 175 cups

Area	Definition	Amount	% of body wt		
			Females	Males	Elderly
Intracellular (ICF)	Water inside cells	28,000 ml 117 cups	35%	45%	25%
Extracellular (ECF)	Water outside of cells	14,000 ml 58 cups	15%	16%	20%
Interstitial part of ECF	Transports nutrients & wastes, bathes cells	10,500 ml 44 cups	10%	11%	15%
Intravascular part of ECF (plasma)	The fluid in blood outside cells	3,500 ml 14 cups	5%	4%	5%

- The adult gains and loses about 2,400 ml of fluid/day

Water losses in the adult body

Amount/day	Route
800-1500 ml	Urine
250-350 ml	Stool
100-250 ml	Perspiration
250-350 ml	Skin
350 ml	Lungs
1900-2800 ml	All sources total

Water gains in the adult body

Amount/day	Route
1000-1250 ml	Ingested liquids
625-1250 ml	Ingested foods
200-400 ml	Metabolic oxidation
1825-2900 ml	All sources total

$$50ml \times 5\ Kg = \underline{\quad 250ml \quad}$$
$$1250ml/day$$

#2   60Kg, 35-year-old women would require how much fluid/day?

$$100ml \times 10Kg = 1000ml$$
$$50ml \times 10Kg = \underline{\quad 500ml}$$
$$20ml \times 40Kg = \underline{\quad 800ml}$$
$$2300ml/day$$

Replacement of Fluids
- Fluids are replaced during hospital stays using this breakdown
    - 7-3 shift — 3/6 of the total fluid intake is given
    - 3-11 shift — 2/6 of the total fluid intake is given
    - 11-7 shift — 1/6 of the total fluid intake is given
- When forcing fluids you double maintenance fluid needs
- Remember that IV replacement of fluids does not meet the caloric needs of your patient.

Fluid imbalance
- Assessment of fluid imbalance is important as it can be life threatening
    - Hypovolemia is too little fluid in the body
    - Hypervolemia is too much fluid in the body
- Symptoms of these two conditions are:

Hypovolemia	Hypervolemia
Dry Skin	Edema
Dry mucous membranes	Puffy eyelids
Decreased urine output	Moist lung rales
Weight Loss	Weight Gain
Fatigue	Dyspnea
Tachycardia	Bounding pulse
Tachypnea	Shortness of breath
Elevated RBCs	Decreased RBCs
Elevated hemoglobin	Decreased hemoglobin
Elevated hematocrit	Decreased hematocrit

INTRAVENOUS (IV) FLUID REPLACEMENT
- For technique for starting an IV see Cardiovascular section
- IV infusion is widely used to treat fluid imbalances, the type of solution used depends on the patients needs

Solution	Kcal/L	Indications	Osmolarity	Na	Cl	K	Ca	NCO₃
D5W Has 50g/L dextrose	170	Prevent dehydration Promotion diuresis of sodium	Isotonic	—	—	—	—	—
D10W Has 100g/L dextrose	340	Hypoglycemia	Hypertonic	—	—	—	—	—
NS 0.9%	—	Diabetic acidosis	Isotonic	154	154	—	—	—
1/2 NS 0.45%	—		Hypotonic	77	77	—	—	—
D5 1/4 NS	170	Fluid maintenance	Hypotonic	34	34	—	—	—
D5 1/2 NS	170	Fluid loss Sodium loss Promote diuresis	Hypotonic	77	77	—	—	—
D5 NS	170		Isotonic	154	154	—	—	—
Lactated Ringers (LR)	<10	Metabolic acidosis Dehydration Burns Infection	Isotonic	130	109	4	3	27
D5 LR	80	Diarrhea Loss of bile or pancreatic juice	Isotonic	130	109	4	3	27
Ringers solution		Fluid maintenance	Isotonic	147	156	4	4.5	

- NS, NaCl, 0.9% are all names for normal saline solution
- Ringers Solution and Lactated Ringers are not the same

Calculating Drip Rates

- Most IV infusions are given via a pump system, however it is still necessary to calculate drip rates to be sure patient is receiving ordered amount
- Formula for calculating drops per minute

$$\text{Drops/min} = \frac{\text{Amount to be infused}}{\text{Minutes to infuse}} \times \text{Drop factor}$$

- Find drop factor of IV tubing on tubing box or package usually 10 gtts/min, 20 gtts/min or 60 gtts/min (micro drops)
- Sample order — D5 1/2 NS to run at 120cc/hr (drop factor is 10)

Drops/min = $\dfrac{\text{Amount to be infused (120cc)}}{\text{Minutes to infuse (60)}}$ X   Drop factor (10)

Drops/min = $\dfrac{120}{60}$ X   10 or 2   X   10 or 20 drops per min

NASOGASTRIC TUBES

Indications:
- Gastric decompression (suction)
- Gastric gavage (feeding)
- Gastric lavage (washing out)

Types of NG tubes
- Check order for purpose of gastric intubation and select appropriate type of NG tube if not ordered
- Select appropriate size of NG tube (usually 16-18 F in adults)

Tube type	Primary purpose	Comments
Cantor tube	Intestinal decompression	Single-lumen tube Balloon tip filled with mercury so balloon will descend into small bowel Do not tape to nose or tube will not descend
Keofeed or other feeding tube	Gastric gavage	Single-lumen tubes Generally less irritating to patient May be weighted
Levin	Gastric decompression	Single-lumen tube Perforated tip and side holes Has radiopaque markings Available in 10-18 french
Miller-Abbott	Intestinal decompression	Double-lumen tube Balloon tip is filled with mercury so that it will descend into the small bowel One lumen is for aspiration, the other lumen is for mercury Do not tape to nose or tube will not descend
Salem-Sump	Gastric lavage or decompression	Double-lumen tube Small tube is air intake vent Has radiopaque markings
Sengstaken-Blakemore tube	Stop bleeding from esophageal varices	Triple-lumen tube One lumen is for aspiration, one for gastric balloon, and the third is for esophageal balloon

Insertion of NG tube
- Assemble equipment needed
  - Appropriate NG tube type and size
  - Lubricant (water soluble)
  - 50 cc irrigating syringe
  - Stethoscope
  - Suction equipment or appropriate feeding solution with primed tubing
  - Emesis basin, tissue, towel, adhesive tape, gloves
- To insert NG tube first position patient in high-Fowler's if possible
- Explain procedure to patient
- Place towel on patient's chest, give basin to patient
- Measure tube from nose to earlobe to xiphoid process, place piece of adhesive tape around tube at mark
- Lubricate tip of tube
- Gently, steadily insert tube along nasal passageway floor
- If resistance is met, ask the patient to swallow small amounts of cold water through a straw while tube is passed
- When adhesive mark is at the nose, stop and aspirate with syringe for gastric contents to assure stomach placement
- Another option to check for placement is to instill 15 cc of air while listening with stethoscope for rush of air over the gastric area
- Tape to nose securely once placement is confirmed
- Begin suction, gavage or lavage as ordered
- Chart the procedure

Care of NG tube after insertion
- Rotate insertion site from nostril to nostril to prevent tissue damage from pressure necrosis
- Provide meticulous mouth care to decrease dryness and irritation
- Petroleum jelly may be applied at nares insertion site to decrease irritation
- Throat lozenges or spray may help with an irritated throat
- Check position of tube at least once per shift if on continuous feeds or suction

Complications of tube feeding:
- The two major complications are diarrhea and nausea
- Diarrhea is generally caused by:

- Bacterial contamination
- Feeding too quickly
- Feeding too cold
- Allergic reaction
- Too much lactose
- Osmolarity too high
- Nausea is generally caused by delayed gastric emptying

TOTAL PARENTERAL NUTRITION (TPN)

Definition:

- TPN provides the caloric needs, via the intravenous route for patients who cannot or will not ingest enough food
- Provides protein, carbohydrates, lipids, electrolytes and trace elements to prevent malnutrition
- Can be provided via peripheral vein, however, long-term TPN should be given via central vein catheter
- TPN may be ordered in hospital or home setting

Prior to initiating TPN, assess:

- Current nutritional status usually performed by a registered dietitian or the primary health care provider
- Baseline vital signs (pulse, respirations, temperature, BP)
- Admission weight
- Current weight

- Ordered TPN solution and rate
    - 1 Liter/day = 43 cc/hour
    - 2 Liter/day = 86 cc/hour
    - 3 Liter/day = 125 cc/hour
- Ordered lipids (fat emulsion solution) and rate if applicable
- Check TPN solution carefully against physician's orders for correct dextrose solution, eectrolytes, and trace minerals
- Check solution for precipitate, do not hang if present

During TPN administration, monitor:

- Rate of infusion, begin TPN infusion slowly usually at 25-50 cc/hour and monitor for glucose tolerance problems
- Vital signs every 4-8 hours depending on agency policy
- Weight, at least every other day and assess for changes

- Blood glucose levels for any elevation, usually checked 2-4 times daily until patient stable
- K+, Na+, Cl-, HCO_3, and BUN levels daily until stable
- Monitor for congestive heart failure due to fluid overload, arrhythmias may result from electrolyte imbalances
- Check catheter site with dressing changes for signs of detachment or infection, change dressing per agency policy
- Check all tubing connections to avoid accidental catheter detachment with possible blood loss or air embolism
- Tubing should be checked for fractures or tears in catheter, change per agency policy
- Strict aseptic technique should be used at all dressing and tubing changes to prevent sepsis especially in central lines
- TPN should not be discontinued suddenly, wean from the solution per primary care providers orders

Chart:

- Date TPN begun, times of rate changes and patient response
- Contents of TPN solution and rate of flow
- Current wt and admission wt, desired wt if known
- All lab work, time done and response of primary care provider

Section V — CONDITIONS

Gastric Ulcer

Definition
- Chronic ulcerative condition of the upper GI tract
- An ulcer is a lesion located in the gastrointestinal mucosa that penetrates through to the muscularis mucosa
- Includes mainly duodenal ulcers and gastric ulcers, may also include ulcers in the esophagus

Prevalence
- 5-10% of the population will have peptic ulcers at one point in their lifetime
- 350,000 new cases of peptic ulcer are reported yearly in USA
- The peak incidence for gastric ulcers is between 40-70 years
- Gastric ulcers occur more frequently in males than females
- The peak incidence for duodenal ulcers is between 25-55 years
- 10-20% of patients with gastric ulcers have duodenal ulcers

Etiology
- The primary cause appears unclear, however it is believed to be related to the action of gastric acid and pepsin on the mucosa of the esophagus, stomach or duodenum
- Factors that have been identified as playing possible roles in the etiology of ulcers include:
  - Heredity or a genetic predisposition
    Duodenal ulcers are more common in relatives of known patients and in those with blood type O
  - Abnormal secretion of acid and pepsin, higher than normal rates have been found in 30-40% of patients with duodenal ulcer disease
  - Reflux
  - Emotional stress, certain emotions such as anger, resentment, guilt and frustration have been linked with increased acid secretion and ulcers
  - Cigarette smoking, nonsteroidal anti-inflammatory drugs (NSAIDs) and adrenocorticosteroids have all been associated with ulcers

- Helicobacter pylori a gram-negative bacteria has been found in 90-95% of patients with duodenal ulcers and 60-70% of patients with gastric ulcers
- No conclusive evidence exists relating alcohol and diet to the development of ulcers
- Duodenal ulcers are rarely malignant, 2-5% of gastric ulcers contain some malignant cells (gastric carcinoma)

Signs and symptoms of peptic ulcers
- Dyspepsia (painful digestion) may be expressed by
  - Abdominal discomfort or pain (see below)
  - Fullness after eating, bloating, belching, and heartburn
  - Nausea and vomiting
- Burning or gnawing episodes of pain in epigastrium
  - Onset of pain is usually 1-3 hours after a meal
  - Pain may awaken patient at night
  - Usually relieved by eating or antacids
  - Pain usually lasts only minutes
  - Episodes of pain occur for days or weeks followed by a pain-free intermission of weeks or years before recurrence
- Bleeding is the most common complication of peptic ulcer and results from erosion of the ulcer into a blood vessel
  - Occurs in 10-20% of patients
  - Mortality rate of 5-10% so early recognition is important
  - Melena or black tarry stools is the most common sign, in severe hemorrhage stool may be bright red
  - Hematemesis or vomiting blood may occur
- Perforation and spillage of gastric or duodenal contents is another complication
  - Occurs in 6-11% of patients with duodenal ulcer
  - Occurs in 2-5% of patients with gastric ulcer
  - Mortality rate of 5-15% so early recognition is important
  - Severe constant abdominal pain is the most common sign Abdomen may be board-like and rigid
  - Accompanied by significant bleeding in some cases

Components of initial examination for peptic ulcer
- *Complete medical history to include:*

- Personal and family history of ulcers including previous and current treatments (over the counter antacid use) and lifestyle changes (any foods known to cause discomfort to the patient)
- Patient's understanding of diagnoses and treatment
- Patient's willingness to make lifestyle changes
- History of dyspepsia to include location of pain, onset of pain in relationship to meals, the number of epidoses of pain per day, week and month and response of pain to eating or antacids
- Assessment of any changes in the quality or frequency of pain which may indicate a complication
- Current or past report of blood in stools or black tarry stools
- *Physical examination to include:*
  - General appearance and current comfort level
    - Pallor may occur with acute or chronic blood loss
  - Location of epigastric tenderness (often is nonspecific) if severe with marked pain and rigidity perforation may be present
  - In uncomplicated peptic ulcers (without perforation or bleeding), physical examination is usually not helpful
  - Vital signs to assess for complications
    - Sytolic blood pressure <100 mm Hg and pulse >100 bpm may suggest a major blood loss due to bleeding or intraperitoneal fluid loss due to perforation
- *Laboratory and diagnostic testing:*
  - Upper GI x-rays with contrast barium
  - Endoscopic visualization with or without biopsy of the ulcer to rule out malignancy
  - Serum gastrin levels if Zollinger-Ellison syndrome is suspected
  - Biopsy of mucosa for H. pylori
  - Hemoglobin and hematocrit if bleeding peptic ulcer is suspected to assess blood loss

Treatment of peptic ulcer

- Goal of treatment is for the ulcer to heal and to prevent the recurrence of future ulcerations
  - Foster the mucosal defense system
  - Reduce the presence of acid and pepsin
  - Allow for cell regeneration to take place

- Medications are the first line therapy for peptic ulcers
- Diet, no specific diet is advocated, all foods are allowed except for foods the patient knows causes them discomfort
  Bland, soft or diets free of spices have not proven effective
- Cigarette smoking is associated with slower healing of ulcers and should be avoided
- If hemorrhage occurs blood transfusion for replacement
- Surgical therapy is used only if ulcers fail to heal or complications such as hemorrhage, perforation or obstruction occur, surgical procedures may include:
  - Subtotal gastrectomy
  - Truncal vagotomy and pyloroplasty

Medications for peptic ulcers

- Antisecretory agents to reduce or block gastric acid secretion these include:
  - H2-Receptor antagonists such as Cimetidine (Tagamet), Ranitidene (Zantac), famotidine (Pepcid) or nizatidine
  - Antacids, usually an aluminum hyrodxide and/or magnesium hydroxide combination are used
- Coating agents such as Sucralfate (Carafate)
- Medication therapy may require 4-6 weeks of treatment before ulcer is healed, once healed maintenance medication therapy may be given to prevent recurrence
- Bismuth, metronidazole and an antibiotic has produced healing of ulcers by eradication of H. Pylori with long ulcer remissions in some patients
- Nonsteroidal anti-inflammatory drugs (NSAID's) should be avoided in patients with peptic ulcers

Section VI — DIETS

- All patient's who are hospitalized will have some type of dietary order
- A patient who is unable to take in fluids or food by mouth will have an NPO order (Latin for non per os) or nothing by mouth
- Patient's not requiring any dietary modification will receive a general or regular diet
- Hospital progression diets are designed to serve the needs of patients who must alter their diet for physical or psychological reasons in order to restore or maintain their health
- The usual hospital progression diet begins with clear liquid diet and progresses as tolerated by patient and ordered by physician to full liquid, soft and finally a regular diet
- Diet is important in the treatment of gastrointestinal disease
- Some individuals with disorders that affect their ability to chew or swallow foods require an alteration in the preparation of their diet (pureed or mechanical soft diet)

CLEAR LIQUID DIET

General description	Foods and fluids that are clear Easily absorbed with minimal residue in GI tract Minimizes stimulation of GI tract Liquids provided may depend upon patients needs
Indications	Common first post-operative diet First step from NPO to regular diet Required for some laboratory and diagnostic tests Ordered pre-operative for some bowel surgeries
Allowable items	Coffee, decaffeinated coffee or teas Artificially flavored fruit drinks Fruit juices without pulp or nectar Carbonated beverages (not for surgical patients) Clear, fat-free broth, bouillons, or consomme Gelatin, Fruit Ices, Popsicles, Hard clear candy
Restricted items	All solid foods Milk products Fruit juices with pulp or nectar Carbonated beverages depending on pt. condition
Nutritional value	Inadequate in calories (600 kcal/day) Usual hospital clear liquid diet provides: 8 g Protein, 3 g Fat, 130 g Carbohydrate 38 mEq Sodium & 16 mEq Potassium Due to limited nutritional value use for 1-3 days
Other comments	Pull privacy curtain during meals if roommate has a more advanced diet Offer fluids frequently

FULL LIQUID DIET

General description	Foods and fluids that are liquid or semiliquid at room temperature Often used for those unable to digest solid foods Type of foods provided may vary with diagnosis
Indications	Second step from NPO to regular diet Patients who are incapable of chewing, swallowing or digesting solid foods Esophageal or gastrointestinal strictures Moderate gastrointestinal dysfunction
Allowable items	All clear liquid diet items plus: Vegetable juices, milk, milk beverages, cocoa Blenderized or cream soups, strained soups Yogurt without fruit, nuts or seeds Refined cooked cereals Pudding, sherbet, ice cream, custard Vegetable puree in soups, seasonings as tolerated Butter, margarine or cream
Restricted items	Carbonated beverages and juices may be restricted in some surgical patients Some surgical patients may have a temporary lactose intolerance postoperatively Meats and other foods requiring chewing Solid foods
Nutritional value	Inadequate in all nutrients except protein, Ca+, and ascorbic acid, provides about 1,100 calories Usual hospital full liquid diet provides: 40 g Protein, 30 g Fat, 170 g Carbohydrate 66 mEq Sodium & 57 mEq Potassium Due to limited nutritional value use for 1-3 days
Other comments	Provides more satisfaction that clear liquid diet Blenderized foods may be used to improve the nutritional adequacy Next step in surgical progression is soft diet

SOFT DIET

General description	Soft foods which are moderately low in fiber Transition between liquid and regular diet
Indications	Third step from NPO to general (regular) dietary plan Patients with mild gastrointestinal problems
Allowable items	All full liquid diet items plus: Any beverages Mildly seasoned soups, soft casseroles Moist, tender meats, fish, poultry, eggs, cheese Peanut butter, oils, gravy, crisp bacon Potatoes, rice, pasta, breads, rolls, crackers Soft cooked vegetables, lettuce, tomatoes Cooked or canned fruit, soft fresh fruits Cake or cookies without nuts or coconut Candy without nuts or coconut Lightly seasoned foods

Restricted items	Gas-forming vegetables (cabbage) Gas-forming lentils Whole kernel corn Products with nuts, seeds or coconut Fresh crisp fruits or vegetables Strong seasonings
Nutritional value	If patient is able to consume adequate amounts of food, this diet will meet RDA of nutrients Usual hospital soft diet provides 1,800 kcal, 65 g Protein, 75 g Fat, 225 g Carbohydrates, 150 mEq Sodium and 90 mEq Potassium
Other comments	Last step for surgical patients on progression diet before general (regular) diet is ordered Small volume meals are offered until patient's tolerance to solid food is regained or known

GENERAL OR REGULAR DIET

General description	Hospital diet based upon the Food Guide Pyramid, Dietary Guideline Americans, American Dietetic Association Exchange Lists and the American Diabetes Association, or other guides for meal planning
Indications	Patient who does not need require any dietary interventions
Allowable items	All foods are allowed Meal plan is consistent with RDA of nutrients
Restricted items	No restrictions unless patient has allergy to any foods
Nutritional value	Usual general diet provides 1,600-2,200 kcal/day, 60-80 g Protein, 60-80 g Fat, 200-300 g of Carbohydrates
Other comments	Meal plan items may be selected by patient

PUREED DIET

General description	Strained, pureed, and liquid foods that are easily swallowed
Indications	Patients with no teeth or who are unable to chew Patients with inflammation or ulceration Patients with structural or motor deficit in oral cavity or esophagus Post-operative esophageal or oral surgical pts After radiation of the oral or pharyngeal region
Allowable items	All items from clear liquid and full liquid diets Any beverages Strained or pureed meats and poultry Cheese sauces, soups, cottage cheeses Blended or pureed casseroles, mashed potatoes
Restricted items	All solid foods (require chewing)

Nutritional value	If patient is able to consume adequate amounts of food this diet will meet RDA nutrient requirement Usual hospital pureed diet provides 1,700 kcal, 60 g Protein, 55 g Fat, 250 g Carbohydrates, 100 mEq Sodium & 95 mEq Potassium
Other comments	Extreme food temperatures may be poorly tolerated Syringe, straw, or spoon may be used for feeding Additional liquid may be required to thin foods for straw or syringe feedings

MECHANICAL SOFT DIET

General description	General diet modified for ease of chewing
Indications	Patients with poorly fitting dentures or no teeth Patients who are unable to chew Esophageal, oral, or laryngeal disorders/surgery Intestinal tract strictures Radiation treatment to oral cavity Sometimes used as diet progression step between enteral or parenteral nutrition to solid foods
Allowable items	Any moist, easy to chew and swallow food All pureed diet items plus: Ground or finely diced meats, moist meats or poultry, flaked fish eggs, cheeses, peanut butter Soft casseroles, rice, pasta Graham crackers as tolerated Vegetables cooked soft without hulls or skin Cooked or canned fruit without seeds or skins Bananas, citrus fruits without membrane
Restricted items	Restrictions are based on individual assessment Usually include: Raw or undercooked vegetables Peas, corn or other vegetables with hulls or skin Nuts, seeds, onions or pieces of hard peppers Breads and rolls may not be well tolerated, may be ordered based on dietary assessment
Nutritional value	Generally more protein than pureed diet If patient is able to consume adequate amounts of food, this diet will meet RDA of nutrients Usual hospital mechanical soft diet provides: 1,700 calories, 60 g Protein, 55 g Fat, 250 g carbohydrate, 100 mEq Sodium & 95 mEq Potassium
Other comments	Milk products may be restricted if increased salivation is a contributing factor in swallowing disorders

Section VII — DRUGS

The tables supply only general information, a drug handbook or the physicians desk reference (PDR) should be consulted for details. Each classification includes detailed information about the Example drug, this drug is representative of the other drugs in the classification and can be used as a model.

Every effort has been made to include the major classes of drugs used in the treatment of gastrointestinal diseases.

ANTACIDS
Action: Reduce acid concentration and pepsin activity within the stomach
Indications: Heartburn, esophageal reflux, peptic ulcers, hiatal hernia
Example: Aluminum hydroxide (*AluCap, Alugel, AluTab, Amphojel, Dialume*)
Also available as Aluminum carbonate or Aluminum phosphate
Route: PO
Pharmacokinetic: Duration 2-3 hours
Contraindications: Low serum phosphate
Common adverse effects: Constipation
Other adverse effects: Hypophosphatemia, dialysis dementia, hypomagnesemia
Interventions:
Administer with water, chewable tablets should be well chewed
Recommended that no other oral drugs are given within 1-2 hours
Assess bowel elimination patterns, stools may be speckled or whitish
Monitor serum calcium and phosphorus levels, report any abnormalities
Examples of other drugs in this classification:
Calcium carbonate (*Calcite-500, Caltrate, Equilet, Nu-Cal, Os-Cal, Tums*), Chronic use may cause milk-alkali syndrome when taken with milk products

Magaldrate (*Lowsium, Riopan*), Used in patients who need to restrict sodium, Shake well before administration
Example: Magnesium hydroxide (*Magnesia, Milk of Magnesia, MOM*)
Route: PO
Contraindications: Abdominal pain, nausea, vomiting, diarrhea, obstruction, renal dysfunction, colostomy, ileostomy
Common adverse effects: diarrhea in excessive dose

Other adverse effects: Hypermagnesemia which can be life-threatening

Interventions:
Administer with water, monitor for hypermagnesemia S&S to include, nausea, weakness, vomiting, lethargy, mental depression, hyporeflexia, hypotension, respiratory depression and coma

Examples of other drugs in this classification:
Magnesium Oxide (*Mag-Ox*)

Sodium Bicarbonate (*Baking soda, Alka-Seltzer, BromoSeltzer, Gaviscon*), Discourage regular use of baking soda as antiacid, OTC preparations are safer for routine use, may cause sodium retention

ANTIDIARRHEAL
Action: Reduces the fluid content of the stool, decreases peristalsis and intestinal motility, decreases digestive secretions and provides a coating to protect the intestinal mucosa

Indications: Diarrhea

Example: Diphenoxylate HCI and atropine (*Lomanate, Lomotil, Nor-Mil*)

Route:PO

Pharmacokinetics: Onset 45-60 minutes, Peak 2 hrs, Duration 3-4 hrs

Contraindications: Sensitivity to diphenoxylate or atrophine, dehydration or electrolyte imbalance, jaundice, poisoning until poison has cleared system, glaucoma, advanced liver disease

Adverse effects: Headache, sedation, drowsiness, dizziness, lethargy, dry mouth, restlessness, euphoria, depression, weakness, malaise, flushing, palpitations, increased heart rate, nystagmus, mydriasis, blurred vision, nausea, vomiting, anorexia, abdominal discomfort, paralytic ileus, urinary retention, swollen gums

Interventions:
Tablets may be crushed and taken with food or fluid

Monitor I&O, assess for dehydration and hold drug if present

Assess for and report dry mouth, flushing, tachycardia and urinary retention these may be related to atropine toxicity

Examples of other drugs in this classification:
Bismuth subsalicylate (*Pepto-Bismol*), PO in chewable or liquid forms, do not use with sensitivity to aspirin, darkens stools

Calcium polycarbophil (*FiberCon, Mitrolan*), PO, take with fluid

Kaolin and Pectin (*Kao-tin, Kapectolin, Kaypectol, K-P, Pecto Kay*), PO, Shake well before administration

Loperamide (*Imodium, Imodium AD*), PO, May cause drowsiness, dry mouth is a common side effect

Octreotide acetate (*Sandostatin*), SC, For severe diarrhea, monitor I&O and fluid electrolytes for imbalances

Paregoric (*Camphorated opium tincture*), PO, Administer with water, check label and dose carefully — not the same as opium tincture, for severe diarrhea, Schedule III drug

ANTIFLATULENTS
Action: Breaks up gastrointestinal gases to enhance expulsion and reduce gastric pain
Indications: Bloating and excessive flatulence. May be used for post-operative gas pain relief.
Example: Simethicone (*Gas-x, Mylicon, Phazyme, Silain*)
Route: PO
Contraindications: sensitivity to this product
Interventions:
If suspension shake thoroughly before administration, tablets should be chewed well before swallowing
Inform patient that they will have an increase in belching or flatulence

DIGESTIVE ENZYMES
Action: Replace enzymes needed for digestion
Indications: A lack of digestive enzymes, may occur in cystic fibrosis, pancreatic disease, obstruction of the bile or pancreatic ducts, or with gastrointestinal bypass surgery
Example: Pancrealipase (Cotazym, Cotazym-S, Festal II, Ilozyme, Ku-Zyme-Hp, Pancrease, Viokase)
Route: PO
Contraindications: sensitivity to pork proteins or enzymes
Adverse effects: With high doses nausea, vomiting, diarrhea may occur
Interventions:
Powder may be sprinkled on food, do not crush enteric-coated tablets
Antacid may be prescribed with digestive enzyme to decrease gastric acid
Dose is dependent upon dietary intake of fat
Monitor I&O, weight, excessive thirst, hunger or polyuria

EMETICS
Action: To induce vomiting
Indications: Ingestion of toxic substances or drug overdose, emetics are used to remove poisons from stomach before they can be absorbed
Example: Ipecac Syrup
Route: PO
Pharmacokinetics: Onset 15-30 minutes, Duration 25 minutes
Contraindications: Unconsciousness, inebriation, sedation, shock, absence or depressed gag reflex, seizures, impaired cardiac function, ingestion of strong alkali poisons or acids, ingestion of strychnine, volatile oils, petroleum distillates or rapid acting central nervous system depressants
Common adverse effects: Persistent vomiting
Other adverse effects: Diarrhea, stomach upset, lethargy
Overdose may be fatal with convulsions, coma, hypotension and arrhythmias
Interventions:
Check label carefully Ipecac syrup is not the same as Ipecac fluid extract fatal Route errors have occurred
Administer with warm water or other clear liquid
If vomiting does not occur within 20 minutes contact primary care provider for further instructions, may be cardiotoxic if absorbed
Assess if ingestion was accidental or deliberate and provide counseling or referral as indicated

HISTAMINE RECEPTOR ANTAGONISTS
Action: To reduce gastric acid by blocking histamine and inhibiting the secretion of gastric acid
Indications: Duodenal ulcers, peptic esophagitis, benign gastric ulcers, and stress ulcers
Example: Cimetidine (Novocimetine, Peptol, Tagamet)
Route: PO, IM, IV
Pharmacokinetics: Peak 60-90 min
Contraindications: sensitivity to cimetidine
Adverse effects: Drowsiness, dizziness, lightheadedness, depression, headache, confusion, paranoia, diarrhea may be mild to severe, abdominal distention, constipation, gynecomastia, breast soreness, galactorrhea, impotence, rash
Life-threatening adverse effects: Aplastic anemia, cardiac arrhythmias or arrest can occur if IV administration is too rapid
Interventions:
Administer PO medication with meals, if antacid is ordered administer it 1 hour before or 2 hours after meals

Administer IV infusion diluted with 50ml of D5W over 15-20 minutes

Administer IV push in at least 20ml of NS over no less than 2 minutes

Monitor pulse and BP, report bradycardia or hypertension

Monitor bowel pattern, assess for bowel sounds, report if absent, report any abdominal discomfort or distention, bleeding or black tarry stools

Monitor blood counts and liver function studies, report if abnormal

Patient should avoid tyramine-rich foods such as cheddar cheese, yogurt, aged meats, soy sauce, red wine or beef extract as these may lead to a transient elevation of blood pressure and headache

Examples of other drugs in this classification:

Famotidine (*Pepcid*), PO/IV, used for short-term treatment

Nizatidine (*Axid*), PO, usually X1 daily at night

Ranitidine hydrochloride (*Zantac*), PO, IV injection should be mixed with 20ml and given at a rate of 4ml/min

LAXATIVES — BULK FORMING

Action: To aid in the passage of stool by absorbing water which increases the bulk and moisture content of the stool which stimulates peristalsis.

Indications: Constipation, hard infrequent stools

Example: Psyllium hydrophilic mucilloid (*Hydrocil, Konsyl, Metamucil, Modane bulk, prodiem plain, reguloid, serutan, siblin, syllact, V-Lax*)

Route: PO

Pharmacokinetics: Onset 12-24 hours, Peak 1-3 days

Contraindications: Intestinal obstruction, fecal impaction, abdominal pain of undetermined origin

Adverse effects: Eosinophilia, nausea, vomiting, diarrhea

Interventions:

Mix well with 8 full ounces of cool water, milk, fruit juice or compatible liquid, do not administer dry

For best results follow with an additional full glass of water

Provide teaching on prevention of constipation to include increased fluids, increased fiber in the diet and a regular time for bowel evacuation

Examples of other drugs in this classification:

Calcium polycarbophil (*FiberCon, Mitrolan*), PO, tablets should be chewed well before swallowing followed by 6-8 ounces of water

Methylcellulose (*Citrucel, Cologel, Maltsupex*), PO, tablets should be chewed well before swallowing followed by 1-2 glasses of water

Polycarbophil (*FiberCon, Mitrolan*), PO, chew tablets well, follow
   with 1 glass of water

LAXATIVES — FECAL SOFTENERS (STOOL SOFTNERS)
Action: To aid in the passage of stool by lowering the surface
tension of the stool allowing the stool to be penetrated by intestinal
fluids
Indications: Constipation, hard infrequent stools. Stool softners
may be particularly helpful in patients where straining at stool is
contraindicated such as hernia, heart disease or post-rectal surgery
Example: Docusate sodium (*Colace, Dio-Sul, Disonate, DGSS,
Lax-gel, Modane, Regutol, Therevac Plus*)
Route: PO
Contraindications: fecal impaction, abdominal pain, nausea,
vomiting, structural anomalies of colon and rectum, intestinal
obstruction
Common adverse effects: Diarrhea
Other adverse effects: Nausea, bitter taste, irritation to throat, rash
Interventions:
Administer with 8 ounces of fluid if possible
Monitor I&O for adequate fluid intake, encourage fluids as allowed

LAXATIVES — SALINE
Action: To aid in the passage of stool by drawing water into the
small intestine as well as the colon.
Indications: Short term constipation, hard, infrequent stools
Example: Magnesium hydroxide (*Magnesia, Milk of Magnesia*)
Route: PO
Pharmacokinetics: Onset: 3-6 hours
Contraindications: Abdominal pain, nausea, vomiting, fecal
impaction
Common adverse effects: diarrhea
Other adverse effects: nausea, vomiting, abdominal cramps,
dehydration, hypermagnesemia
Life-threatening effects: hypermagnesemia
Interventions:
Shake well before administration, administer with full glass of water
Examples of other drugs in this classification:
Magnesium citrate (*Citrate of Magnesia, citroma, citro-nesia*) PO
Magnesium oxide (*Mag-Ox, Maox, Par-Mag, Uro-Mag*), PO

LAXATIVES — STIMULANT
Action: To aid in the passage of stool by preventing absorption of

fecal fluid by the colon thereby producing a softer and more lubricated stool

Indications: Constipation, hard infrequent stools, may be particularly helpful in patients where straining at stool is contraindicated such as with myocardial infarction, hernia, post-rectal surgery or hemorrhoids

Example: Bisacodyl (*Bisacolax, Dacodyl, Dulcolax, Fleet Bisacodyl*)

Route: PO

Pharmacokinetics: Onset 6-8 hours PO, 15-60 minutes per rectum

Contraindications: Nausea, vomiting, intestinal obstruction, impaction

Adverse effects: Rare — nausea, vertigo, diarrhea, fluid and electrolyte imbalances

Interventions:

Administer in evening or before breakfast, do not crush or chew tablets give with a full glass of water, do not administer with milk or antacids

Examples of other drugs in this classification:

Cascara sagrada, PO

Castor oil (*Alphamul, Emulsoil, Fleet Castor oil stimulant laxative, Neoloid, Unisoil*), PO, Best tolerated if chilled prior to administration

Phenolphthalein (*Alophen, Correctol, Espotabs, Evac-U-Gen, Evac-U-Lax, Ex-Lax, Feen-a-mint, Lax-pill, Modane, Phenolax, Prulet*), PO, administer at bedtime

Senna (*Black Draught, Gentlax B, Senexon, Senokot, Senolax*), PO

Section VIII — GLOSSARY OF TERMS

Accessory organ   An organ that assists other organs to perform their functions

Amino acids   The basic building blocks of protein

Antagonists   Counteracts the action of something else

Ascites   The accumulation of fluid in the peritoneal cavity

BEE   Basal energy expenditure is the amount of energy required to maintain life at rest

Bitot's spots   Shiny, gray spots on the conjunctiva, due to a vitamin A deficiency

Bolus   A portion of chewed food ready to be swallowed

Borborygmi   The loud rumbling, gurgling sound heard when gas is moved down the intestinal tract

Bruits   Sound heard during auscultation, arises from an arterial or venous source; always abnormal

cal or Kcal   Calorie

Cheilosis   Reddened lips with fissures at the angles due to a deficiency of vitamin B complex

Chyme   A mass of partially digested food with digestive enzymes, found in the stomach and small intestine during digestion

cm   Centimeter, a unit of measure, 1 in = 2.54 cm

Constipation   Dry, hard, infrequent stools that are difficult to expel from the body

D5W, D10W   Dextrose solution in water, intravenous solutions available in a wide range of concentrations

Deglutition   The act of swallowing

Diabetes mellitus   A condition where insulin is either inadequate or totally absent

Diarrhea   Loose, watery, and frequent stools

Digestion	The chemical and mechanical breakdown of food so that it can be absorbed
Disaccharides	A carbohydrate made up of two monosaccharides (simple sugars)
DNA	Deoxyribonuclecic acid; genetic material
Edema	Swelling in the body tissues
Elimination	Removal of wastes from the body
Emesis	Vomit
Feces	Product of bowel elimination
Force fluids	To increase fluid intake, usually to twice the normal fluid requirement
Gastrointestinal	Pertaining to the stomach and intestinal tract
Gastric decompression	To remove pressure from the GI tract via decompression suction, also remove gastric contents that are irritating
Gastric gavage	Feeding provided through a nasogastric tube when patient is NPO or refuses food
Gastric lavage	To wash out the stomach done through a nasogastric tube
GI	Gastrointestinal
Glossitis	Inflammation of the tongue that is characterized by redness, pain and swelling
GT tube	Gastrostomy tube, a tube surgically placed through the abdominal wall, used to provide gastric gavage or lavage
Hemorrhoid	An external or internal dilated vein in the anal area
Hernia	The abnormal protrusion of a partial or whole organ through the wall of a body cavity
Hepatitis	Inflammation of the liver, may be accompanied by jaundice
ht	Abbreviation for height

Romanski, Suzanne O'Leary: "Interpreting ABGs," **Nursing 86**, September 1986, page 56.

Rudy, Susan F.: "Take A Reading On Your Blood Pressure Techniques," **Nursing 86**, August 1986, Vol. 16 No. 8, pages 46-49.

Scherer, Priscilla: "Coma, Assessing The Logic of Coma," **AJN**, May 1986, Vol. 86 No. 5, pages 541-557.

Signor, Ginger: "A Sinfully Easy Way to Interpret ABGs," **RN**, September 1982, pages 45-49.

Solomon, Jacqueline: "Managing a Failing Heart," **RN**, August 1991, pages 46-50.

Stiesmeyer, Johanna K.: "What triggers a ventilator alarm?," **AJN**, October 1991.

Stopford, Jane Lloyd: "Static Exercise — Physiologic Dangers and Proper Training Techniques," **Nurse Practitioner**, April 1988, Vol. 13 No. 4, pages 7-18.

Wienke, V. Kay: "Pressure Sores: Prevention is the Challenge," **Orthopaedic Nursing**, July/August 1984, Vol. 6 No. 4, pages 26-30.

Yacone-Morton, Linda Ann: "Cardiac assessment," **RN**, December 1991, pages 28-34.

Hyperkalemia	More potassium than normal in the bloodstream
Hypervolemia	Increased fluid in the bloodstream
Hyponatremia	Decreased sodium in the bloodstream
Hypovolemia	Decreased fluid in the bloodstream
Indigestible	Not digestible
Ingestion	The process of taking food into the body via the mouth
Jaundice	A sign of excess bilirubin in the blood, characterized by yellowness in the sclera of the eyes, skin and mucous membranes
K+	Symbol for potassium
kg	Kilogram, a unit of measure 1 kg = 2.2 pounds
Lipids	Fat or fatty substance that is insoluble in water
Mastication	Chewing
Monosaccharides	A simple sugar such as fructose, galactose or glucose
Na++	Symbol for sodium
NaCl	Symbol for sodium chloride
Nasogastric tube	A soft flexible tube passed from the nostril to the stomach or intestine
Necrosis	Death of an area of tissue that is generally caused by an insufficient blood supply
NG	Nasogastric
NPO	Non per os (Latin) or nothing by mouth
NS	Normal saline or 0.9% sodium chloride
Nutrient	Substance necessary for life such as water, minerals, vitamins, carbohydrates, fats, proteins and electrolytes

Osmolarity	The ion concentration of a solution, isotonic solution being osmotically the same as tissue fluids
Osteomalacia	Softening of the bone caused by vitamin D deficiency in adults, symptoms may include pain in bones, anemia and weakness
Osteoporosis	Condition of Ca^{++} loss from the bone, seen in elderly population: results in porous or weak bone structure
Pellagra	A disorder due to the deficiency of niacin
Pepsin	An enzyme found in gastric juice that breaks down proteins into peptone and proteose
Peristalsis	Wavelike contractions of the gastrointestinal tract to move the products of digestion
Pureed food	Ground or blenderized food that is semisolid without lumps
Salivary gland	Glands which produce saliva to lubricate food and start digestion
Scurvy	A disorder characterized by fatigue, anemia, weakness, bleeding gums and hemorrhage
Skin turgor	Normal tension found in well-hydrated healthy skin. Measured by pinching up a small area of skin, if turgor is good skin returns immediately back to position
Sprue	A disorder characterized by weakness, weight loss and impaired digestion
Striae	A stretching of the skin's outermost layer, often in pregnancy, known as "stretch marks"
Synergists	A helper, as in vitamins, one that aids or potentiates functioning
Synthesize	To form a complex structure from smaller parts
Total parenteral nutrition	TPN, an intravenous solution that provides some essential nutrients and calories

Tube feedings	Feedings provided via the nasogastric or gastrostomy tube when normal ingestion of food is insufficient
Ulcers	A sore found in the mucous membranes (GI tract) or skin with inflammation and a gradual disintegration of surrounding tissue
Vesicles	A blister-like sac that contains fluid
Vitamin	An organic compound derived from the diet needed in very small quantities to promote growth and maintain life
wt	Abbreviation for weight
Xerophthalmia	Dryness of the conjunctiva due to a deficiency of vitamin A

APPENDIX 1

THE BASIC ASSESSMENT

General Information:
- Name, age, sex, marital status, race
- Referring physician
- Source of information (patient, parent, significant other)
- Persons present
- Known allergies
- Name of translator, if needed, and native language

Example:
Jeremy Smith, 16-year-old black male, single
Referred by Dr. C. O'Niell
Information obtained from parents: Bob and Neta Smith
Persons present: Both parents and patient

Chief complaint:
- Stated by the patient in a direct quote
- Concise and brief statement
- Recorded in quotation marks if direct quote
- Time reference

Example:
Parents state, "Blacked out after breakfast and started an epileptic fit." Lasted until EMS. arrived.
Patient states, "Dr. O'Niell sent me over for a CAT scan."

Present illness:
- What happened?
- When did it begin?
- How did it begin?
- Has the problem changed over time? Why does the patient think it changed?
- What treatments have been given?
- Medications: dose, frequency, result?
- What physicians has the person seen and with what result?

- What are the symptoms right now?
- Chart in chronological order whenever possible

  Example:

  States seizure activity began after breakfast, and involved only the right side of the body. This is the third seizure in seven years; two previous seizures (May 1990 and November 1996) involved the entire body and were related to high temperatures. No anticonvulsants were prescribed. A CT scan in November of 1996 was normal, ordered by Dr. R. Graham of Atlanta General Hospital. At present, the only complaint is headache and generalized weakness on the right side.

Past medical history:
- Illnesses, hospitalizations (include name), surgeries
- Current medications
- Allergies
- Past blood transfusions and reactions, if any
- Tobacco, alcohol and drug use
- Significant childhood illness

Social history:
- Educational level
- Marital status and/or history
- Vocation, work hours, occupation hazards
- Usual sleep pattern, routines, elimination patterns

Family history:
- Members of immediate family to include age, sex and general health status
- Cause of death for any deceased, immediate family members
- History of cancer, heart disease, lung, kidney or neurological disorders in blood relatives
- Determine if other family members have similar problems

Review of symptoms:
- Each of the major body systems are reviewed for past problems
- See assessment forms for each system
- Includes a general section where weight changes, fever, chills and allergies can be documented

Interview tips:

- Use open ended questions to obtain information. Example: "Tell me about your pain."
- Avoid judgmental questions such as, "You don't have more than two drinks a day, do you?"
- Ask visitors to step out of room to provide confidentiality and to avoid embarrassing the patient
- If possible, provide quiet environment for the interview with few distractions, turn off television, close the curtain

Physical examination tips:

The physical examination is composed of several factors that can be equally important. These are observation, palpation, and auscultation.

- Always provide for privacy prior to the exam. Ask visitors to step outside, pull the curtain or shut the door
- Always leave the patient properly gowned, assisting in tying gowned and putting on pajamas
- Begin with the presenting problem, unless a full head-to-toe physical is to be performed

Example:

- If your patient has just returned from surgery, check the dressings, bowel sounds, level of consciousness, respirations, blood pressure, and lung sounds first. If surgery was for a brain tumor you would concentrate on the neurological area for reduction of a fracture you would assess peripheral pulses of affected extremity
- Chart areas assessed that are of significance; negative assessments can be just as vital as positive ones.

Example:

A negative Babinski is an important finding in a child with a suspected brain tumor and should be charted if performed.

APPENDIX 2

HOSPITAL PROGRESSION DIETS

The following are diets that may be ordered for a patient on any hospital unit. The diets are listed in progressive order beginning with the most restrictive diet and ending with a general or regular diet.

The rate of dietary progression depends upon the patient's diagnosis and response to treatment or surgical options.

The sodium value of the diets is for usual foods and does not include salt added in preparation or on the tray.

Post-Operative Diets

Oral intake is resumed as soon as the gastrointestinal tract is functioning (auscultated bowel sounds and/or passage of flatus).

* Progression of diet may be rapid

> Breakfast = clear liquid
> Lunch = full liquid
> Dinner = soft

> or dietary progression may be slow (abdominal surgery)

> Monday = clear liquid
> Tuesday = full liquid
> Wednesday = soft
> Thursday = general

* If abdominal distension or cramping occur, the diet should revert back to earlier stage.

See Gastrointestinal Diet Section for diet details.

BIBLIOGRAPHY

BOOKS

American Heart Association: **Textbook of Advanced Cardiac Life Support**, 2nd ed., American Heart Association, 1990.

Bates, Barbara: **A Guide to Physical Examination**, 5th. ed., Philadelphia, J.B. Lippincott Co., 1991.

Benenson, Abram S.: **Control of Communicable Diseases in Man**, 15th ed., American Public Health Association, 1990.

Berkow, Robert, editor-in chief: **The Merck Manual**, 15th ed., Rahway, N.J., Merck Sharp & Dohme Research Laboratories, 1992.

Brunner, Nancy A.: **Orthopedic Nursing A Programmed Approach**, St. Louis, C.V. Mosby Co., 1983.

Carpenito, Lynda Juall: **Handbook of Nursing Diagnosis**, 4th edition, Philadelphia, J.B. Lippincott Company, 1991.

Cloherty, John P. and Ann R. Stark: **Manual of Neonatal Care,** Boston, Little, Brown and Company, 1991.

Edmunds, Marilyn W: **Nursing Drug Reference A Practitioner's Guide**, Bowie Maryland, Brady Communications Co., 1985.

Gioiella, Evelynn Clark and Catherine Waechter Bevil: **Nursing Care of the Aging Client, Promoting Healthy Adaptation**, Norwalk Connecticut, Appleton-Century-Crofts, 1985.

Gomella, Leonard G., G. Richard Braen and Michael Olding: **Clinician's Pocket Reference**, 5th ed., Norwalk, Connecticut, Appleton-Century-Crofts, 1991.

Govoni, Laura E. and Janice E. Hayes: **Drugs and Nursing Implications**, 6th ed., Norwalk, Connecticut, Appleton-Century-Crofts, 1992.

Green, Marilyn L. and Joann Harry: **Nutrition in Contemporary Nursing Practice**, New York, Wiley Medical Publication, 1981.

Henry, John Bernard: **Clinical Diagnosis and Management by Laboratory Methods** 17th ed., W.B. Saunders Co., 1984.

Isselbacher, Kurt J., et al: **Harrison's Principles of Internal Medicine**, 13th ed., New York, McGraw-Hill, Inc., 1994.

Jaffe, Marie, Linda Skidmore-Roth, and Rebecca Rayman: **Procedure Cards for Clinical Use**, Norwalk Connecticut, Appleton-Century-Crofts, 1986.

Kee, Joyce LeFever: **Laboratory and Diagnostic Tests with Nursing Implications** 2nd ed., Norwalk Connecticut, Appleton & Lange, 1987.

Lebovitz, Harold E., editor: **Therapy for Diabetes Mellitus and Related Disorders**, Alexandria, Virginia, American Diabetes Association, Inc., 1991.

Malasanos, Lois, et al: **Health Assessment**, St. Louis, Mosby-Yearbook Company, 1990.

Marino, Lisa Begg: **Cancer Nursing**, St. Louis, C.V. Mosby, 1981.

Meheny, Norma M.: **Fluid and Electrolyte Balance — Nursing Considerations**, Philadelphia, J.B. Lippincott Company, 1992.

McLane, Audrey M.: **Classification of Nursing Diagnoses, Proceedings of the Seventh Conference**, St. Louis, C.V. Mosby Co., 1987.

Pagana, Kathleen D. and Timothy J. Pagana: **Mosby's Diagnostic and Laboratory Test Reference**, 2nd ed., St. Louis, Mosby Co., 1995.

Patrick, Maxine L., et al: **Medical-Surgical Nursing, Pathophysiological Concepts**, Philadelphia, J.B. Lippincott Co., 1986.

Phipps, Wilma J., Barbara C. Long and Nancy Fugate Woods: **Medical-Surgical Nursing, concepts and clinical practice**, St. Louis, C.V. Mosby Co., 1991.

Porth, Carol: **Pathophysiology, Concepts of Altered Health States**, 3rd ed., Philadelphia, J.B. Lippincott Co., 1990.

Powers, Margaret A., editor: **Nutrition Guide for Professionals, Diabetes Education and Meal Planning**, American Diabetes Association, Inc., 1988.

Pritchard, Jack A., Paul C. MacDonald and Norman F. Gant: **Williams Obstetrics** 18th ed., Norwalk Connecticut, Appleton-Century-Crofts, 1985.

Schroeder, Steven A, Marcus A. Krupp and Lawrence M. Tierney Jr.: **Current Medical Diagnosis &Treatment**, Norwalk, Connecticut, Appleton & Lange, 1992.

Taber's Cyclopedic Medical Dictionary 17th ed., edited by Clayton L. Thomas, Philadelphia, F. A. Davis Company, 1993

Wyngaarden, James B., Lloyd H. Smith, Jr. and J. Claude Bennett: **Cecil Textbook of Medicine**, 19th ed., Philadelphia, W. B. Saunders Company, 1992.

JOURNALS

Adelman, Eleanore McGowan: "When the Patient's Blood Pressure Falls...What Does it Mean? What Should You Do?" **Nursing 87**, October 1987, pages 66-73.

"AIDS: A guide for survival," **The Harris County Medical Society and The Houston Academy of Medicine**, 1987.

Anastasi, Joyce K., and Julie Linksman Rivera: "AIDS drug update, ddI and ddC," **RN**, November, 1991.

Anderson, Barbara Jo: "Tube Feeding: Is Diarrhea Inevitable?" **AJN**, June 1986, Vol. 86 No. 6, pages 704-706.

Barrick, Bill: "Light at the end of a decade", **AJN**, November 1990, pages 37-40.

Bassett, Frank H., et al.: "Optimal Care for Acute Knee Injuries," **Patient Care**, February 28, 1987.

Bavin, Terry K. and Marjorie A. Self: "Weaning from intra-aortic balloon pump support," **AJN**, October 1991.

Bergfeld, John A., et al. "Women in Athletics: Five Management Problems," **Patient Care**, February 28, 1987, pages 60-82.

Bockus, Sherry: "Trouble shooting your tube feedings", **AJN**, May 1991, pages 24-28.

Braun, Anne E.: "Drugs that dissolve clots", **RN**, June 1991, pages 52-57.

Byrnes, Carol A.: "What's New In The Diabetic Diet," **Nursing 87**, August 1987, pages 58-59.

Carroll, Patricia Fuchs: "The Ins and Outs of Chest Drainage Systems" **Nursing 86**, December 1986, pages 26-33.

Carroll, Patricia: "What's new in chest-tube management", **RN**, May 1991, pages 34-40.

Clark-Mims, Barbara: "Interpreting ABG's," **RN**, March 1991, pages 42-46.

Cohen, Stephen: "How to Work With Chest Tubes," **AJN**, April 1980, pages 685-712.

Conn, Robert D. and Henry S. Miller: "Which Adults Need Preexercise Stress Tests?" **Patient Care**, February 28, 1987.

Dirubbo, Nancy E.: "The Condom Barrier," **AJN**, October 1987, Vol. 87, No. 10, pages 1306-1309.

Dunn, Melinda M.: "Guidelines for an Effective Personal Fitness Prescription," **Nurse Practitioner**, September 1987, Vol. 12 No. 9, pages 9-23.

Fitzgerald, Margaret Ann: "The physical exam," **RN**, November 1991, pages 34-38.

Fischer, Andrew A., et al.: "Mobilizing the sedentary patient," **Patient Care**, February 28,1987, pages 14-31.

Gehring, Patsy Eileen: "Physical assessment begins with a history," **RN**, November 1991, pages 27-31.

Greifzu, Sherry: "Helping cancer patients fight infection," **RN**, July 1991, pages 24-28.

Hansell, Mary Jo: "Fractures and the Healing Process," **Orthopaedic Nursing**, January/February 1988, Vol. 7 No. 1, pages 43-50.

Hefti, Deanne: "Chest trauma," **RN**, May 1991, pages 28-32.

Hill, Martha N. and Carlene Minks Grim: "How to take a precise blood pressure," **AJN**, February 1991, pages 38-42.

Hoffman, Leslie A., Marion C. Mazzocco and James E. Roth: "Fine Tuning Your Chest PT," **AJN**, December 1987, Vol. 87 No. 12, pages 1566-1573.

Howard, Patricia: "Elevated cholesterol: A nurse's guide to drug therapy," **RN**, August 1991, pages 26-29.

Jones, Sandra: "L-E-A-D Drugs for Cardiac Arrest," **Nursing 88**, January 1988, Vol. 18 No. 1, pages 34-42.

King, Carole: "Checking The Patient's Neurological Status," **RN,** December 1982, page 57-60.

King, Carole: "Examining the Thorax and Respiratory System," **RN**, August 1982, page 55-64.

Klass, Kathleen: "Troubleshooting Central Line Complications," **Nursing 87**, November 1987, Vol. 17 No. 11, pages 58-61.

Koeckeritz, Jane Large: "Assessing the Heart: What's Normal and What's Not," **RN**, September 1982.

"Latest Protocols for Blood Transfusions, The," **Nursing 86**, October 1986, Vol. 16 No. 10, page 34-41.

Loucks, Arlene: "Chlamydia, Unheralded Epidemic," **AJN**, July 1987, Vol. 87 No. 7, pages 920-922.

Malkiewicz, Judy: "For a Really Thorough Abdominal Exam...," **RN**, October 1982, pages 59-64.

Malkiewicz, Judy: "What Assessing the Mouth Can Tell You," **RN**, May 1982, page 65-70.

Martinez, Geralyn: "Hypertension and Electrolyte Therapy," **Progress in Cardiovascular Nursing**, Summer 1994, pages 32-37.

Meyer, Charles: "Nursing and AIDS: A decade of caring," **AJN**, December 1991, pages 26-31.

McHugh, Jeannette: "Perfecting the 3 Steps of Chest Physiotherapy," **Nursing 87**, November 1987, pages 54-57.

Meola, Donna R.:"Responding Quickly to Tachydydrhythmias," **Nursing 87**, November 1987, pages 34-41.

Miracle, Vickie A.: "Anatomy of a Murmur," **Nursing 86**, July 1986, Vol. 86 No. 7, page 26-31.

Mutnick, Alan H.: "Cardiac Drugs, Inotropic and Chronotropic Agents," **Nursing 87**, October 1987, pages 58-60.

National Institutes of Health: "The 1988 Report of the Joint National Committee on Detection, Evaluation, and Treatment of High Blood Pressure," **NIH Publication** No. 88-1088, U.S. Government Printing Office.

Nehme, Alexander E.: "Nutritional Support of the Hospitalized Patient, the Team Concept," **JAMA**, May 16,1980, Vol. 243 No. 19, pages 1906-1908.

Phipps, Marion, et al: "Staging Care for Pressure Sores," **AJN**, August 1984, Vol. 84 No. 8, pages 999-1003.

Practical Briefings: "What's best to quench the athlete's thirst?," **Patient Care**, February 28,1987, page 13.

Quinn, Andrea: "Thora-Drain III, Closed Chest Drainage Made Simpler and Safer," **Nursing 86**, September 1986, pages 46-50.

INDEX

A

ORDER FORM

Qty.	Title	Qty.	Title
____	Handbook of Long-Term Care (2nd ed.) $18.00	____	Pediatric Nursing Care Plans $32.95
____	Nurse Assistant Handbook (2nd ed.) $18.00	____	RN NCLEX Review Cards $26.95
____	The Nurse's Survival Guide (2nd ed.) $29.95	____	PV/VN Review Cards $26.95
____	The Body in Brief (3rd ed.) $31.95	____	Geratric Nursing Care Plans (2nd ed.) $32.95
____	Nurses Trivia Calendar $9.95 ea.	____	Geriatric Outline $22.95
		____	Infection Control $85.00
____	Diagnostic and Laboratory Cards $24.95	____	OBRA $85.00
____	Geriatric Nutrition and Diet Therapy (2nd ed.) $17.95	$_____	Order Total*

Name
Address
City   StateZip
Phone   (   )
❏ Visa   ❏ MasterCard   ❏ American Express   ❏ Check/Money Order
Card #   Expiration Date
Signature (required)

MAIL OR FAX ORDER TO:
SKIDMORE-ROTH PUBLISHING, INC.
2620 S. Parker Rd., Suite 147
Aurora, Colorado 80014

(800) 825-3150   **FAX (303) 306-1460**

*Prices subject to change.
Please add $4.00 each for postage and handling.
Include local sales tax.
Visit our website at http://www.skidmore-roth.com